MW00837287

Laser and Lights: Volume 1

Vascular • Pigmentation • Scars • Medical Applications

Procedures in Cosmetic Dermatology

Series Editor: Jeffrey S. Dover MD FRCPC
Associate Editor: Murad Alam MD

Botulinum Toxin 
Alastair Carruthers MABM BCh FRCPC FRCP(Lon) and
Jean Carruthers MD FRCS(C) FRC(OPHTH)
ISBN 1 4160 2470 0

Soft Tissue Augmentation 
Jean Carruthers MD FRCS(C) FRC(OPHTH) and
Alastair Carruthers MABM BCh FRCPC FRCP(Lon)
ISBN 1 4160 2469 7

Cosmeceuticals
Zoe Diana Draelos MD
ISBN 1 4160 0244 8

Laser and Lights: Volume 1 
Vascular • Pigmentation • Scars • Medical Applications
David J. Goldberg MD JD
ISBN 1 4160 2386 0

Laser and Lights: Volume 2 
Rejuvenation • Resurfacing • Hair Removal • Treatment of Ethnic Skin
David J. Goldberg MD JD
ISBN 1 4160 2387 9

Photodynamic Therapy
Mitchel P. Goldman MD
ISBN 1 4160 2360 7

Liposuction 
C. William Hanke MD MPH FACP and Gerhard Sattler MD
ISBN 1 4160 2208 2

Treatment of Scars
Kenneth A. Arndt MD

Chemical Peels
Mark Rubin MD

Hair Restoration
Dowling B. Stough MD and Robert S. Haber MD

Leg Veins 
Tri H. Nguyen MD

Blepharoplasty 
Ronald L. Moy MD

Face Lifting 
Ronald L. Moy MD

PROCEDURES IN COSMETIC DERMATOLOGY

Series Editor: Jeffrey S. Dover MD FRCPC

Associate Editor: Murad Alam MD

Laser and Lights

Vascular • Pigmentation • Scars • Medical Applications

Volume 1

Edited by

David J. Goldberg MD JD

Director, Skin Laser & Surgery Specialists of New York and New Jersey, Hackensack, NJ; Clinical Professor of Dermatology and Director, Laser Research and Mohs Surgery, Mount Sinai School of Medicine; Clinical Professor of Dermatology and Director of Dermatologic Surgery, UMDNJ-New Jersey Medical School; Adjunct Professor of Law, Fordham Law School, New York, NY, USA

DVD Editor

Thomas E. Rohrer MD

Clinical Associate Professor of Dermatology, Boston University School of Medicine, Chestnut Hill, MA, USA

Series Editor

Jeffrey S. Dover MD FRCPC

Associate Professor of Clinical Dermatology, Yale University School of Medicine, Adjunct Professor of Medicine (Dermatology), Dartmouth Medical School, Director, SkinCare Physicians of Chestnut Hill, Chestnut Hill, MA, USA

Associate Editor

Murad Alam MD

Chief, Section of Cutaneous and Aesthetic Surgery, Department of Dermatology, Northwestern University, Chicago, IL, USA

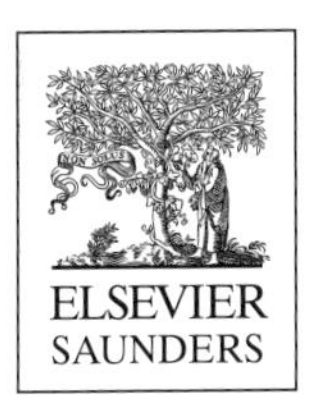

ELSEVIER
SAUNDERS

An imprint of Elsevier Inc.

First published 2005

ISBN-13: 978–1–4160–2386–9
ISBN-10: 1–4160–2386–0

British Library Cataloguing in Publication Data
A catalogue record of this book is available from the British Library

Library of Congress Cataloging in Publication Data
A catalog record of this book is available from the Library of Congress

Notice

Medical knowledge is constantly changing. Standard safety precautions must be followed, but as new research and clinical experience broaden our knowledge, changes in treatment and drug therapy may become necessary or appropriate. Readers are advised to check the most current product information provided by the manufacturer of each drug to be administered to verify the recommended dose, the method and duration of administration, and contraindications. It is the responsibility of the practitioner, relying on experience and knowledge of the patient, to determine dosages and the best treatment for each individual patient. Neither the Publisher nor the editor assumes any liability for any injury and/or damage to persons or property arising from this publication.

The Publisher

Printed in China
Last digit is the print number: 9 8 7 6 5 4 3

Commissioning Editors: **Sue Hodgson, Shuet-Kei Cheung**
Project Development Managers: **Martin Mellor Publishing Services Ltd, Louise Cook**
Project Managers: **Naughton Project Management, Cheryl Brant**
Illustration Manager: **Mick Ruddy**
Design Manager: **Andy Chapman**
Illustrators: **Richard Prime, Tim Loughhead**

Contents

Series Foreword vii

Preface ix

List of Contributors xi

1 **Lasers and Light Tissue Interactions** 1
Richard J. Barlow, George J. Hruza

2 **Vascular Lesions** 11
Karen H. Kim, Thomas E. Rohrer, Roy G. Geronemus

3 **Leg Veins** 29
Jeffrey T.S. Hsu, Robert A. Weiss

4 **Pigmented Lesions and Tattoos** 41
Chrysalyne D. Schmults, Ronald G. Wheeland

5 **Laser Treatment for Scars** 67
Keyvan Nouri, Sean W. Lanigan, Maria Patricia Rivas

6 **Treatment of Actinic Keratoses and Nonmelanoma Skin Cancer** 75
Ramsey F. Markus, Janna Kate Nunez-Gussman, Paul T. Martinelli

7 **Acne** 89
E. Victor Ross Jr, Nathan Uebelhoer

8 **Psoriasis** 103
Ming H. Jih, Paul M. Friedman

9 **Cooling** 127
E. Victor Ross Jr, Dilip Paithankar

10 **Anesthesia** 137
Suzanne L. Kilmer

Index 143

Series Foreword
Procedures in Cosmetic Dermatology

While dermatologists have been procedurally inclined since the beginning of the specialty, particularly rapid change has occurred in the past quarter century. The advent of frozen section technique and the golden age of Mohs skin cancer surgery has led to the formal incorporation of surgery within the dermatology curriculum. More recently technological breakthroughs in minimally invasive procedural dermatology have offered an aging population new options for improving the appearance of damaged skin.

Procedures for rejuvenating the skin and adjacent regions are actively sought by our patients. Significantly, dermatologists have pioneered devices, technologies and medications, which have continued to evolve at a startling pace. Numerous major advances, including virtually all cutaneous lasers and light-source based procedures, botulinum exotoxin, soft-tissue augmentation, dilute anesthesia liposuction, leg vein treatments, chemical peels, and hair transplants, have been invented, or developed and enhanced by dermatologists. Dermatologists understand procedures, and we have special insight into the structure, function, and working of skin. Cosmetic dermatologists have made rejuvenation accessible to risk-averse patients by emphasizing safety and reducing operative trauma. No specialty is better positioned than dermatology to lead the field of cutaneous surgery while meeting patient needs.

As dermatology grows as a specialty, an ever-increasing proportion of dermatologists will become proficient in the delivery of different procedures. Not all dermatologists will perform all procedures, and some will perform very few, but even the less procedurally directed amongst us must be well-versed in the details to be able to guide and educate our patients. Whether you are a skilled dermatologic surgeon interested in further expanding your surgical repertoire, a complete surgical novice wishing to learn a few simple procedures, or somewhere in between, this book and this series is for you.

The volume you are holding is one of a series entitled "Procedures in Cosmetic Dermatology." The purpose of each book is to serve as a practical primer on a major topic area in procedural dermatology.

If you want make sure you find the right book for your needs, you may wish to know what this book is and what it is not. It is not a comprehensive text grounded in theoretical underpinnings. It is not exhaustively referenced. It is not designed to be a completely unbiased review of the world's literature on the subject. At the same time, it is not an overview of cosmetic procedures that describes these in generalities without providing enough specific information to actually permit someone to perform the procedures. And importantly, it is not so heavy that it can serve as a doorstop or a shelf filler.

What this book and this series offer is a step-by-step, practical guide to performing cutaneous surgical procedures. Each volume in the series has been edited by a known authority in that subfield. Each editor has recruited other equally practical-minded, technically skilled, hands-on clinicians to write the constituent chapters. Most chapters have two authors to ensure that different approaches and a broad range of opinions are incorporated. On the other hand, the two authors and the editors also collectively provide a consistency of tone. A uniform template has been used within each chapter so that the reader will be easily able to navigate all the books in the series. Within every chapter, the authors succinctly tell it like they do it. The emphasis is on therapeutic technique; treatment methods are discussed with an eye to appropriate indications, adverse events, and unusual cases. Finally, this book is short and can be read in its entirety on a long plane ride. We believe that brevity paradoxically results in greater information transfer because cover-to-cover mastery is practicable.

Most of the books in the series are accompanied by a high-quality DVD, demonstrating the procedures discussed in that text. Some of you will turn immediately to the DVD and use the text as a backup to clarify complex points, while others will prefer to read first and then view the DVD to see the steps in action. Choose what suits you best.

We hope you enjoy this book and the rest of the books in the series and that you benefit from the many hours of clinical wisdom that have been distilled to produce it. Please keep it nearby, where you can reach for it when you need it.

Jeffrey S. Dover MD FRCPC and Murad Alam MD

To the women in my life

My grandmothers, Bertha and Lillian
My mother, Nina
My daughters, Sophie and Isabel
And especially to my wife, Tania

For their never-ending encouragement, patience, support, love, and friendship

To my father, Mark
A great teacher and role model

To my mentor, Kenneth A. Arndt for his generosity, kindness, sense of humor, joie de vivre, and above all else curiosity and enthusiasm

At Elsevier, Sue Hodgson who conceptualized the series and brought it to reality

and

Martin Mellor for polite, persistent, and dogged determination.

Jeffry S. Dover

The professionalism of the dedicated editorial staff at Elsevier has made this ambitious project possible. Guided by the creative vision of Sue Hodgson, Martin Mellor and Shuet-Kei Cheung have attended to the myriad tasks required to produce a state-of-the-art resource. In this, they have been ably supported by the graphics team, which has maintained production quality while ensuring portability. We are also deeply grateful to the volume editors, who have generously found time in their schedules, cheerfully accepted our guidelines, and recruited the most knowledgeable chapter authors. Finally, we thank the chapter contributors, without whose work there would be no books at all. Whatever successes are herein are due to the efforts of the above, and of my teachers, Kenneth Arndt, Jeffrey Dover, Michael Kaminer, Leonard Goldberg, and David Bickers, and of my parents, Rahat and Rehana Alam.

Murad Alam

Preface

In 1983 Anderson and Parrish published in the journal *Science* their newly developed concept of selective photothermolysis (SPTL). Selective photothermolysis revolutionized laser medicine and dermatology. This original concept originally explained how laser physicians could safely and effectively treat children with port wine stains using laser light. SPTL also led to the development of a specific laser, the pulsed dye laser, to treat a specific condition, port wine stains in children. This concept has now also been used to develop more effective treatments of many other cutaneous problems including the treatment of tattoos, benign pigmented lesions, and the removal of unwanted or excessive hair. Our understanding of SPTL defined a way to localize thermal injury to the tissue being treated while minimizing collateral thermal damage to the surrounding non-targeted tissue. This is accomplished by choosing the proper wavelength of light that will be absorbed by the specific targeted chromophore and delivering the right amount of energy with the proper pulse duration, known as the thermal relaxation time (TRT). The TRT is based on the physical size of the target.

It is these basic concepts of laser physics that have led in the short period of two decades to the transformation of laser dermatology. The breadth of this field is evidenced by the need for a two volume series dedicated to laser skin surgery. Each chapter is dedicated to a specific topic. In all there are 17 chapters. Chapters are written to give both the beginning and experienced laser physician a practical clinical everyday approach to using cutaneous lasers. Appropriate patient selection and choice of lasers is emphasized. An overview of treatment strategies, indications and contraindications is stressed. Where appropriate advanced treatment tips are provided. All chapters contain selected further readings and clinical photographs. Many chapters contain useful treatment videos.

This volume begins with a chapter discussing a practical approach to laser tissue interaction. Subsequent chapters discuss laser treatment of vascular lesions, leg veins, pigmented lesions and tattoos, scars, pre-cancerous and cancerous changes of the skin, acne, and psoriasis. The final chapter in this volume discusses the unique issues of anesthesia and skin cooling.

Laser and Lights represents the definitive practical guide to use of lasers on the skin.

David J. Goldberg, MD

List of Contributors

Richard Barlow MBBCh MD FRCP
Consultant Dermatologist, Dermatological Surgery and Laser Unit, St John's Institute of Dermatology, St Thomas' Hospital, London, UK

Paul M. Friedman MD
Clinical Assistant Professor of Dermatology, University of Texas Medical School, Houston, TX, USA

Roy G. Geronemus MD
Director, Laser and Skin Surgery Center of New York; Clinical Professor, New York University Department of Dermatology, New York, NY, USA

George J. Hruza MD
Clinical Associate Professor of Dermatology and Otolaryngology, Head and Neck Surgery, St Louis University, St Louis, MO, USA

Jeffrey T.S. Hsu MD
Director of Vein Treatment Center, SkinCare Physicians of Chestnut Hill, Chestnut Hill, MA, USA

Ming H. Jih MD PhD
Fellow, Derm Surgery Associates, Houston, TX, USA

Suzanne L. Kilmer MD MS
Director, Laser and Skin Surgery Center of Northern California; Assistant Clinical Professor, Department of Dermatology, University of California, UC Davis Medical Center, Sacramento, CA, USA

Karen H. Kim MD
Director of Research, Laser and Skin Surgery Center of New York, New York, NY, USA

Sean W. Lanigan MD FRCP DCH
Consultant Dermatologist and Group Medical Director, Lasercare Clinics, Sickle Cell Centre, City Hospital, Birmingham, UK

Ramsey F. Markus MD
Assistant Professor of Dermatology, Department of Dermatology, Baylor College of Medicine, Houston, TX, USA

Paul T. Martinelli MD
Dermatology Resident, Department of Dermatology, Baylor College of Medicine, Houston, TX, USA

Keyvan Nouri MD
Director of Mohs Micrographic Surgery, Dermatologic and Laser Surgery; Director of Surgical Training; Assistant Professor, Department of Derm and Cutaneous Surgery, University of Miami School of Medicine, Miami, FL, USA

Janna Kate Nunez-Gussman MD
Mohs Micrographic Surgery Fellow, Baylor College of Medicine, Houston, TX, USA

Dilip Paithankar PhD
Director of New Applications, Candela Corporation, Wayland, MA, USA

Maria Patricia Rivas MD
Research Fellow, Department of Dermatology and Cutaneous Surgery, University of Miami, FL, USA

Thomas E. Rohrer MD
Clinical Associate Professor of Dermatology, Boston University School of Medicine; Director of Mohs Fellowship, SkinCare Physicians of Chestnut Hill, Chestnut Hill, MA, USA

E. Victor Ross Jr MD
Residency Program Director, Dermatology Department, Naval Medical Center, San Diego, CA, USA

Chrysalyne D. Schmults MD
Assistant Professor of Dermatology, University of Pennsylvania School of Medicine, Philadelphia, PA, USA

Nathan Uebelhoer DO
Dermatologic and Laser Surgery Fellow, SkinCare Physicians of Chestnut Hill, Chestnut Hill, MA, USA

Robert A. Weiss MD
Associate Professor, Department of Dermatology, Johns Hopkins University School of Medicine, Baltimore, MD, USA

Ronald G. Wheeland MD
Professor and Chief, Section of Dermatology, University of Arizona Health Sciences, Tucson, AZ, USA

1 Lasers and Light Tissue Interactions

Richard J. Barlow, George J. Hruza

History

The first laser of clinical significance, introduced in 1960 by Maiman, contained a ruby rod and emitted light with a wavelength of 694 nm. Other lasers followed, importantly the neodymium : yttrium-aluminium-garnet laser (Nd : YAG) in 1961, the argon laser in 1962, and the carbon dioxide (CO_2) laser in 1964. By 1965, Goldman had reported use of the ruby laser in removing tattoos with minimal associated scarring. This was followed by work with the Nd : YAG laser in managing tattoos and superficial vascular malformations. The argon laser was first used to treat vascular lesions during the mid 1970s but was limited by a high risk of scarring. It was only in 1983, with the publication of the theory of selective photothermolysis (as discussed below), that a fuller understanding of laser–tissue interactions was possible. This in turn has facilitated the design and manufacture of lasers for specific uses in medicine.

Laser Light

The term 'laser' is an acronym for 'light amplification by stimulated emission of radiation'. Stimulated emission is made possible through an understanding of spontaneous emission and the quantum mechanics of matter. Atoms (or molecules) consist of a nucleus (or nuclei) surrounded by orbiting electrons. In their resting state, electrons are usually at the lowest energy level. By absorbing energy in the form of a photon (i.e. a quantum of electromagnetic radiation or light), an electron will move to an orbit at a greater distance from the nucleus (Fig. 1.1). This represents an excited, unstable state, the tendency of which is to revert to the resting position by dropping back to the original orbit. A photon of energy is released during this process which is called spontaneous emission of radiation.

Stimulated emission occurs when an already excited electron absorbs a further photon of equal energy and then reverts to the resting orbit. In this

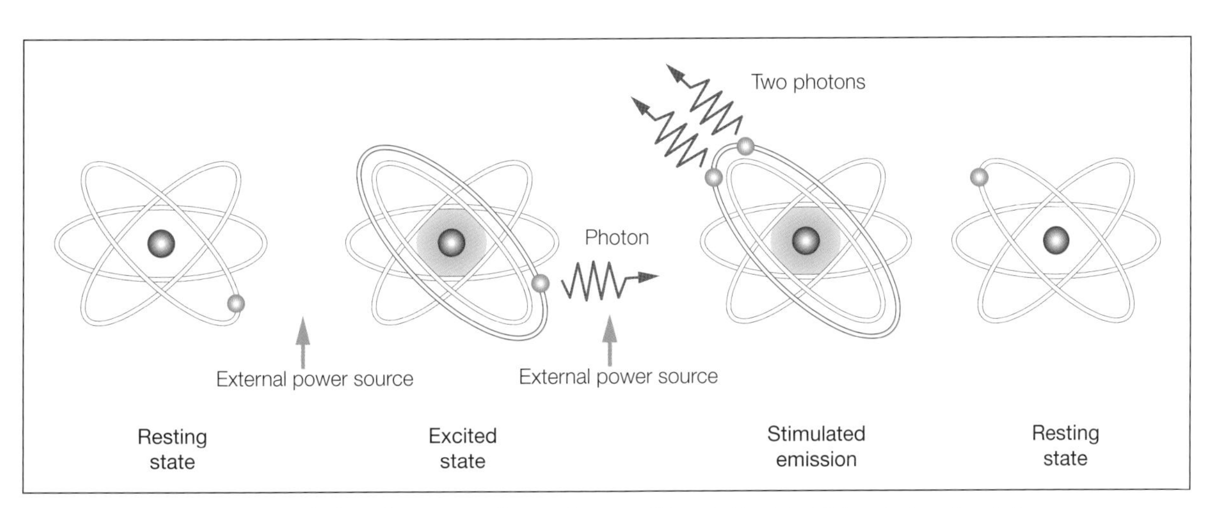

Fig. 1.1 Representation of excitation of an atom with spontaneous (**A**) and stimulated (**B**) emission of radiation

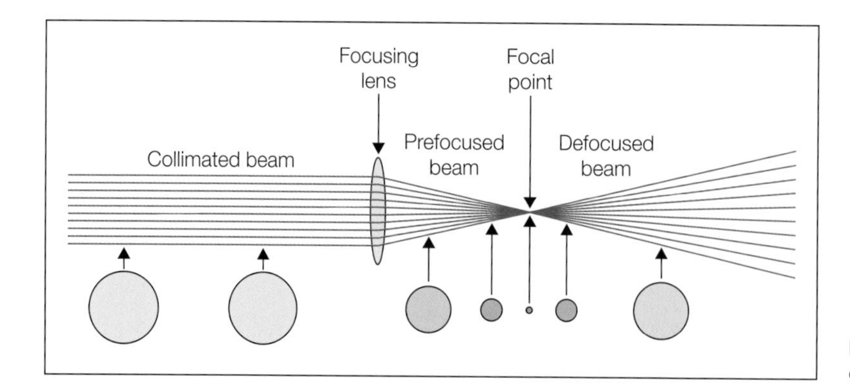

Fig. 1.2 Representation of a collimated beam of light

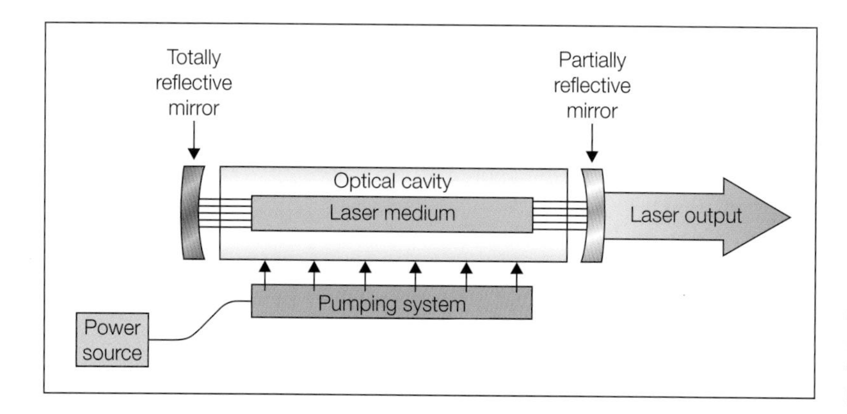

Fig. 1.3 Diagram of a laser showing external power source, the active medium within the resonator cavity, and a system of fully and partly reflective mirrors

process, two photons of light are released, both with the wavelength, phase and direction of the absorbed photon. The energy which is required for this process is provided to a laser by an external power source. Each time the process is repeated, the number of photons within the laser cavity increases. When the majority of electrons are no longer in their resting orbits but in an excited state, they are described as having undergone population inversion. The significance of this is that stimulated emission becomes more probable and light amplification more significant.

In addition to intense brightness, laser light differs from light emitted by conventional light sources in that it has the following characteristics:

1. **Monochromaticity**. The identity of the atom or molecule which is being excited determines the wavelength of the radiation produced. More precisely, this is a narrow band in a Gaussian distribution around the characteristic wavelength of the laser. The argon laser is unusual in that it emits light of two wavelengths (488 and 514 nm), a consequence of there being intermediate orbits between the excited and resting states.
2. **Coherence**. Light can be considered as a sine wave. The light emitted by a laser has the distinction of being both temporally and spatially coherent, i.e. the waves are in phase in time and space.
3. **Collimation**. This is a direct consequence of coherence and refers to the nondivergent and energy conserving properties of light in which the waves are parallel. It means that the diameter of the beam changes only minimally over distance, unless it is focused by a lens (Fig. 1.2). Both forms may be useful, such as in CO_2 laser surgery where a focused beam is required for excisional applications and where a scanner is used with a focused or collimated beam for resurfacing.

Lasers

Lasers are usually named after the constituents of the medium (laser medium) (Fig. 1.3). This may be a gas (e.g. argon, CO_2, and excimer lasers), a liquid (e.g. pulsed dye laser), a solid (e.g. alexandrite,

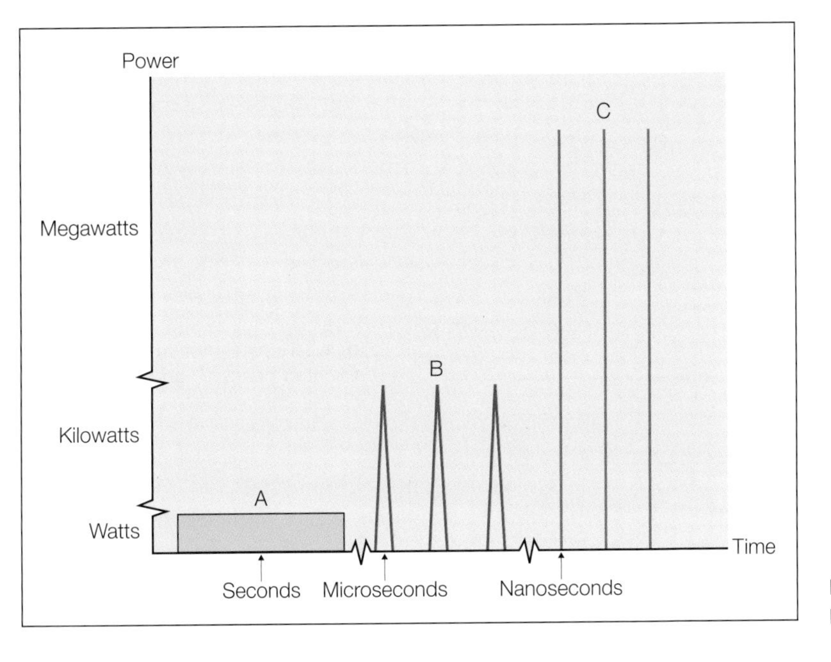

Fig. 1.4 Simplified representation of pulse types

diode, erbium : yttrium-aluminium-garnet (Er : YAG), Nd : YAG, and ruby lasers) or solid state (diode laser), and is excited by an external source of energy such as a flashlamp. The laser medium is contained within the optical (or resonator) cavity and determines the wavelength of the light created by stimulated emission of radiation. Photons which are moving parallel to the axis of the optical cavity are reflected between two opposing mirrors, in turn stimulating emission on the same axis. One of the mirrors is fully and the other partly reflective. Light is amplified until such time as it is emitted through the latter. It then enters a delivery system for transmission to the operator handpiece. Delivery systems may take the form of fiberoptic cables or articulated arms through which light is reflected by mirrors. Fiberoptic cables have the advantage of being lighter and easier to operate and maintain. However, they may break when bending or twisting the fiber beyond its tolerance during operation, movement, or cleaning. This can add significantly to operating expenses as each fiber may cost up to several thousand dollars to replace and is not usually covered by the manufacturer's warranty or service contract. Fibers are not sufficiently robust to transmit light emissions from systems such as CO_2, Er : YAG, or short pulse Q-switched lasers, where articulated arms containing multiple mirrors are required. Each delivery system ends in a handpiece in which light can be focused by a lens or transmitted as a collimated beam. Either type can be scanned over a predetermined area of skin in order to limit the time to which the skin is irradiated.

Lasers are also classified according to the pulse characteristics of the beam. This may be continuous, pulsed, or quality switched (Q-switched) (Fig. 1.4A, B and C respectively). Continuous wave light consists of an uninterrupted beam of relatively low power, such as is emitted by the CO_2 laser. This continuous beam can be shuttered to deliver individual pulses of energy. However, mechanical shuttering alone may not be beneficial as these 'pulses' do not have sufficient energy to be clinically useful. Another modification, superpulsing, was developed so that the laser emitted a rapid train of higher peak power pulses of energy. However, these so called 'quasi-continuous' lasers release pulses which are so close together that there is insufficient time for cooling between pulses. The effect of this on the skin appears very similar to a continuous wave laser beam. It was only with the development of high peak power lasers with true individual pulses containing enough energy in each pulse that clinically significant tissue effects were achieved. Examples include the pulsed dye laser, normal mode alexandrite, diode and the UltraPulse CO_2 laser with pulse durations in the millisecond or high microsecond range. Quality switching or Q-switching is a means of creating very

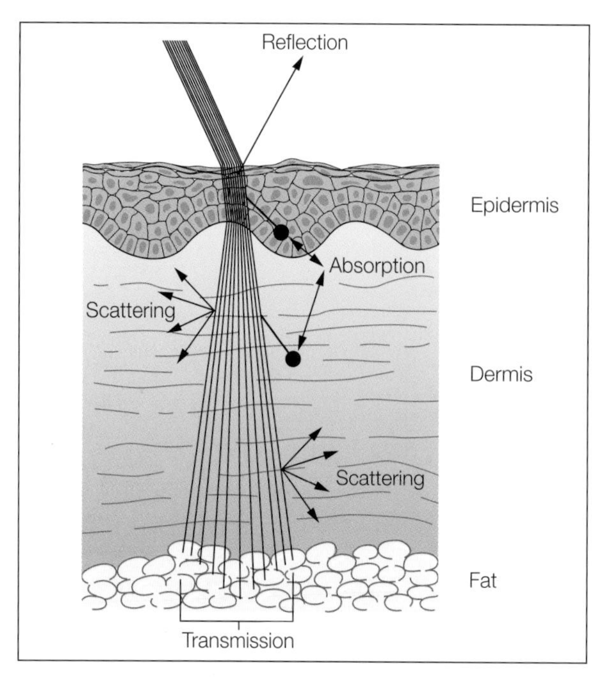

Fig. 1.5 Fate of incident light on skin

short pulses (5–100 ns) with extremely high peak powers. This is achieved by means of an electro-optical switch which consists of two polarizers. Depending on their alignment, these will either transmit or block light. The pulse width is varied so that it approximates the thermal relaxation time (see below) of the target chromophore.

Tissue optics

The fate of incident light on skin can be discussed under four headings (Fig. 1.5):

1. Reflection
2. Absorption
3. Scattering
4. Transmission.

Reflection

About 4–6% of light is reflected at the level of the stratum corneum.

Absorption

Absorption of photons is described by Beer's law. This states that the intensity of light of a particular wavelength which is transmitted through tissue (ideally a uniform medium) depends on its initial intensity as well as on depth of penetration and extinction length (the distance over which 90% of the beam is absorbed). Without absorption of light, there can be no effect on tissue. When a photon is absorbed by a target molecule or chromophore, all of its energy is transferred to that molecule. The basis for selective skin laser surgery is that light can be manipulated in terms of its wavelength, energy content, and pulse duration so that a particular target chromophore absorbs light and is damaged or destroyed whereas other chromophores are not.

The endogenous chromophores of importance are melanin, hemoglobin, water, and collagen (Fig. 1.6). Melanin is present normally in the epidermis and hair follicles. Its principal function is to protect against sunlight and its absorption includes ultraviolet (UV) and visible light, with decreasing absorption into the near-infrared spectrum. Hemoglobin has absorption peaks in the UVA, blue (400 nm), green (541 nm), and yellow (577 nm) wavelengths, collagen in the visible and near-infrared spectra and water in the mid- and far-infrared regions. There are also a number of exogenous chromophores, of which the most important in this context is tattoo ink.

Scattering

In skin, this is largely due to collagen in the dermis. Because the collagen molecule is similar in size to the wavelength of visible and near-infrared light, scatter is mainly forward in direction, but enough backscatter occurs to increase the energy density in the upper dermis beyond that of the incident light in certain situations. Two other types of scattering also occur in the skin, namely the weak scatter in all directions (Rayleigh scatter) that is caused by molecules smaller than the incident light wavelength and that caused by objects larger than the incident light, which is also forward in direction. Scattering is important as it rapidly reduces the energy fluence that is available for absorption by the target chromophore and therefore the clinical effect in tissue. Scattering decreases with longer wavelengths, making these the ideal vehicle for targeting deep dermal structures such as hair follicles. The wavelength range of 600–1200 nm is an optical window into the skin because there is not only low scattering but also limited absorption by endogenous chromophores at these wavelengths.

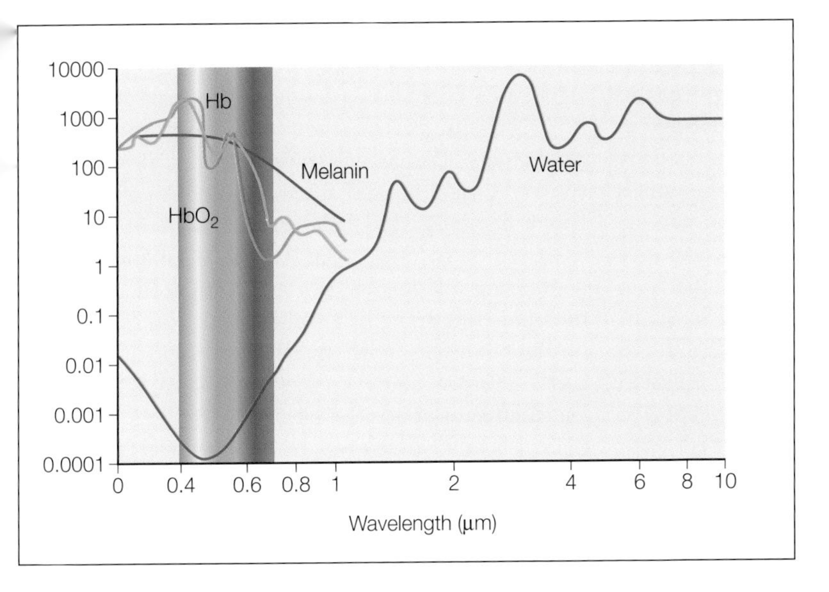

Fig. 1.6 Absorption spectra of principal tissue chromophores

Transmission

Residual light is transmitted to subcutaneous tissue. This is largely dependent on wavelength, with shorter wavelengths (300–400nm) being scattered and penetrating less than 0.1 mm. Wavelengths in the 600–1200 nm range penetrate deeper because they are scattered less.

Light–Tissue Interaction

The wavelength of light influences the extent to which it is absorbed by one or more tissue chromophores. In addition to being absorbed, light must also have sufficient energy if it is to alter the target structure. Energy is measured in Joules (J), though it is usually more useful to consider its 'fluence' or energy density (J/cm^2). 'Power' is the rate at which energy is delivered and is measured in Watts (i.e. W or J/s). The term 'irradiance' refers to the 'power density' or the rate at which energy is delivered per unit area and is therefore measured in W/cm^2.

Depending on these qualities, light may affect tissue in the following ways:

1. Photostimulation
2. Photodynamic reactions
3. Photothermolytic and photomechanical reactions.

Photostimulation

There is equivocal evidence to suggest that low energy lasers expedite wound healing. The mechanism for this is unclear.

Photodynamic reactions

This forms the basis of photodynamic therapy and involves the topical or systemic administration of a photosensitizer or precursor thereof. Subsequent irradiation with an appropriate light source elicits two types of photo-oxidative reaction and an immediate cytotoxic effect. Photodynamic therapy can also use endogenous chromophores such as those found in *Pityrosporum acnes* where the *P. acnes* organisms are killed with blue light irradiation with subsequent clinical improvement of acne.

Photothermolytic and photomechanical reactions

The theory of selective photothermolysis has been applied to the removal of superficial vascular malformations, exogenous tattoos, certain benign pigmented lesions, and hair. It postulates that light can be used to selectively damage or destroy a target chromophore if its wavelength is selected so that there is as big a difference as possible between the absorption coefficient of the target and the surrounding tissue, the energy fluence is sufficiently high to damage the target, and the pulse duration is less than or equal to the thermal relaxation time (TRT). The TRT is the time taken for the target to dissipate about 63% of the incident thermal energy. These factors are considered in more detail below.

1. **Wavelength**. The absorption spectra of important tissue chromophores are shown in Figure 1.6 in relation to the wavelengths of the lasers widely used in dermatology. Hemoglobin has a number of

different absorption peaks whereas absorption by melanin gradually diminishes with longer wavelengths of incident light. Consideration must also be given to the depth of the target structure, as scattering in the dermis is strongly influenced by wavelength, making a longer wavelength, which may be relatively poorly absorbed, often preferable, to a short wavelength with the opposite characteristics. In some situations, particularly in relation to melanin, a single wavelength may not be necessary and it may even be preferable to use flashlamps because of their broad emission spectrum (500–1200 nm). These are cheaper to manufacture than lasers and can be used with light filters (515–755 nm) to allow a potentially wide range of applications. It is possible to vary their pulse durations from 0.5 to 88.5 ms and to introduce intervals between pulses of 1–300 ms. At present they cannot substitute for lasers where focused, high energy beams are required.
2. **Energy fluence**. The energy contained within light is expressed in Joules (J) and its fluence or energy density per unit area in J/cm^2.
3. **Thermal relaxation time (TRT)**. The TRT is related only to the size of the target chromophore, being proportional to the square of the target diameter squared, and varies from a few nanoseconds (tattoo particles) through several hundred milliseconds or more (leg venules).

Some tissue targets, notably the hair follicle, are not uniform in their absorption of light, and it is possible that light assisted hair removal is better explained by an 'extended theory of selective photothermolysis'. This distinguishes between an 'absorber' chromophore (in which heat is generated) and a distant 'target', to which heat is transmitted and which is damaged as a result. In the context of hair removal, melanin in the hair shaft, and matrix cells may act as the absorber, whereas the stem cells of the isthmus (and possibly the blood vessels in the papilla) represent the distant target. The time to achieve selective damage of the target is the thermal damage time (TDT). This is the time for the entire target, including the primary chromophore (e.g. melanin) and the surrounding target (e.g. hair follicle), to cool by about 63% and includes cooling of the primary chromophore as well as the entire target. The TDT is longer than the TRT as it allows for heat diffusion from the chromophore throughout the entire target.

A practical outcome of this theory has been termed 'thermokinetic selectivity'. Because large structures cool more slowly than small structures, it is proposed that they will reach higher and potentially damaging temperatures if the light source is manipulated appropriately. An example of this is light assisted hair removal where a pulse is used which is longer than the TDT of the melanin containing epidermis (1 ms) compared with the melanin containing hair follicle (30–100 ms). Lasers or light sources with pulse durations of 5–50 ms can therefore allow energy to accumulate in and thermally coagulate the hair follicle. Even while the energy is being delivered, the epidermis is protected as it cools and its temperature is therefore kept below its thermal coagulation threshold.

Tissue Cooling

Light wavelengths between 500 and 1200 nm are preferentially but not specifically absorbed by either hemoglobin or melanin, depending on the wavelengths employed. Epidermal melanin will therefore absorb both direct and back scattered light from all such devices, whether or not it is the intended chromophore. Heat damage to the epidermis may result in blistering, dyspigmentation, or scarring, and is particularly likely in pigmented skin. To reduce this risk, the wavelength should be optimized with respect to the absorption characteristics and depth of the target chromophore. The use of long pulses and cooling of the epidermis further enhances safety in these patients. The latter may be done before, during, or after the light pulse, or all three.

Cooling may take three forms:

1. **Cold air convection**. Air, chilled to temperatures as low as –30°C, is directed onto the area to be treated.
2. **Contact cooling**. This may involve simple application of ice-packs or more sophisticated systems which pass chilled water between colorless and transparent plates which are usually sapphire as it is a far more efficient conductor than glass. Although an excellent method of cooling during light delivery, in humid environments condensate on the plates can obscure the skin and require frequent wiping.
3. **Cryogen spray (dynamic) cooling**. A frozen gas is sprayed onto the skin immediately before the laser pulse. Evaporative cooling has a high heat

transfer coefficient and this is therefore the most efficient way of precooling. With timed, automated control this method is also relatively predictable and reproducible.

One important benefit of epidermal cooling has been to allow treatments at higher energy fluences than would otherwise be considered safe, and thereby enhanced treatment efficacy, which has made it possible to reduce the number of treatments required. Cooling has also made it possible to safely treat patients with all skin types. Furthermore, cooling decreases the pain associated with treatment, thus reducing the need for topical or local anaesthetic. However, if used excessively, cooling may cause cryogen injury.

Light and Tissue Interactions: Clinical Relevance

Superficial vascular lesions

A wavelength of 577 nm was used in early pulsed dye lasers for selective photothermolysis of superficial blood vessels because of its highly selective absorption by oxyhemoglobin. This was subsequently replaced with 585–600 nm light which has the advantage of deeper dermal penetration though with reduced oxyhemoglobin absorption at the longer wavelengths. A pulse duration of approximately 0.45 ms was included in the design of early pulsed dye lasers (PDLs), on the basis of a calculated TRT of <1 ms for vessel diameters of 10–50 μm. The theoretical models may have slightly underestimated the TRT, and indeed this was measured in a subsequent in vivo study as 1–10 ms for vessel diameters of 30–150 μm. As a consequence, newer pulsed dye lasers allow pulse durations of up to 40 ms. The 585 nm short pulse PDL is probably the treatment of choice for pediatric port wine stain (PWS) because vessel diameters are relatively small. At 595 nm, the absorption coefficient of oxyhemoglobin is a factor of five lower than at 585 nm and, used in conjunction with longer pulses of 1.5–6 ms, may be the most suitable for treating the larger ectatic vessels seen in resistant or adult PWS. The use of cryogen spray cooling with higher energy fluences in both short and long pulse (1.5–4.0 ms) PDL has expedited treatment of PWS. Lesions immediately become purpuric if treated with adequate fluences and pulse durations of 10 ms or less. Although reduced by both cooling and long pulsing, a degree of post-treatment purpura formation is thought to be necessary for effective treatment of lesions.

Another laser useful for vascular anomalies is the potassium titanyl phosphate (KTP) laser (532 nm). KTP lasers may be flashlamp or diode pumped and are characterized by trains of short pulses which summate to give a wide pulse effect (quasicontinuous) that is not associated with purpura. Light produced by KTP lasers is highly absorbed by hemoglobin (and melanin) but its wavelength penetrates only superficially. The main advantage of KTP lasers is their lack of purpura.

Flashlamps have large spot sizes and are used with contact cooling, allowing rapid treatment and reduced likelihood of purpura. The alexandrite (755 nm) and Nd : YAG (1064 nm) lasers emit light with longer wavelengths and therefore relatively deep dermal penetration, the latter absorbed by a small hemoglobin absorption peak at 900–1000 nm.

Leg venules are probably best treated with sclerotherapy because of their relatively high hydrostatic pressure. Nevertheless, long pulse (1.5–4.0 ms) PDLs with wavelengths in the 585–600 nm range and energy fluences of 7–9 J/cm^2 may sometimes be useful for small superficial vessels. If sclerotherapy is contraindicated, the bigger and deeper vessels should respond best to large spot sizes of 3–4 mm, high energy fluences (relative to wavelength), and long pulse durations, used in conjunction with effective cooling devices. Wavelength should be chosen according to the depth of the target vessel. The 3 ms alexandrite laser (755 nm), used with a fluence of 86 J/cm^2, has been reported to clear as many as 75% of leg vessels less than 3 mm in diameter. Nd : YAG lasers, with energy fluences higher than 100 J/cm^2 and with pulse durations of up to 1 second, have also been used and may be useful for larger vessels.

Tattoos and benign pigmented lesions

Melanin absorbs light in the ultraviolet-1200 nm range (Fig. 1.6). At the longer wavelengths, absorption is lower and penetration deeper than at the shorter wavelengths. For example, the Q-switched Nd : YAG (1064 nm) laser emits light that penetrates 2–3 mm into the dermis and is therefore suitable for the removal of deeper dermal pigmentation such as found in nevus of Ota. By passing the beam through a KTP crystal the frequency is doubled and the wavelength halved (532 nm). The shorter wavelength penetrates less deeply and is therefore more useful for the removal of epidermal pigment, such as in ephelides. The ruby (694 nm) laser, which penetrates less than 1 mm into skin, is also of most use in treating superficial lesions such as in freckles or café-au-lait macules.

The Q-switch is an electro-optical device which is used to produce pulses of only a few nanoseconds. These are designed to be within the estimated TRT of melanosomes (0.5–1 μs) although longer than that of tattoo particles, which is in the low nanosecond domain. Flashlamps can pulse within a millisecond range, which is relatively long in this context. Nanosecond light may fragment and disperse melanin and tattoo ink, thereby altering its optical properties. Most of the lightening occurs due to gradual uptake and removal of the fragmented particles by activated macrophages through the lymphatic system. Some may also be removed by transepidermal elimination.

Black or blue tattoo pigments absorb radiation across a broad range of wavelengths in the visible and near-infrared spectrum. Green inks respond optimally to the Q-switched ruby (694 nm) and Q-switched alexandrite (755 nm) lasers but often persist. Conversely, red pigments respond best to the green light emitted by the frequency doubled Nd : YAG (532 nm). The Nd : YAG laser is effective for blue-black tattoos but is relatively poorly absorbed by green pigments. It has been used successfully to treat tattoos in pigmented skin. Red, brown, white, or skin colored inks that contain iron or titanium oxides can be chemically reduced to a permanent slate-grey or black color during laser treatment. This may be faded with subsequent treatments. As these pigments may be used in cosmetic camouflage tattoos, test patches are important. Yellow and pastel colors are difficult to treat and complete resolution is unusual. Amateur tattoos usually require fewer treatments than professional tattoos.

Hair reduction

The mechanism for light assisted hair reduction remains incompletely understood. It is likely that the theory of selective thermolysis applies in this context. However, the targets are likely to be stem cells (mainly in the lower isthmus) and blood vessels in the papilla whereas the absorbing chromophore is melanin in the hair shaft and matrix cells. For this reason, fair or white hair is largely resistant to treatment. Radiation in the 600–1200 nm spectrum is absorbed by melanin and penetrates the dermis further at longer wavelengths. The normal mode ruby (694 nm), alexandrite (755 nm), diode (800 nm), and Nd : YAG (1064 nm) lasers have all been used with fluences of 20–60 J/cm^2, depending on spot size. The TRT of a 200–300 μm follicle is about 25–50 ms but much shorter pulse durations seem to be effective. It has recently been demonstrated that considerably longer pulses (30–400 ms) may be more effective in damaging the stem cells and papillary vessels, neither of which contains melanin nor is in direct contact with the melanin rich components of the follicle. This observation has been explained in terms of an 'extended theory of selective photothermolysis'. By using long pulses and by limiting the power of the light source, the heat generated by the 'absorber' (i.e. melanin in the hair shaft) can be kept below levels which would alter its structural and optical properties and thus interfere with further absorption of light. On the other hand, the heat generated may be high enough to diffuse into and denature the distant 'target' (i.e. the stem cells and papillary vessels). The delay between heating of the absorber chromophore and the distant target is referred to as the thermal damage time (TDT) and is significantly longer than the TRT.

In patients with pigmented skin, long wavelengths (i.e. 1064 nm) and cooling devices are particularly important in reducing the risk of epidermal damage with subsequent dyspigmentation or scarring. A small proportion of patients seem to experience a paradoxical increase in hair growth.

Resurfacing

Ablative laser resurfacing

This was performed initially with pulsed or scanned CO_2 lasers, the immediate effect of which is ablation (or vaporization) of the epidermis and often the upper dermis. There is also thermal damage to a band of underlying dermis, together with collagen denaturation and contraction. In the healing period, there is re-epithelialization from the hair follicles and other adnexal tissue in addition to a band of upper dermal fibrosis, or 'collagen remodeling'. CO_2 lasers produce light (10 600 nm) which is relatively poorly absorbed by the chromophore, water, and which therefore has a relatively high penetration

(30 μm). Unless the irradiance is high, the effect of this is to elicit less ablation and more thermal damage than was initially thought desirable. As a consequence, Er : YAG lasers were developed and marketed because they emit light (2940 nm) which is highly absorbed by water and has a low penetrance (3 μm). This in turn is associated with more ablation and less thermal damage. It soon became apparent, however, that a degree of thermal damage was necessary for hemostasis and probably also for greater efficacy. Er : YAG lasers were then adapted to cause more rather than less thermal damage. Attention then switched from ablation, which by now was considered undesirable on account of the unpleasantness and complications of what were, in effect, second degree facial burns.

Nonablative resurfacing

This procedure aims to wound the upper dermis without damaging the epidermis. Prerequisites to this are therefore epidermal cooling systems and wavelengths which are sufficiently long to penetrate and injure the dermis. A variety of lasers and light sources have been studied, including some originally developed for other purposes.

Further Reading

Altshuler GB, Anderson RR, Manstein D, et al 2001 Extended theory of selective photothermolysis. Lasers in Surgery and Medicine 29:416–432

Anderson RR, Parrish JA 1981 Microvasculature can be selectively damaged using dye lasers: a basic theory and experimental evidence in human skin. Lasers in Surgery and Medicine 1:263–276

Anderson RR, Parrish JA 1983 Selective photothermolysis: precise microsurgery by selective absorption of pulsed radiation. Science 220:524–527

Ara G, Anderson RR, Mandel KG, et al 1990 Irradiation of pigmented melanoma cells with high intensity pulsed radiation generates acoustic waves and kills cells. Lasers in Surgery and Medicine 10: 52–59

Bennet WR Jr, Faust WL, McFarlane RA, et al 1962 Dissociative excitation transfer and optical laser oscillation in NeO_2 and ArO_2 RF discharges. Physiological Reviews 8:470–473

Chang C-J, Kelly K, van Gemert MJC, Nelson JS 2002 Comparing the effectiveness of 585 nm vs. 595 nm wavelength pulsed dye laser treatment of port wine stains with cryogen spray cooling. Lasers in Surgery and Medicine 31:352–358

Chang C-J, Nelson JS 1999 Cryogen spray cooling and higher fluence pulsed dye laser treatment improve port-wine stain clearance while minimizing epidermal damage. Dermatologic Surgery 25:767–772

Dierickx CC, Alora MB, Dover JS 1999 A clinical overview of hair removal using lasers and light sources. Dermatologic Clinics 17:357–366

Dierickx CC, Casparian JM, Venugopalan V, et al 1995 Thermal relaxation of portwine stain vessels probed in vivo: the need for 1–10 millisecond laser pulse treatment. Journal of Investigative Dermatology 105:709–714

Garden JM, Bakus AD 1997 Laser treatment of portwine stains and haemangiomas. Dermatologic Clinics 15:373–383

Geronemus RG, Lou WW 2001 Treatment of port-wine stains by variable pulse width pulsed dye laser: a preliminary study. Dermatologic Surgery 27:903–905

Geronemus RG, Quintana AT, Lou WW, Kauvar AN 2000 High-fluence modified pulsed dye laser photocoagulation with dynamic cooling of port-wine stains in infancy. Archives of Dermatology 136:942–943

Goldman L, Nath G, Schindler G, et al 1973 High power neodymium-YAG laser surgery. Acta Dermato-Venereologica (Stockholm) 53:45–49

Goldman L, Wilson R, Hornby P 1965 Radiation from a Q-switched ruby laser: effect of repeated impacts of power output of 10 megawatts on a tattoo of man. Journal of Investigative Dermatology 44:69–71

Goyal S, Arndt KA, Stern RS, et al 1997 Laser treatment of tattoos; a prospective, paired comparison study of the Q-switched Nd : YAG (1064 nm), frequency doubled Nd : YAG (532 nm) and Q-switched ruby lasers. Journal of the American Academy of Dermatology 36:122–125

Johson LF 1961 Optical maser characteristics of rare earth ions in crystals. Journal of Applied Physiology 34:897–909

Jones A, Roddey P, Orengo I, Rosen T 1996 The Q-switched Nd : YAG laser effectively treats tattoos in darkly pigmented skin. Dermatologic Surgery 22:999–1001

Kienle A, Hibst R 1997 Optimal parameters for laser treatment of leg telangiectasia. Lasers in Surgery and Medicine 20:346–353

Kilmer SL, Lee MS, Grevelink JM, et al 1993 The Q-switched Nd : YAG laser effectively treats tattoos: a controlled dose–response study. Archives of Dermatology 129:971–978

Maiman T 1960 Stimulated optical radiation in ruby. Nature 187:493–494

Patel CKN, McFarlane RA, Faust WL 1964 Selective excitation through vibrational energy transfer and optical laser action in N_2CO_2. Physiological Reviews 13:617–619

Tan OT, Murray S, Kurban AK 1989 Action spectrum of vascular specific injury using pulsed irradiation. Journal of Investigative Dermatology 92:868–871

Tse Y, Levine VJ, McClain SA, Ashinoff R 1994 The removal of cutaneous pigmentary lesions with the Q-switched ruby laser and the Q-switched neodymium : yttrium-aluminium-garnet laser: a comparative study. Journal of Dermatology and Surgical Oncology 20: 795–800

Waner M, Suen JY 1996 Lasers in head and neck cancer. In: Suen JY, Myers E (eds) Cancer of the head and neck. WB Saunders, New York

Weiss RA, Weiss MA 1999 Early clinical results with a multiple synchronized pulse 1064 nm laser for leg telangiectasias and reticular veins. Dermatologic Surgery 25:399–402

2 Vascular Lesions

Karen H. Kim, Thomas E. Rohrer, Roy G. Geronemus

Introduction

Cutaneous vascular lesions are one of the most common indications for laser treatment in dermatology. Vascular lesions require proper diagnoses and a clear understanding of their biologic behavior.

This chapter discusses the evaluation and treatment of acquired and congenital vascular lesions of the face including telangiectasia, erythema, and vascular anomalies. Significant developments in laser and light based technology have had tremendous impact on the therapeutic options for these conditions, making it the preferred treatment for vascular lesions. Treatment of these common conditions is efficacious, well tolerated, and can be tailored for all skin types.

The theory of selective photothermolysis is the ability to target a specific chromophore in the skin without damaging surrounding structures through the selection of the proper wavelength, pulse duration, and fluence. Treatment parameters therefore can be optimized, permitting precise treatment of the intended structure while minimizing collateral injury to other tissues. The target chromophore in the treatment of vascular lesions is oxyhemoglobin. The peaks of oxyhemoglobin absorption are at 18 nm, 542 nm, and 577 nm. By selecting oxyhemoglobin, the surrounding vessel absorbs sufficient energy and is coagulated (Fig. 2.1). To minimize thermal injury to surrounding structures, the laser pulse duration should be equal to or shorter than the thermal relaxation time of the intended target. The thermal relaxation time is the cooling time of the target and is proportional to the square of the target diameter. For example, a port wine stain contains blood vessels that average 50–100 µm in diameter. The thermal relaxation time is approximately

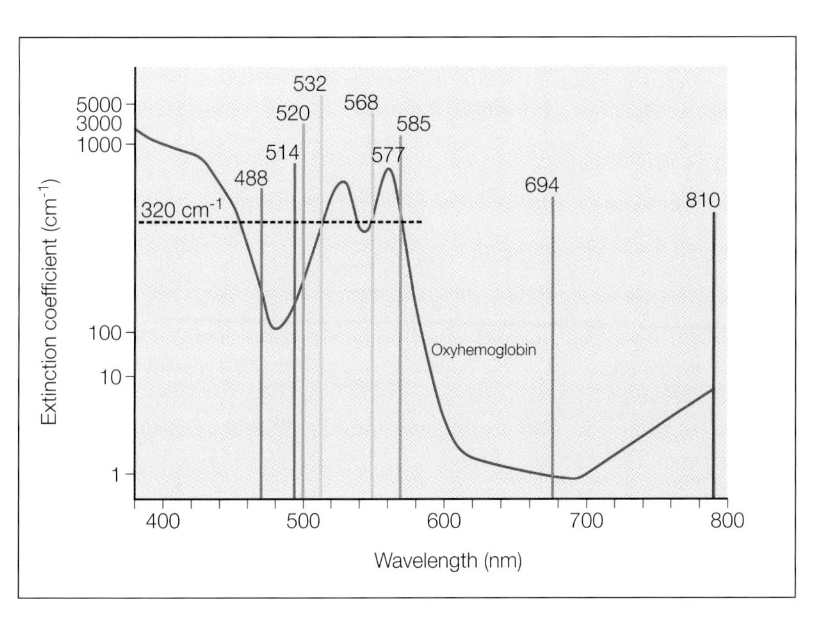

Fig. 2.1 Oxyhemoglobin absorption curve

1–10 ms. Longer pulse durations than the thermal relaxation time can lead to thermal diffusion and resultant damage to other structures.

Many lasers have been described for the treatment of vascular skin disorders with variable efficacy and safety. The first major advancement in laser treatment for vascular lesions was the 488 nm and 514 nm continuous argon laser in the 1970s. Early reports were very promising. The blue-green light emitted by the argon laser is well absorbed by oxyhemoglobin. Unfortunately, the continuous wave laser system (producing a continuous beam of light with little or no variation in power output over time) caused nonspecific coagulation necrosis of the superficial dermis that often led to subsequent scarring and depigmentation. Twenty one per cent of adult patients and 38% of patients under 12 years old had permanent hypopigmentation and scarring.

The argon pumped tunable dye, with wavelengths adjusted to the yellow range (577 or 585 nm), was more selective for blood vessels. It is a quasicontinuous wave mode laser with wavelengths ranging from 488 to 638 nm but which could be operated in the 577–585 nm range. The laser could be modified to deliver pulse widths of 20 ms, but the majority of clinical applications require a minimum of 100 ms pulse duration. There was minimal postprocedure purpura and hyperpigmentation, compared to traditional dye but unfortunately, the risk of atrophic or hypertrophic scarring was as high as 25% in treatment groups.

Commercially available in 1981, copper vapor and copper bromide lasers are quasicontinuous wave mode lasers that deliver yellow light with a wavelength of 578 nm. Also available at 510 nm, they can be utilized for the treatment of cutaneous pigmented lesions. Light is emitted as 20 ns pulses at a repetition rate of 6000–15 000 pulses per second. Various types of vascular lesions have been treated with good efficacy by these heavy metal vapor lasers. Facial telangiectasias, cherry angiomas, and pyogenic granulomas have been successfully treated with copper vapor and copper bromide lasers. Large blood vessels with longer thermal relaxation times are well suited for treatment by these lasers. However, energy is also absorbed by epidermal and dermal melanin and therefore should be restricted to patients of lighter skin types, namely, Fitzpatrick skin types I and II. Patients with darker skin types are at high risk of postinflammatory pigmentary changes and should not be treated with this laser system. Other adverse effects include crusting and blistering.

The introduction of the pulsed dye laser (PDL) in 1989 revolutionized the treatment of vascular lesions. It quickly became the treatment of choice for port wine stains, hemangiomas, and telangiectasias given its safety and efficacy. The first PDL emitted laser light at 577 nm, coinciding with the last peak of the oxyhemoglobin absorption spectrum (418, 542, 577 nm). By lengthening the wavelength to 585 nm, the PDL had deeper penetration into the dermis without compromising vascular selectivity. Currently available pulsed dye lasers emit a wavelength of 585 or 595 nm with longer pulse durations. Although there is deeper penetration of energy at 595 nm compared to 585 nm, the absorption of oxyhemoglobin is less after 585 nm. In order to compensate for decreased absorption, the longer wavelength PDL (595–600 nm) requires an additional 20–50% fluence compared to 585 nm PDL systems. Fluence is energy per unit area and is measured as joules/cm^2. Clinical studies of port wine stains treated with 595 nm PDL have demonstrated excellent clinical efficacy, comparing favorably with the results of the 585 nm PDL, and improving the clearance of resistant port wine stains previously treated with the 585 nm PDL. This effect is further enhanced by cooling systems that chill the skin prior to treatment, thereby protecting the epidermis. Skin cooling also allows higher energy to be delivered to target vessels and provides anesthetic relief during treatment.

On determining the thermal relaxation time of blood vessels in port wine stains to be between 1 and 10 ms, modified PDLs with pulsed durations of 1.5 ms were designed. These systems permit the use of higher fluences with lower peak energies, thereby decreasing adverse effects while enhancing efficacy.

Other laser and light systems that are currently used to treat vascular lesions include the intense pulsed light, KTP, diode, alexandrite, and Nd : YAG (1064 nm) lasers. The intense pulsed light source (IPLS) laser emits polychromatic, noncoherent light from 515 to 1200 nm. This light system has been described to be effective in the treatment of a variety of conditions including facial telangiectasia, poikiloderma of Civatte, superficial hemangiomas, and port wine stains.

Intense pulsed light systems emit broadband light that is capable of targeting vessels at various depths. IPLs is also based on the principle of selective photothermolysis. By using cut-off filters to filter out shorter wavelengths and permitting the emission of blue-green to yellow wavelengths, selective damage of cutaneous vessels can be seen.

The longer wavelengths can penetrate deeper to affect deeper blood vessels. A limiting factor of PDL is the depth of penetration. Histological studies have shown poor coagulation of dermal vessels beyond 1.16 mm in depth after PDL treatment. As longer wavelengths penetrate deeper, however, laser energy absorption in oxyhemaglobin decreases. Therefore, higher fluences are necessary to compensate for the decreased absorption. IPLs uses long wavelengths and high fluences for effective heating of superficial and deep vasculature. It also has large spot sizes that enable treatment of vascular abnormalities covering broad areas. Another potential advantage of IPLs is the delivery of laser energy over longer pulse durations, leading to more uniform heating and coagulation throughout the vessel in its entirety.

The frequency doubled Nd : YAG (or KTP) is a continuous wave laser using a neodymium : yttrium-aluminum-garnet (Nd : YAG) crystal with a wavelength of 1064 nm that is frequency doubled with a potassium titanyl phosphate crystal (KTP), such that green light with a 532 nm wavelength is emitted with good absorption by hemoglobin. The active medium in Nd : YAG lasers is a yttrium-aluminum-garnet (YAG) crystal doped with 1–3% neodymium ions. Doping is a process whereby crystals are grown with intentional impurities such that the YAG crystal lattice contains the Nd impurity. Nd : YAG lasers are typically powered by an incoherent light source such as a xenon arc lamp, using a curved surface to concentrate light on the Nd : YAG crystal rod, or diode lasers. Sufficient energy emitted in a single pulse lasting 10–50 ms leads to slow heating of vessels with minimal collateral damage and no resultant purpura. Facial vessels respond very well with the KTP laser with minimal morbidity.

Lasers with longer wavelengths such as the alexandrite laser, emitting light at 755 nm and pulse durations of 2–20 ms, as well as Nd : YAG lasers with a wavelength of 1064 nm and pulse durations up to 500 ms, have also been used for vascular lesions with good results. They can be useful for the treatment of facial reticular veins that are often recalcitrant to treatment with the shorter wavelength lasers including the PDL and KTP. Notably, one report had 100% resolution of all eight facial reticular veins 1 month after one treatment session. These results are rather exceptional, however, as the authors' clinical experiences have shown that multiple treatments are necessary.

Vascular Anomalies (Hemangiomas and Port Wine Stains)

Vascular lesions are the most common cutaneous abnormalities in the neonate (Table 2.1). Vascular anomalies should be properly identified, since the diagnosis predicts the biologic course and affects decisions about the interventions that can be implemented. Most of the time, the clinical appearance and clinical course are sufficient in determining an accurate diagnosis. Lesions that are present at birth and appear to grow at the same rate as the rest of the body are usually vascular malformations, whereas lesions that develop within the first few weeks of life that increase in size asynchronously are typically hemangiomas.

Diagnosis of hemangiomas and port wine stains					
	Present at birth?	**Growth out of proportion to rest of body?**	**Spontaneous involution?**	**Increase in size with high venous pressure?**	**Palpable thrill?**
Hemangiomas	No	Yes	Yes	No	No
Vascular malformation	Yes	No	No	Yes—venous malformation No—arterial, arteriovenous or lymphatic malformation	No—venous malformation Yes—arterial or arteriovenous malformation

Table 2.1 Diagnosis of hemangiomas and port wine stains

The classification of vascular anomalies has evolved through the years. Virchow and Wegener developed the first classification system of vascular lesions in the late 1800s, based on histologic features, in which vascular tumors were separated into angiomas and lymphangiomas, and subdivided into 'simplex', cavernous', and 'racemosum'.

Mulliken and Glowacki later developed a classification system that took into account the biologic behavior of vascular lesions in addition to the physical and microscopic appearance. According to their classification, there are two main subtypes: hemangiomas and vascular malformations. Vascular lesions are distinguished by their presence or absence at birth and their proliferation pattern. Vascular malformations are present at birth and grow proportionately with the rest of the body. They persist throughout life and many develop nodularity during adulthood that can become more burdensome, particularly in areas prone to trauma.

By contrast, hemangiomas are absent at birth. They appear in the first few weeks of life and grow at a much faster rate than the rest of the body within the first year. After the first year, they undergo slow involution. Mulliken further classified hemangiomas into 'capillary', 'cavernous', and 'capillary cavernous', based on their depths in the dermis and subcutaneous fat. Capillary hemangiomas (previously called strawberry hemangiomas) refer to lesions in the papillary dermis; cavernous hemangiomas are located in the deeper reticular dermis and/or subcutaneous fat. 'Capillary cavernous' hemangiomas are lesions involving the papillary and reticular dermis and subcutaneous fat. Waner and Suen invoked a slightly modified approach to hemangioma classification, dividing them into 'superficial', 'deep', and 'combined' based on the clinical depth of involvement.

Hemangiomas

Hemangiomas are the most common vascular anomaly, affecting up to 12% of all children by 1 year of age. There is a female predominance, with a 3 : 1 ratio compared to affected males. Sixty per cent of all hemangiomas are found in the head and neck region. The majority (80%) of hemangiomas appear as single lesions. Usually radiographic imaging is not necessary with single hemangiomas. In the presence of multiple hemangiomas, magnetic resonance imaging scans may be recommended to rule out visceral involvement.

One third of hemangiomas are present at birth, usually as solitary lesions on the head and neck. The majority of hemangiomas appear shortly after birth, typically within the first few weeks of life. They subsequently undergo rapid growth in the first year when the lesion grows much faster than the rest of the body. Some begin to involute by the end of the first year. By age five, 50% of hemangiomas spontaneously involute. Each year thereafter, an additional 10% involute. Unfortunately, even after lesions have involuted, 40–50% of children are still left with residual fibrofatty tissue. Parents and physicians should be cognizant of this, as it may have important cosmetic, functional, and psychosocial consequences.

Clinical features are useful for hemangioma classification. According to Waner and Suen, hemangiomas can be described as superficial, deep, or combined based on their depth in the skin. Cellular markers have also been used to distinguish proliferating and involuting hemangiomas. Such markers include elevated levels of basic fibroblast growth factor, type IV collagenase, vascular endothelial growth factors, urokinase, and proliferating cell nuclear antigen in proliferating hemangiomas. Involuting hemangiomas exhibit tissue inhibitor metalloproteinase, angiostatin, endostatin, interleukin 12, and thrombospondin metalloproteinase inhibitors. Another useful laboratory finding is urinary bFGF (basic fibroblast growth) factor levels. They were found to be elevated in children with proliferating hemangiomas and were low or not present in children with vascular malformations.

In evaluating hemangiomas, the anatomic location and constellation of other clinical findings should alert the physician to consider rare, multisystem syndromes including PHACES and diffuse neonatal hemangiomatosis and recommend a work-up as necessary. PHACES is an acronym for the following associated features: ***p***osterior fossa malformation, ***h***emangiomas (especially segmental), ***a***rterial anomalis, ***c***oarctation of the aorta, ***e***ye abnormalities, and ***s***ternal or supraumbilical raphe. Large hemangiomas may be associated with Kasabach–Merritt syndrome. This syndrome contains the following findings: hemolytic anemia, consumptive coagulopathy, and platelet destruction.

Complications that may be associated with hemangiomas include ulceration, bleeding, scarring, and infection. Ulcerated hemangiomas can be very tender and usually occur in the setting of rapid proliferation. Rapidly proliferating hemangiomas on the face can be concerning because they can obscure vision or compromise vital structures.

Treatment of hemangiomas

Given the course of spontaneous involution, clinical observation is advisable in many circumstances. Therapeutic intervention should be considered for the following reasons: compromised airway, visual axis impairment, oral/gastrointestinal tract obstruction, and auditory involvement. Bleeding, ulceration, and facial involvement are other indications for aggressive intervention. We believe early intervention during the proliferative phase offers the potential of reducing the overall eventual size of the hemangioma. It may halt the progression or rapid growth of hemangiomas. This is important in hemangiomas located in cosmetically sensitive areas or areas that may be more susceptible to injury and ulceration, such as the face, chest (especially in females), and anal-genital region.

Various therapeutic options have been explored for the treatment of hemangiomas (Table 2.2). Cryosurgery and sclerotherapy have been utilized but cases were often fraught with high degrees of scarring and inconsistent results. Intralesional and high dose systemic steroid therapy (2–4 g/kg/day) has been effective in the treatment of rapidly growing hemangiomas. However, if the hemangioma continues to grow after 8–10 days of systemic treatment, it is recommended that steroids be halted and another therapy be implemented. Interferon alpha has been used with clinical efficacy. Unfortunately, the adverse effects of spastic diplegia and other neurologic complications affecting gait, speech, and fine motor skills seen in up to 26% of treated patients severely limit the practical utility of this therapy.

Surgical excision may be appropriate in certain cases, especially in combination with laser therapy for larger lesions. In these instances, it is important to determine whether functionally and cosmetically the resultant postsurgical scar will be superior to the hemangioma, in light of its eventual natural resolution. After involution, the residual fibrofatty tissue can be surgically excised.

Lasers provide an important therapeutic approach for hemangiomas. The flash lamp pulsed dye, the KTP, argon, alexandrite, and Nd : YAG lasers have been reported to be quite effective. The wavelength, power output of the laser system, spot size, and exposure times are important factors in determining the effectiveness. Given the excellent safety profile and good efficacy, the flash lamp pulsed dye laser is regarded as the treatment of choice for superficial

Treatment table							
System	**Wavelength (nm)**	**Fluence (J/cm^2)**	**Pulse duration (ms)**	**Spot size (mm)**	**Epidermal cooling?**	**Vascular condition**	**Comments**
PDL	585–595	6.5–7.5	10	10	Cryogen spray	Facial Erythema/ Telangiectasia	Pulse stacking
		7.5	1.5	10	Cryogen spray	Port wine stain	Pulse stack in nodular areas only
		12	1.5	7	Cryogen spray	Hemangioma	
KTP	532	15–18	20	3	Contact cooling	Telangiectasia Hemangiomas	Do not pulse stack for telangiectasia
IPL	550–1200	30–50 28–42 25–35	3 2.5–3.5 2.5		Contact Contact Contact	Hemangiomas Vascular malformation Erythema/poikiloderma	590 nm filter 570 nm filter 570 nm filter
Nd : YAG	1064	130				Reticular vein	Do not pulse stack
Alexandrite	755	60–80	3	8	Cryogen	Hemangiomas	Do not pulse stack

Table 2.2 Treatment table. Note: these are treatment settings used at our institutions; results may vary with different laser models and calibrations

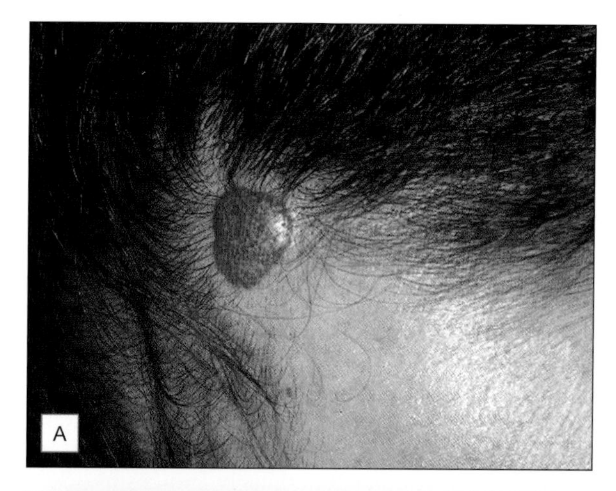

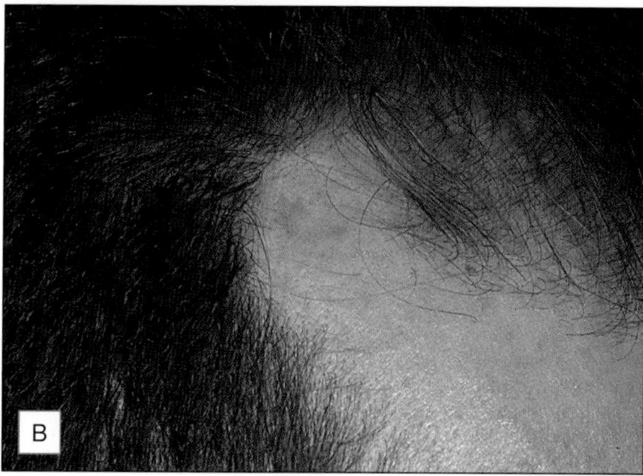

Fig. 2.2 Hemangioma. (**A**) Pretreatment. (**B**) Post-treatment with PDL

hemangiomas. The 585 nm wavelength has a depth of penetration to 1.2 mm and is a limiting factor for thicker lesions. Ninety-four per cent lightening in lesions with a thickness of 3 mm or less has been achieved after four treatment sessions with the PDL, whereas mixed hemangiomas with greater than 3 mm thickness had 85.1% lightening but a mild reduction in thickness. In another study, 86% of superficial hemangiomas achieved good to excellent results after an average of two treatments, compared to 39% of mixed hemangiomas with good response after two sessions. A study comparing the 585 nm PDL and the 532 nm KTP demonstrated that the PDL achieved a higher regression rate (93% in PDL vs. 70% with KTP after 3.0 and 2.6 treatments, respectively) (Fig. 2.2)

Longer wavelength lasers can penetrate deeper and may be better suited for thicker lesions and deeper, larger vessels. The Nd : YAG laser, emitting a wavelength of 1064 nm, has several theoretical advantages. The longer wavelength can enable deeper penetration into the dermis. Oxyhemoglobin absorption has a peak at 1064 nm while melanin absorption decreases at longer wavelengths, so the risk of post-treatment hyperpigmentation is decreased at 1064 nm. This is especially helpful in the treatment of darker skin types, where the risk of pigmentary alteration is high.

The Nd : YAG laser is available as continuous or pulsed beams and can penetrate to a depth of 4–6 mm to coagulate deeper, larger vessels. Continuous wave Nd : YAG lasers cause shrinkage of hemangiomas primarily by nonspecific thermal damage and have an inherent risk of scarring. They have been used to treat mixed or deep hemangiomas. Deeper hemangiomas have been reported to reduce by 50% after one treatment. The long pulsed Nd : YAG laser system, Coolglide (Altus, Burlingame, CA, USA), has a pulse duration range of 0.1–300 ms, maximum fluence of 300 J/cm^2 with spot size ranging from 3 to 10 mm. Using this system, after one treatment, all 13 hemangiomas reportedly improved with 50–99% resolution. Unfortunately, the precise details of the type and locations of these lesions were not specified.

Interstitial Nd : YAG laser therapy, in which a probe is inserted into the hemangioma, has been reported to be helpful, especially for deep subcutaneous hemangiomas. However, the high risk of scarring makes it a less favorable approach for most hemangiomas.

The intense pulsed light system is a noncoherent polychromatic light source emitting wavelengths from 515 to 1200 nm. Although the Photoderm VL (ESC Medical, Needham, MA, USA) was the earliest IPL system, numerous other systems are in wide use today. The pulse durations can range from 1.0 to 100 ms. It can target superficial vessels with the shorter wavelengths while penetrating to deeper vessels with the longer wavelengths. The long pulse durations enable delivery of energy with uniform heating of the vessels. Single, double or triple pulses can be emitted with intervals in between pulses to allow the epidermis and smaller vessels to cool down while heat remains in the deeper vessels, leading to selective thermal injury. The large spot size used with the IPL systems enhances penetration of energy with less scatter. By changing the parameters of the system, a variety of vascular lesions can be treated effectively. Hemangiomas that have been resistant to other treatments, including deep lesions, have been reported to respond with this system. Between 75% and 100% clearance has been reported after one to four treatments. The disadvantages of this system are the generally greater number of treatment sessions necessary for clearance, higher potential for adverse effects including scarring, and higher degree of discomfort during the procedure.

When evaluating a patient, it is important to consider the depth of the hemangioma. Superficial hemangiomas respond very well to laser therapy. If the majority of the hemangioma is deep, the response to laser intervention is poor. In combination hemangiomas, the superficial portion responds well with minimal effect on the deep component. Patients and the patient's family must understand that post-treatment purpura will occur and typically lasts 7–10 days. Multiple treatments are required, usually at 3 week intervals. Faster growing lesions may need more frequent sessions. The degree of improvement after each treatment can be variable. If the hemangioma continues to proliferate rapidly after several treatment sessions, alternative therapeutic options should be explored.

Port wine stains (capillary vascular malformation)

Vascular malformations may be localized or diffuse and occur as errors of embryonic development. They are subdivided into arterial, arteriovenous, venous, capillary, or lymphatic malformations. Capillary malformations (port wine stains) and lymphatic malformations are usually noticed at birth, whereas venous malformations can appear congenitally or become apparent during adulthood. Arterial and arteriovenous malformations often manifest during hormonal fluctuations such as pregnancy or puberty.

Port wine stains (nevus flammeus) are a type of capillary vascular malformation and, by definition, are present at birth. They do not resolve. Occurring in 0.3% of the population, they have an equal incidence in males and females. Port wine stains are composed of ecstatic vessels in the papillary dermis. They can vary in size from a few millimeters in diameter to greater than 50% of the body surface area. Any part of the body may be affected, but the head and neck is the most common site of involvement. Fifty per cent of port wine stains affecting the face are restricted to one of the three trigeminal sensory regions. The more extensive the cutaneous involvement, the more likely that there is underlying neurologic, ophthalmologic, or other systemic abnormalities.

A complete history and physical examination are usually sufficient to distinguish port wine stains from other vascular malformations or hemangiomas. Sometimes, a nevus simplex (salmon patch) or hemangioma in its early stage of development can be mistaken for a port wine stain. In those cases, close observation of their clinical course can be helpful. Clinical features are also tremendously helpful. Venous and lymphatic malformations are typically soft and compressible. Venous malformations increase in size with increased venous pressure. This can be assessed by positioning the lesion in a dependent fashion to look for size fluctuations. Arterial and arteriovenous malformations are firm to touch, usually have a palpable thrill, and feel warmer than the surrounding skin.

Vascular malformations can also be categorized based on radiographic features. Angiography delineates malformations as 'low flow' or 'high flow'. Capillary, venous and lymphatic malformations have low flow characteristics, and arterial malformations including aneurysms, ectasia, stenosis, and arteriovenous fistulas are considered high flow.

A main distinguishing feature of port wine stains is that they persist throughout life, in comparison to hemangiomas. They are usually located on the face, most commonly in the V2 distribution. In two thirds of patients with port wine stains, the soft tissue of involved areas hypertrophy and the initial flat pink-red patches evolve into 'cobblestoned' purple plaques and nodules as a result of progressive vascular ectasia by the fifth decade. Consequently, they are more prone to bleeding and susceptible to trauma during adulthood. Pyogenic granulomas can occasionally also develop. These features have strong implications in the treatment plan.

Syndromes that must be considered during the evaluation of vascular malformations include Sturge–Weber syndrome, Olser–Weber–Rendu syndrome, blue rubber bleb syndrome, Parkes–Weber syndrome, Klippel–Trenaunay syndrome, Servelle–Martorell syndrome, Cobb's syndrome, and Maffucci's syndrome. Patients with port wine stains in the first branch of the trigeminal nerve (V1) are at risk of Sturge–Weber syndrome. Additionally, patients with port wine stains involving the upper or lower eyelid should be seen regularly by an ophthalmologist, as they are at increased risk of having glaucoma. Those patients with port wine stains affecting the lower extremity should also get periodic leg length measurements to evaluate for limb hypertrophy. Appropriate radiographic and systemic work-up is advised based on the anatomic location, extent of surface area involvement, and level of clinical suspicion.

Treatment of port wine stains

The flash lamp pulsed dye laser is an excellent treatment option for port wine stains, as the emitted wavelength (585 or 595 nm) is well absorbed by the target chromophore, oxyhemoglobin, such that blood vessels are selectively targeted and injury to other components of the epidermis is minimized (Table 2.3). Pulsed dye lasers contain rhodamine dye dissolved in methanol and emit light in the yellow portion of the visible spectrum. Oxyhemoglobin is the target chromophore in vascular lesions and has absorption peaks at 420, 540, and 577 nm. Although the highest peak in oxyhemoglobin absorption and the greatest difference in absorption between oxyhemoglobin and the competing chromophore melanin occurs at 420 nm, the light energy at 420 nm does not penetrate to reach vessels in the dermis. The depth of light penetration increases in a somewhat linear form from 400 nm out to 1000 nm. By using a wavelength of 585 nm, early pulsed dye lasers are able to preferentially heat oxyhemoglobin at a depth necessary to treat port wine stains. The first pulsed dye lasers utilized a pulse duration of 0.45 ms. Although the ideal pulse duration for the treatment of port wine stains was determined to be at least 1 ms, engineers were unable to develop a flashlamp that could deliver pulsed laser energy with pulse durations longer than 0.45 ms. As technology progressed, it became possible to create flashlamps capable of delivering pulse durations of 1.5 ms and the second generation pulsed dye lasers utilized this pulsed duration. The wavelength was increased out to 600 nm to increase the depth of penetration in an attempt to treat slightly deeper vascular lesions such as superficial leg veins. Commercially available PDLs that are in wide use today include the Candela V Beam and the Cynosure V Star, both emitting wavelengths at 595 nm and having pulse durations that may be adjusted from 0.45 to 40 ms. Although the energy absorption of oxyhemoglobin is slightly less at 595 nm compared to 585 nm, the longer wavelength PDL systems have the advantage of enabling deeper penetration into the dermis for deeper vessels. In fact, using a 595 nm PDL with 1.5 ms pulse duration at 11–12 J/cm^2, there was greater than 75% clearance of port wine stains in 63% of patients achieved after four treatments. This was an improvement over previous reports of 75% clearance in 40% of patients with the 585 nm PDL.

An important consideration for laser therapy is skin type. Patients with skin of a darker color were previously described to have poor results because of the presence of a competing chromophore, melanin, in their darker skin. However, the availability of epidermal cooling, larger spot size, and variable pulse widths has provided a safe and effective means of treating vascular conditions in people with skin of a darker color with less risk of epidermal injury and pigmentary alteration and high patient satisfaction.

Multiple studies have demonstrated the safety and efficacy of the pulsed dye laser and it is widely accepted as the treatment of choice for port wine stains. However, despite over 20 years of clinical experience, less than 25% of port wine stains have complete clearing after multiple PDL treatments. There have been suggestions that optical properties of vascular lesions change after laser irradiation. In vivo measurements before and after PDL therapy with reflectance spectroscopy have confirmed the

Pulsed dye lasers				
	Manufacturer	**Wavelength (nm)**	**Pulse width (ms)**	**Cooling**
C beam	Candela	585	0.45	Cryogen
Sclero HP	Candela	595	1.5	Cryogen
V beam	Candela	595	0.45–40	Cryogen
V Star	Cynosure	595	0.5–40	Air
N Light	USA Photonics	585	0.45	None

Table 2.3 Pulsed dye lasers

formation of methemoglobin after PDL therapy at fluences higher than 5 J/cm^2. It is thought that methemoglobin formation correlates with hemoglobin denaturation and vessel wall destruction. By addressing the optical properties of methemoglobin, treatment parameters may be further optimized to yield improved clearance of port wine stains.

Our experience suggests that the early treatment of port wine stains yields the best response (Box 2.1). Likely factors that contribute to the favorable response are thinner skin in infants, smaller and more superficial vessels, and a smaller affected surface area leading to improved clearance in fewer treatment sessions (Figs 2.3, 2.4)

Hypertrophic and nodular port wine stains, with larger and deeper vessels, do not respond as well as flat lesions with pulsed dye lasers. Other laser and light source systems have helped improve lesions resistant to PDL. Intense pulsed light systems have been reported to yield good results. An average of four sessions led to complete clearance in pink lesions, while darker, purple lesions achieved 70–99% lightening after four sessions. This may be due to the inclusion of longer and therefore more deeply penetrating light wavelengths in these broadband light sources. Nodular port wine stains were reported to respond better to the 1064 nm Nd : YAG laser than flat port wine stains after one treatment. Early reports of utilizing photodynamic therapy in the treatment of port wine stains have been promising. Future studies with PDT may show higher success rates, especially in resistant cases.

When treating port wine stains, it is important to establish the treatment site prior to laser therapy. Reactive erythema often makes the borders of affected and unaffected skin appear indistinct. Laser irradiation is associated with increased dermal blood volume, partly due to local heat production. Outlining the involved areas with a skin marking pen

Treatment tips and pitfalls

- Purpuric doses are necessary for the successful treatment of vascular malformations and hemangiomas
- The earlier you start treating congenital vascular malformations, the better the result. Treatments ideally should begin in early infancy
- The first three treatments at appropriate settings generally yield the most dramatic results
- Use ocular shields when treating periorbital regions
- Apply Surgilube to hair bearing areas prior to treatment to avoid injury to the hair
- Have patients or patient's parent outline the affected area prior to treatment with a skin marking pen. Area may become less obvious as it lightens after successive treatments. Also, patients may get agitated during treatment causing transient flushing of normal adjacent skin that may be mistaken for affected skin
- The degree of clearance is location dependent. The neck, forehead, chin, and lateral cheek areas respond more quickly than centrofacial areas
- Use caution in the presence of laryngeal masks or intubation. Minimize exposure to potentially flammable substances such as oxygen, hair, make-up, gauze, sponges, and endotracheal tubes. Apply a wet drape over the face mask and remove oxygen or nitrogen from the surgical field when the mask is removed
- If a patient has been on oral isotretinoin, wait at least 6 months after the cessation of isotretinoin prior to initiating laser therapy to avoid the risk of keloids or hypertrophic scarring

Box 2.1 Treatment tips and pitfalls

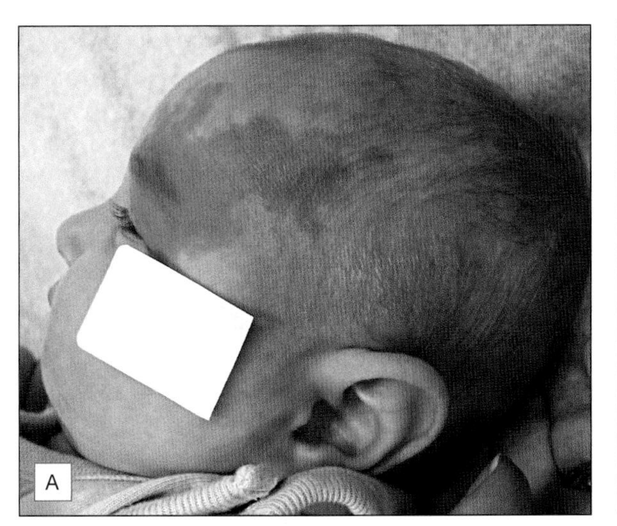

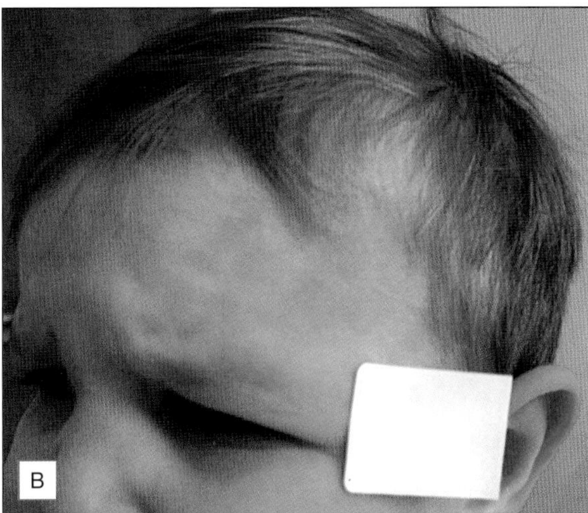

Fig. 2.3 Port wine stain. (**A**) Pretreatment. (**B**) After 12 treatments with PDL

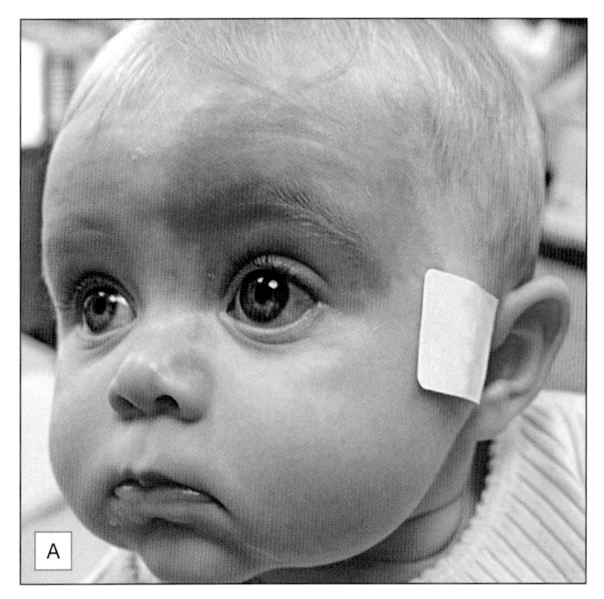

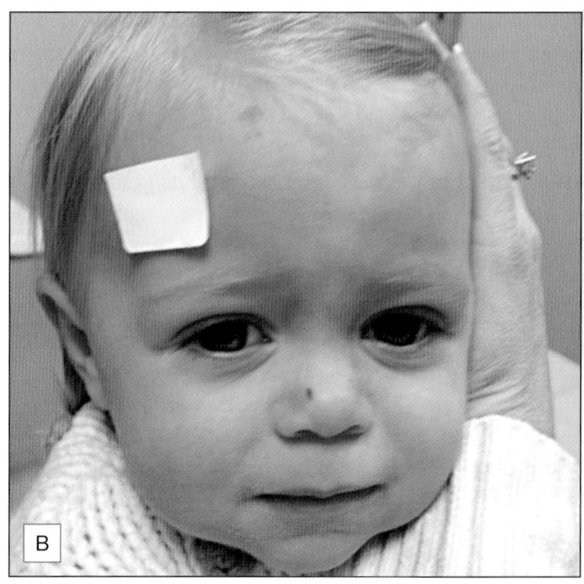

Fig. 2.4 Port wine stain. (**A**) Pretreatment. (**B**) After six treatments with PDL

or treating the edge of the port wine stain first can facilitate the treatment and prevent inadvertent treatment of unaffected adjacent skin. The treatment is associated with temporary purpura that lasts for 7–10 days. Sessions are repeated every 4–8 weeks. For darker skin types, it is recommended to wait as long as 3 months between treatment sessions to appreciate the full benefit of each treatment and permit postinflammatory hyperpigmentation, if present, to resolve.

Venous Malformations

Venous malformations are low flow vascular lesions that typically present as faint blue or soft, blue masses. They occur in a variety of ways, and include varicosities, ectasias, localized spongy masses, and complex lesions infiltrating organ systems, especially muscle. Like port wine stains, they occur at birth and grow proportionally with the rest of the body during infancy and childhood. Rarely, they may grow in adulthood. They are usually asymptomatic; however, occasionally they may swell and become painful. They may enlarge over time and develop phleboliths, thrombosis, or hemorrhage. An extensive venous malformation can cause a localized intravascular coagulopathy.

When a patient presents with a venous malformation, it is generally recommended to obtain additional imaging for further evaluation. Magnetic resonance imaging is the most informative technique for venous malformations, and they are usually seen as T2 hyperintense lesions. Doppler ultrasonagraphy can characterize the presence or type of blood flow (low or high flow).

Venous malformations affecting the head and neck region and those involving limbs may require treatment because of risk to adjacent structures or facial distortion. Treatment of venous malformations include surgery, sclerotherapy, and/or laser therapy. Surgery can be considered for well circumscribed lesions; however, excising extensive lesions can lead to functional motor loss and nerve damage. Sclerotherapy can also be used to reduce the size or as an adjunct with other methods. Sclerosing agents in liquid and microfoam form have been utilized. They include osmotic agents such as hypertonic saline or salicylates, detergents such as sodium tetradecyl sulfate, polidocanol, morrhuate sodium or diatrizoate sodium, or other chemical agents including iodine or alcohol.

Laser therapy is helpful for superficial venous malformations. The PDL and KTP laser have been used. However, multiple treatments are necessary and the limited light penetrance has yielded modest results. The Nd : YAG laser emits infrared light at 1064 nm and can penetrate to depths of 5–7 mm. Percutaneous and intralesional Nd : YAG photocoagulation therapy has been reported to be useful for complex malformations. The IPL system has also been found to be effective in the treatment of small venous malformations. In one report, small venous malformations had 70–100% clearance after between two and eight treatments. The smaller lesions required fewer treatments compared to larger lesions. The cut-off filters used were 550, 570 or 590 nm, depending on the depth of the malformation. Most treatments were sequenced as triple pulses and an average fluence of 80 J/cm^2 was delivered.

Facial Telangiectasia

Significant telangiectasias of the face occur in at least 10–15% of adults and children. Simple telangiectasias are small, dilated vessels that are 0.1–1.0 mm in diameter. They are commonly located on the midface region and appear as linear red or blue vessels. Spider telangiectasias ('spider nevi') consist of red, radial branches emanating from a central arteriole that blanch with pressure. They are especially common in children. Many persist for years, prompting patients and parents to look for treatment options. Exogenous factors can induce or exacerbate telangectasias. Alcohol, estrogen, corticosteroids, and chronic actinic damage can precipitate their onset. Trauma or postoperative tension resulting from excisions, facelifts, or rhinoplasties can also promote neovascularization resulting in telangiectasia. Telangiectatic vessels are a predominant feature of rosacea and enlargement of deeper vessels and increased numbers of smaller vessels can manifest as facial erythema and flushing. Poikiloderma of Civatte is a clinical condition induced by chronic, excessive sun exposure. It presents as reticulated brown pigmentation as well as discrete and confluent vascular ectasias and prominent telangiectasias on the lower face, neck and anterior chest region. Collagen vascular disease can often be associated with telangiectasias occurring on the head and neck region.

The treatment of facial telangiectasias and erythema is one of the most frequent indications for cutaneous laser therapy (Box 2.2). Vessels may be located in conspicuous areas on the face, eliciting unwanted attention. Female patients recount their dependence on heavy cover-up or foundation in attempts to attenuate the erythema and camouflage the telangiectasia. Men and teenage boys often report their frustration and embarrassment with the ruddy appearance and the social stigmata in the mistaken association with the plethora seen in alcoholics.

Postoperative care instructions given to patients following treatment of facial telangiectasia

- Mild redness will occur postprocedure. On occasion, bruising can occur. Some swelling can occur, especially near the eye or lip. Keep the head elevated during sleep. Applying ice packs to the treated area can help with the swelling
- Rarely, if blistering or crusting occurs, apply Aquaphor healing ointment to the area twice a day and cover with a nonstick bandage. The area may get wet while bathing
- Make-up may be worn if no blistering or crusting occurs. Avoid anything that may be too abrasive or irritating

Box 2.2 Postoperative care instructions given to patients following treatment of facial telangiectasia

People with facial erythema and flushing had very few options for amelioration of their condition prior to advances in laser and light based systems. Before the availability of laser therapy, the treatment of facial telangiectasia was largely limited to electrocautery or sclerotherapy. These modalities have the disadvantages of risk of ulceration, atrophy, hyperpigmentation, and high recurrence.

Fortunately, facial telangiectasias are very amenable to laser treatment. Pulsed dye lasers with variable pulse duration ranging from 0.45 to 40 ms are very effective in treating facial ectasias. Improved vessel clearance and reduction of facial erythema can be accomplished with stacking pulses of lower fluence and longer pulse durations, obviating the need for post-treatment purpura. The mean percentage of facial telangiectasia vessel clearing following a single treatment improved from 67% with nonoverlapping pulses to 87% with the pulse stacking technique (Fig. 2.5).

Other laser systems that are useful in the treatment of facial telangiectasia are the KTP, Nd : YAG, and IPL systems (Tables 2.4, 2.5). The KTP laser is a frequency doubled Nd : YAG laser emitting green light at 532 nm. KTP lasers currently in use are the Orion/Aura Gemini (Laserscope, Palo Alto, CA, USA), the Diolite (Iriderm, Mountain View, CA, USA), and the Versapulse (Coherent, Palo Alto, CA, USA). The 532 nm wavelength approximates an absorption peak of hemoglobin, hence it is well suited for the treatment of superficial blood vessels (Fig. 2.6).

The Aura laser is a stable continuous wave KTP doped Nd : YAG laser that can deliver energy in 1–50 ms pulses. Five handpieces in 0.25, 1, 2, and 4 mm sizes, as well as a computerized scanning

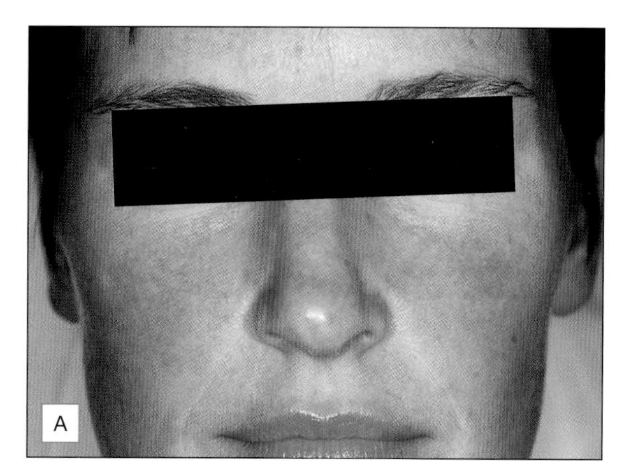

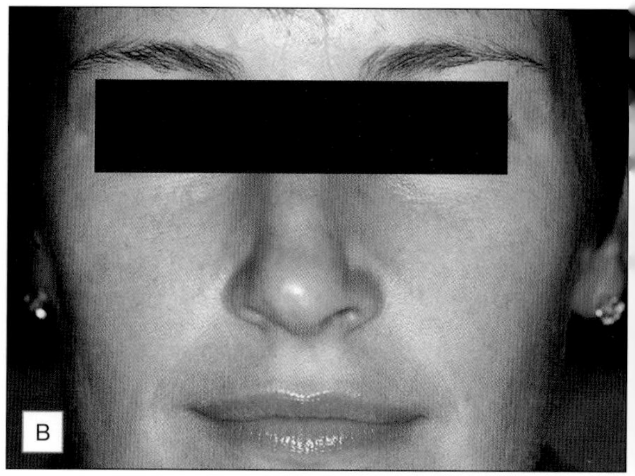

Fig. 2.5 Facial erythema and telangiectasia. (**A**) Pretreatment. (**B**) Post-treatment with PDL

1064 nm Nd : YAG lasers						
	Manufacturer	**Wavelength (nm)**	**Pulse width (ms)**	**Spot size (mm)**	**Fluence (J/cm^2)**	**Cooling**
Lyra	Laserscope	1064	20–100	1.5,3,5,10	5–200	Contact
Cool Glide	Altus	1064	20–100	10	1–300	Contact
Varia	CoolTouch	1064	300–500	2,4,6,8	1–500	Cryogen pre and post
Vasculight	ESC	1064	2–16	6	1–150	Contact
Gentle:YAG	Candela	1064	0.25–300	1.5–18	1–500	Cryogen

Table 2.4 1064 nm Nd : YAG lasers

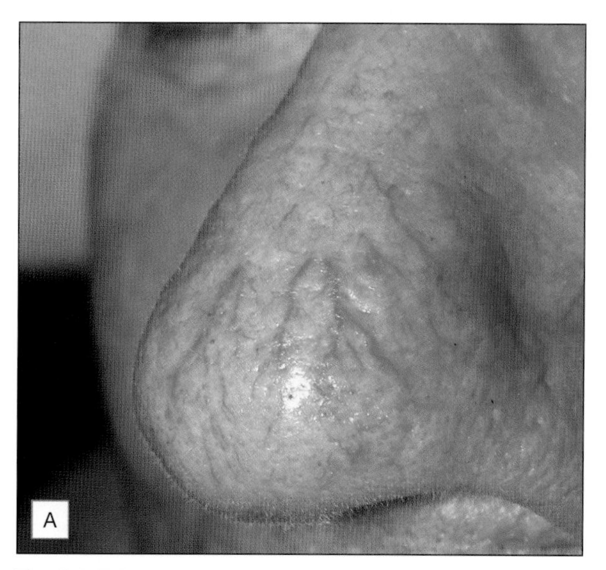

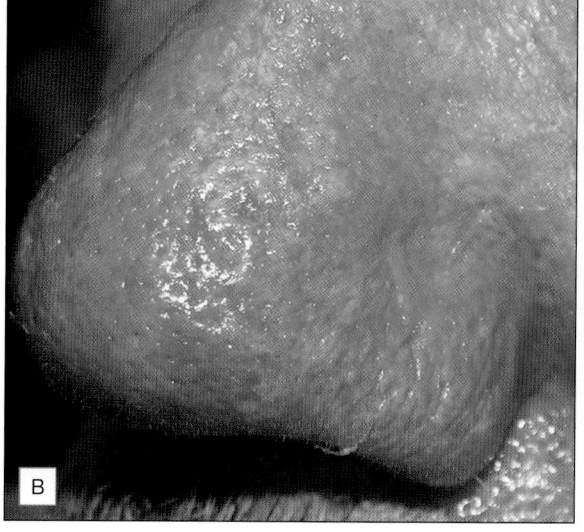

Fig. 2.6 Telangiectasia. (**A**) Pretreatment. (**B**) Post-treatment with KTP

IPL devices							
	Source of light	**Spectrum (nm)**	**Optical filter**	**Fluence (J/cm^2)**	**Pulse sequence**	**Pulse duration (ms)**	**Spot size (mm)**
Photoderm	IPL	515–1200	515/55/570/590/ 615/645/695/755	3–90	1,2,3	1–300	120,280
EpiLight	IPL	590–1200	590/615/645/ 695/755	20–65	2, 3, 4, 5	2.5–7	1–300
VascuLight SR,HR,VX,DL	IPL/Nd : YAG	515–1200/1064	515/550/560/570/ 590/615/640/645/ 695/755	3–90/ 40–150	1,2,3	0.5–25/ 2–16	1–300/ 1–300
AestiLight	IPL	645–1200	Factory setting	24–32	3	Factory setting	Factory setting
IPL Quantum HR	IPL	695–1200	645, 755	Prepro-grammed settings	Prepro-grammed settings	Prepro-grammed settings	272
IPL Quantum SR	IPL	560–1200	560,590,640	Prepro-grammed settings	Prepro-grammed settings	Prepro-grammed settings	272
Ellipe relax light	IPL	400–950	600–950, 550–950, 400–720	21–23	1–7	0.5–88.5	1.5–127
Aurora DS	IPL/RF	680–980		10–30 5–20	10–30 5–20	7–100/200	
Aurora SR	IPL/RF	580–980		10–30 5–20	10–30 5–20	7–100/200	

Table 2.5 IPL devices

handpiece that emits a 1 mm spot size encompassing a 1.3 cm diameter hexagonal shaped pattern, are available. The DioLite delivers energy in pulses lasting 10–50 ms. Fluence can range from 0.1 to 950 J/cm^2 and available spot sizes are 0.2, 0.5, 0.7, 1, and 1.4 mm. Unlike other KTP lasers that group Q-switched pulses into millisecond pulses, the Versapulse is a variable pulse width frequency doubled Nd : YAG laser that produces a true millisecond pulse. Therefore, the Versapulse has a slightly higher energy output compared to the other lasers in this category. It has a water cooled sapphire chill tip for contact cooling and the spot size can be changed from 2 to 10 mm, the pulse duration can vary from 2 to 50 ms, and fluence can be adjusted from 0.6 to 40 J/cm^2. In one study, 93.9% of patients treated for facial telangiectasia with a KTP laser had 75–100% clearance after one treatment. Spider angiomas respond quite favorably. By contrast, perialar telangiectasia are more challenging to clear and often require multiple treatments. After one treatment, 83% of cases of spider angiomas showed good to excellent improvement, while one treatment of telangiectasia in the perialar region yielded good to excellent results in 53% of patients.

Long pulsed alexandrite (755 nm) and diode lasers (800, 810, and 930 nm) have longer wavelengths within a small peak of hemoglobin absorption that make them theoretically suitable for the treatment of deeper, larger vessels. The Gentlelase (Candela, Wayland, MA, USA) is an alexandrite laser with a pulse duration of 3 ms; available spot sizes include 8, 10, 12, 15 and 18 mm and maximum fluence varies between 20 and 100 J/cm^2. The Gentlelase has a cryogen spray for epidermal cooling. The EpiTouch Alex (ESC/Sharplan, Lumenis) is an alexandrite laser with a pulse duration of 2 ms, spot size range of 5, 7, and 10 mm, and fluence range between 1 and 50 J/cm^2. The Apogee (Cynosure, Chelmsford, MA, USA) is an alexandrite laser with pulse durations of 5, 10, or 20 ms and spot sizes of 7, 10, 12.5 and 6 × 10 mm. Maximum fluence ranges from 35 to 50 J/cm^2. The LightSheer (Star Medical Tech., Lumenis Pleasanton, CA, USA) is an Al-Ga-As semiconductor diode laser with a pulse duration ranging from 5 to 30 ms, 9 × 9 mm spot size, 10–40 J/cm^2 maximum fluence, and a chill tip for contact cooling. Cutaneous vessels measuring larger than 0.4 mm in diameter appear to respond well with alexandrite and diode lasers. Although there have been no reports in peer reviewed literature, alexandrite and diode lasers have been used effectively in the treatment of hemangiomas or vascular malformations.

Blue reticular veins previously resistant to the shorter wavelength lasers including the pulsed dye laser and the 532 nm laser have been found to respond to treatments with the Nd : YAG 1064 nm laser. Greater than 75% improvement was seen in 97% of facial telangiectasia and periorbital reticular veins. Reticular veins remain one of the more challenging vascular lesions and multiple treatment sessions are necessary. Another difficult area is the perialar region. Telangiectasis in that area require multiple treatments and they may need retreatment in the future.

The IPL systems are helpful in treating facial telangiectasia and poikiloderma of Civatte, especially when it extends over a large area. Good to excellent clearance of facial telangiectasia was reported after one to ten sessions with the IPL. An improvement of 50–75% was seen after an average of 2.8 treatment sessions for poikiloderma of Civatte. Between 75 and 100% clearance was achieved in 82% of patients with poikiloderma after three treatments with Photoderm VL.

Other Vascular Lesions

Cherry angiomas

Cherry angiomas are well circumscribed, small, red papules composed of vascular ectasias that typically appear in early adulthood and tend to increase with age. They may occur anywhere on the body, especially on the abdomen.

Treatment options for this benign proliferation include electrocautery, shave excision, and laser therapy. A variety of lasers can be used including the KTP, PDL, argon, continuous wave dye, and Nd : YAG lasers. With the PDL, purpuric doses are necessary and patients should be warned that bruising will occur post-treatment lasting 7–10 days. Using the KTP or Nd : YAG laser, the dome shaped papule may develop a small crust. In that event, it should be kept moist with a topical ointment such as Aquaphor healing ointment until the area is completely healed.

Venous lakes

Venous lakes are varicosities or dilated vessels resulting from weakening of pre-existing vessel walls. Elastosis of the vessel wall induced by photodamage weakens the vessel, causing dilatation. They present as blue papules on the face in older people, most commonly on the lips or ears. These lesions are very amenable to laser therapy. The KTP, PDL, argon, continuous wave dye, or Nd : YAG laser and the IPL yield excellent response.

Nevus simplex

Nevus simplex ('salmon patch' or 'stork bite') is a vascular birthmark that is seen in 25–40% of newborn babies. Composed of ectatic capillaries, these lesions are presumably a result of persistence of fetal circulation. Areas of involvement include the nape of the neck (most commonly), the glabella, and the eyelids. In the majority of cases, these lesions fade spontaneously by age 3. The lesions on the nape of the neck tend to persist. For those persistent lesions, treatment with the PDL is very effective. Energy delivery at purpuric doses, similar to port wine stains, is recommended for better efficacy in fewer treatments.

Arteriovenous malformations

Arteriovenous malformations (AVMs) are high flow lesions that, in contrast to other vascular malformations, can go undiagnosed until adulthood. Conditions such as puberty, pregnancy, trauma, or surgery can exacerbate these lesions. When involving the skin, they present as faint blue or pink macules or as a pulsatile mass. They may be painful, have a pulsation or thrill, or have associated hyperhidrosis or hypertrichosis overlying the lesion. They may also feel cool to touch.

AVMs are typically solitary lesions. They can be quite extensive, affecting underlying vasculature.

Bruits can be appreciated with auscultation. In questionable cases, this can help distinguish them from hemangiomas and other vascular malformations. Although magnetic resonance imaging and Doppler studies can be helpful for further assessment, angiography is the study of choice for full evaluation.

Treatment options include arterial embolization with or without surgical excision. Laser therapy has not been found to be helpful in these lesions.

Lymphatic malformations

Lymphatic malformations are abnormalities of lymphatic vessels and can appear localized or diffuse. They are usually congenital and typically manifest in infancy but may appear in adulthood. Acquired lymphatic malformations also occur after radiation, scarring or chronic lymphedema. Cystic hygromas are lymphatic cysts that occur on the neck and commonly communicate with adjacent lymph structures. Localized clusters of multicystic lymphatic malformations are called lymphangioma circumscriptum and clinically present as clear colored fluid filled vesicles, resembling 'frog spawn'. Sites of predilection include the axillae, proximal limbs, chest, and abdomen. Large, extensive lymphatic malformations can present as lymphedema of an extremity and are typically accompanied by superficial vesicles.

Treatment options include laser ablation with carbon dioxide or erbium laser for superficial lymphatic malformations. Extensive lymphatic malformations are best treated with surgical excision. Superficial lymphatic malformations can appear like vascular lesions, especially if there is bleeding of surrounding capillaries. However, unlike true vascular lesions, lymphatic malformations do not respond well to visible light lasers or light sources.

Treatment recommendations

Preoperative and postoperative care instructions are similar in the treatment of facial erythema, telangiectasia, vascular malformations, and hemangiomas. Preoperatively, patients are offered the option of an anesthetic applied to the skin, injected locally, or injected as a nerve block. Most patients being treated for telangiectasias and erythema do not have topical anesthesia applied. In fact, topical anesthesia is discouraged since it causes local vasoconstriction, skin pallor, and lightening of the target chromophore. If topical anesthesia is necessary, we use topical 2.5% lidocaine (lignocaine) and 2.5% prilocaine. Infraorbital, supraorbital and mental nerve blocks can be employed for segmental regions. Children younger than 1 year of age are treated without any anesthesia given the risk of systemic absorption and toxicity. Older children with extensive involvement are treated either with topical lidocaine or under conscious sedation in the operating room.

By using a large spot size, and a pulse width of at least 6–10 ms, the treatment of facial telangiectasia with the pulsed dye laser may now be effectively performed at subpurpuric fluences. A transient purpura lasting less than several seconds may be seen during the treatment when fluences just below true purpura are used and this is often a good visual clue as to when an appropriate energy has been reached. Results may be significantly improved by stacking several nonpurpuric pulses one after another. Stacking should be stopped when the goal of vessel spasm and clearing is achieved, or if purpura occurs or more than four pulses have been delivered. When treating a large area such as the cheek, pulses may be placed next to each other with a 50% overlap. This will effectively give the center of the treatment area a double pulse while leaving the periphery single pulsed and potentially feathered out. This 50% overlap will usually prevent the honeycomb appearance that may occur when treating confluent erythema with purpuric doses or sequentially stacked pulses.

With the KTP and Nd : YAG lasers, the treatment tip is applied along the discrete telangiectatic vessels in nonoverlapping pulses. Immediate lightening or disappearance of the target vessel may be observed. Patients are advised that they need not be alarmed if vessels reappear in a few days as these vessels will then likely gradually fade. Retreatment is common and may be repeated at 4 week intervals. As mentioned earlier, a particularly challenging area that may require multiple treatment sessions is the perialar region. Reticular veins are also difficult and require many sessions.

Postoperatively, a cool gel pack (Second Skin) and/or packed ice may be applied to the treatment area for palliative relief and temporary swelling. Purpura is immediately evident in the treatment of vascular malformations and hemangiomas, and lasts 7–10 days. Mild erythema and swelling can be expected after the treatment of facial telangiectasia or erythema. This typically lasts 1–2 hours post-treatment. Facial telangiectasia treatment with a 532 mm KTP laser can occasionally result in superficial crusting that heals in 3–5 days. Applying an aqueous lubricant such as Surgilube to the treatment site to enhance skin contact with the treatment tip can reduce the risk of crusting, especially in areas where it is difficult to maintain full contact for cooling, such as the perialar region. Crusting is very likely to occur following laser treatment of cherry angiomas and venous lakes. Patients should be warned of this effect prior to treatment and be advised to keep the area moist with an ointment such as Aquaphor healing ointment for 1 week thereafter.

Treatment can be repeated every 4–6 weeks for facial telangiectasia, facial erythema, and vascular malformations. For proliferating hemangiomas, patients return every 3 weeks until clinical regression is observed.

Side Effects, Complications, and Advanced Topics

Complications from pulsed dye laser treatment are uncommon. Prior to the availability of skin cooling, atrophic scarring, hyperpigmentation, hypertrophic scarring, or eczematous dermatitis were reported with an incidence of less than 1% with the PDL. Hypopigmentation occurred in 2.6% of treated patients. Overlapping of treatment pulses or treatment of young children at excessively high fluences can contribute to epidermal atrophy. The current 595 nm pulsed dye lasers with longer pulse durations and cryogen spray cooling have made these complications exceedingly rare. Occasionally, cutaneous depressions have been found 1–2 months after treatment with pulsed dye lasers of port wine stains (PWS). These changes are temporary and resolve in 3–18 months.

Atrophic scarring can occur with all lasers if an area is treated too aggressively, especially with the Nd : YAG (1064 nm) or frequency doubled Nd : YAG (532 nm) lasers. Pulse stacking with these particular laser systems should always be avoided. The target vessel should be traced with nonoverlapping treatment spots. One should look for immediate blanching of the target vessel with no change in the overlying skin. If the overlying skin turns white-gray, crusting will likely occur. In that event, the patient is advised to keep the area moist with topical antibiotic ointment or Aquaphor healing ointment until the area is completely healed (usually within 5–7 days). If the area requires additional treatment, the fluence should be reduced.

Conclusion

Treatment options are constantly evolving as research continues to help to redefine ways in which vascular lesions can be managed optimally. Recent advances in laser and light based technology including longer wavelength systems, varied pulse durations, and epidermal cooling methods have made great strides in the effective treatment of facial hemangiomas, vascular malformations, and telangiectasia. As newer technology emerges with greater understanding of the biologic processes underlying these conditions, complete clearance in even fewer treatment sessions with minimal complications may soon be achieved.

Further Reading

Bernstein LB, Geronemus RG 1995 Keloid formation with the 585 nm pulsed dye laser during isotretinoin treatment. Archives of Dermatology 133:111–112

Bernstein EF, Lee J, Lowery J, et al 1998 Treatment of spider veins with the 595 nm pulsed dye laser. Journal of the American Academy of Dermatology 39:746–750

Cassuto DA, Ancona DM, Emanuelli G 2000 Treatment of facial telangiectasia with a diode-pumped Nd : YAG laser at 532 nm. Journal of Cutaneous Laser Therapy 2:141–146

Chiller KG, Passero D, Frieden IJ 2002 Hemangiomas of infancy: clinical characteristics, morphologic subtypes, and their relationship to race, ethnicity, and sex. Archives of Dermatology 138:1567–1576

Dover JS, Arndt KA 2000 New approaches to the treatment of vascular lesions. Lasers in Surgery and Medicine 26:158–163

Eremia S, Li CY 2002 Treatment of face veins with a cryogen spray variable pulse width 1064 Nd : YAG laser: a prospective study of 17 patients. Dermatologic Surgery 28:244–247

Finn MC, Glowacki J, Mulliken JB 1993 Congenital vascular lesions: clinical application of new classification. Journal of Pediatric Surgery 18:894–900

Garden JM, Bakus AD, Paller AS 1992 Treatment of cutaneous hemangiomas by the flashlamp pumped-dye laser: prospective analysis. Journal of Pediatrics 120:550–560

Geronemus RG 1991 Treatment of spider telangiectases in children using the flash-lamp pulsed dye laser. Pediatric Dermatology 8:61–63

Geronemus RG, Ashinoff R 1991 The medical necessity of evaluation and treatment of port-wine stains. Journal of Dermatologic Surgical Oncology 17:76–79

Goldman MP, Weiss MP 2001 Treatment of poikiloderma of Civatte on the neck with an intense pulse light source. Plastic and Reconstructive Surgery 107:1376–1381

Groot D, Rao J, Johnston P, Nakatsui T 2003 Algorithm for using a long-pulsed Nd : YAG laser in the treatment of deep cutaneous vascular lesions. Dermatologic Surgery 29:35–42

Jacobs, AH, Walton RG 1976 The incidence of birthmarks in the neonate. Pediatrics 58:218–222

Landthaler M, Hohenleutner U, El Raheem TA 1995 Therapy of vascular lesions in the head and neck area by means of argon, Nd : YAG, and flashlamp-pumped pulsed dye lasers. Advances in Otorhinolaryngology 49:81–86

Laube S, Taibjee S, Lanigan SW 2003 Treatment of resistant port wine stains with the V Beam pulsed dye laser. Lasers in Surgery and Medicine 33:282–287

Levine V, Geronemus RG 1995 Adverse effects associated with the 577- and 585-nanometer pulsed dye laser in the treatment of cutaneous vascular lesions: a study of 500 patients. 32:613–617

Loo WJ, Lanigan SW 2002 Recent advances in laser therapy for the treatment of cutaneous vascular disorders. Lasers in Medical Science 17:9–12

Pham RTH 2001 Treatment of vascular lesions with combined dynamic precooling, postcooling thermal quenching, and Nd : YAG 1064 nm laser. Facial Plastic Surgery 17:203–208

Raulin C, Greve B 2001 Retrospective clinical comparison of hemangioma treatment by flashlamp-pumped (585 nm) and frequency-doubled Nd : YAG (532 nm) lasers. Lasers in Surgery and Medicine 28:40–43

Raulin C, Greve B, Grema H 2003 IPL technology: a review. Lasers in Surgery and Medicine 32:78–87

Reid WH, Miller ID, Murphy MJ, McKibben B, Paul JP 1992 Treatment of port-wine stains using the pulsed dye laser. British Journal of Plastic Surgery 45:565–570

Renfro L, Geronemus RG 1993 Anatomical differences of port wine stains in response to treatment with the pulsed dye laser. Archives of Dermatology 129:182–188

Rohrer TE, Chatrath V, Iyengar V 2004 Does pulse stacking improve the results of treatment with variable-pulse pulsed-dye lasers? Dermatologic Surgery 30:163–167

Tan OT, Morrison P, Kurban AK 1990 585 nm for the treatment of port-wine stains. Plastic and Recontructive Surgery 86:1112–1117

Waldorf HA, Alster TA, McMillan K, et al 1997 Effect of dynamic cooling on 585 nm pulsed dye laser treatment of port wine stain birthmarks. Dermatologic Surgery 23:657–662

Weiss RA, Goldman MP, Weiss MA 2000 Treatment of poikiloderma of Civatte with an intense pulsed light source. Dermatologic Surgery 26:823–828

West TB, Alser TS 1998 Comparison of the long-pulse dye (590–595 nm) and KTP (532 nm) lasers in the treatment of facial and leg telangiectasias. Dermatologic Surgery 24:221–226

3 Leg Veins

Jeffrey Hsu, Robert Weiss

Introduction

Venulectasia on legs occurs in 29–41% of women and 6–15% of men in the United States. Lasers have been used to treat leg veins since the 1970s, although laser surgeons did not achieve acceptable results until the advent of the pulsed dye laser in the 1980s. In the 1990s, the development of lasers with longer wavelengths and longer pulse durations ensured a consistent outcome and branded a niche for lasers in the treatment of leg veins. As with other indications, laser treatment of leg veins relies on the principle of photothermolysis. The ideal laser must have the following characteristics: (i) a wavelength that is better absorbed by hemoglobin than the surrounding chromophores; (ii) penetration to the depth of the target blood vessel; (iii) sufficient energy to damage the blood vessel without injuring the epidermis; and (iv) a pulse duration to slowly coagulate the vessel without damaging the surrounding tissue.

Patient evaluation

When larger truncal varicose veins are present, the associated telangiectases cannot be successfully treated without addressing the underlying hydrostatic pressure. In cases of greater saphenous vein incompetence, surgical techniques or endovenous ablative techniques may be required. Ambulatory phlebectomy allows treatment of virtually all large varicose veins, while compression sclerotherapy can be used to treat large varicose veins and reticular varicose veins. Only then should the telangiectases be treated with sclerotherapy or with laser or light based devices. However, in patients with only isolated telangiectases without pressure problems, sclerotherapy or laser/light therapy may be used primarily.

Physicians must diagnose the origin of the reverse flow. Physical examination is necessary to determine whether the surface telangiectases originate from a deeper source of incompetence. One must have adequate knowledge of the basic superficial venous anatomy and proper diagnostic tools. Important superficial venous systems include the greater saphenous vein (GSV), the lesser saphenous vein (LSV), and the lateral subdermic venous system (LSVS) (Figs 3.1–3.3). Younger patients usually present with telangiectatic webs originating from reflux in the lateral venous system. When there is a positive family history of large varicose veins, the physician must consider reflux from the GSV or LSVS.

Patient expectations

Aside from proper counseling regarding the possible side effects, such as dyspigmentation, matting, or even ulceration and scarring, patients must also understand that perfection is not possible, that there will always be veins, albeit very tiny veins, that may not resolve. Once the patient understands the nature and risk of treatment, digital images are recorded. These images are indispensable tools to evaluate treatment progress, and more importantly, to document improvement for the patient. All too often, patients fail to recognize partial resolution. Comparison of the 'before' and 'after' images will enhance patient satisfaction. Patients should also understand that the treatment of leg veins is not a case of instant gratification. When using laser and light devices, 8–12 weeks may be the optimal interval between treatments. Often telangiectases will ultimately improve despite no signs of change within the initial 2 weeks.

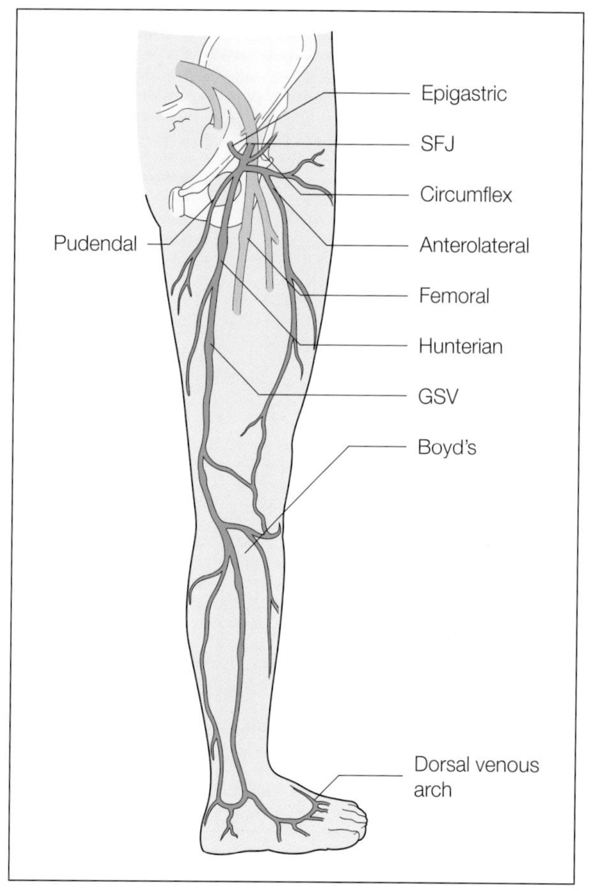

Fig. 3.1 Greater saphenous vein. SFJ = saphenofemoral junction

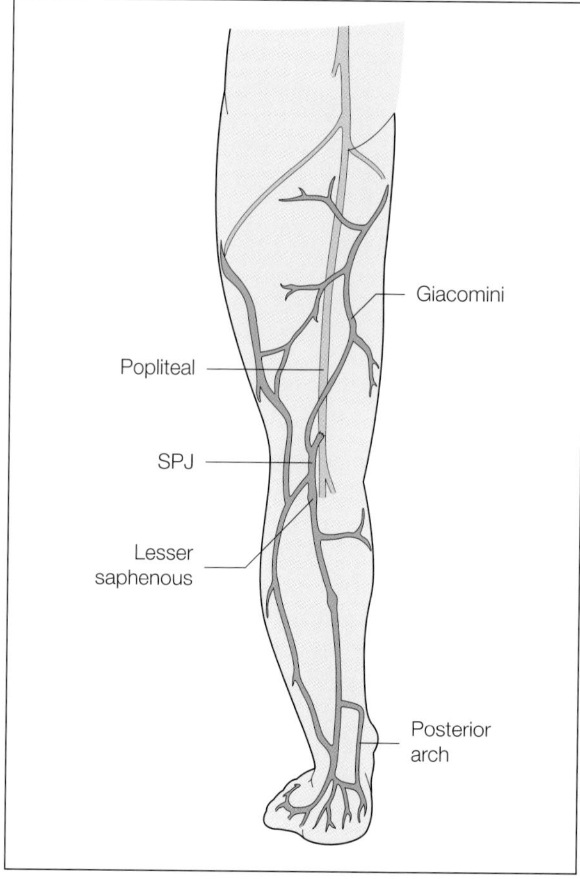

Fig. 3.2 Lesser saphenous vein. SPJ = saphenopopliteal junction

Diagnostic tools

While most physicians are familiar with tools to diagnose cardiac disease, few are familiar with the equivalent tools when it comes to venous disease (Table 3.1). The handheld Doppler is the most common and cost effective tool to detect reflux in the superficial venous system (Fig. 3.4). The optimal frequencies for examining superficial vessels (less than 2 cm below the skin) are 8–10 MHz, while deeper vessels require frequencies of 4–5 MHz. Manual compression of the calf generates an audible signal of flow. When compression is released, reverse flow ensues, but ceases within 0.5–1.0 second when competent valves close. However, when the valves are incompetent, flow continues.

Plethysmography measures pressure or volume changes (Fig. 3.5). Photoplethysmography is the most common variant, taking advantage of hemoglobin absorption of light to calculate change in blood volume. The patient is first asked to dorsiflex several times to allow the calf muscle pump to empty the venous system. The device then measures the change in volume over time as the venous system refills. When reflux is present, refill is rapid. A refill time shorter than 25 seconds indicates significant venous insufficiency.

Analogous tools in the evaluation of the heart and leg veins	
Heart	**Leg vein**
Stethoscope	Handheld Doppler
Electrocardiogram	Photoplethysmography
Echocardiogram	Duplex ultrasound

Table 3.1 Analogous tools in the evaluation of the heart and leg veins

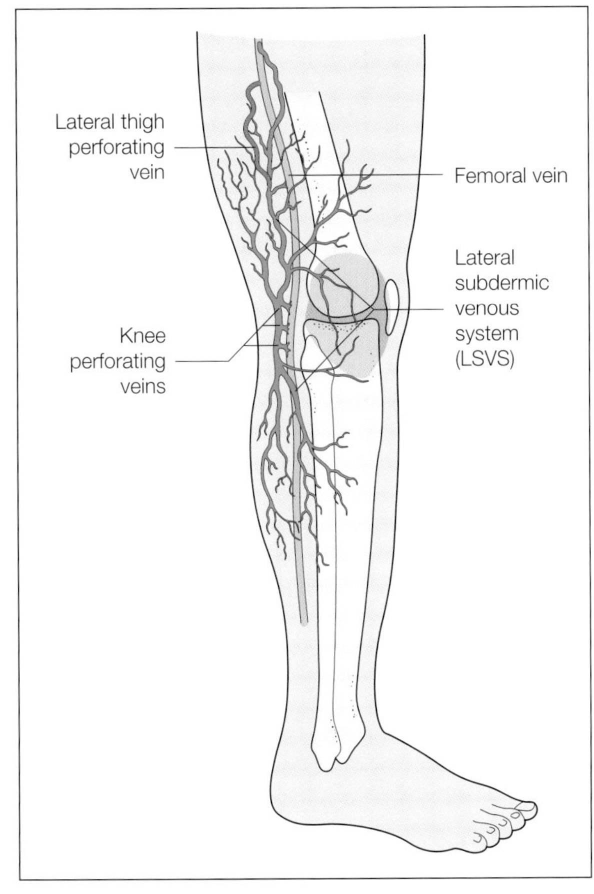

Fig. 3.3 Lateral subdermic venous system

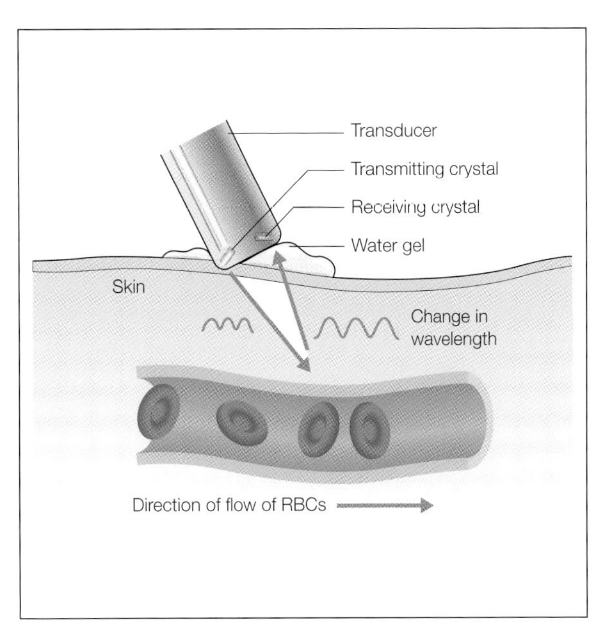

Fig. 3.4 Handheld Doppler

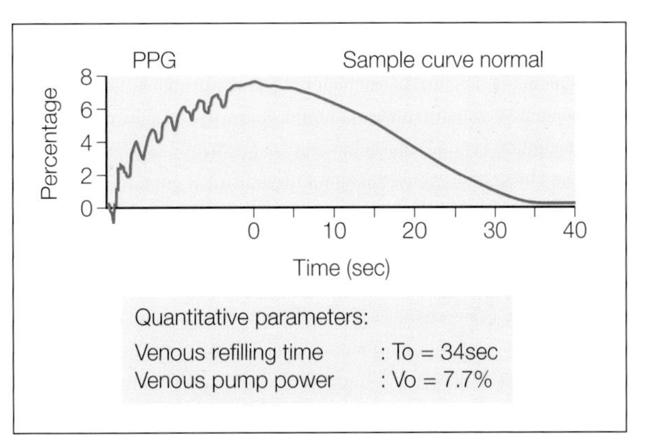

Fig. 3.5 Plethysmography

Duplex ultrasound graphically presents the anatomy of the venous system in two dimensions while superimposing the Doppler flow signal as a color marker (Fig. 3.6). The origin of the reflux can then be identified. The transducer is placed over the vessel in question while compression of the leg is applied distally to increase cephalad flow. When compression is released, functional valves should close to stop reverse flow. Retrograde flow of greater than 0.5 second reveals pathologic reflux.

Treatment Strategy

Target selection

The success of treating varicosities depends on a logical progression of interventions (Fig. 3.7). Reticular or larger varicose veins should be eliminated first surgically or through endovenous ablation, followed by sclerotherapy of the remaining vessels, from largest to smallest (Fig. 3.8). Vessels that do not respond to sclerotherapy, that are too small to be injected, or that remain after sclerotherapy, should be considered for laser and light treatment. Another clear indication for laser and light sources are telangiectatic matting (Fig. 3.9). Matting refers to multiple tiny new telangiectases that appear in patients, often after sclerotherapy. It presents as a patch composed of numerous vessels less than 0.2 mm in diameter located at the site of treatment. The incidence of matting after sclerotherapy is between 15 and 24%. Although it usually resolves spontaneously in 3–12 months, it can lead to dissatisfaction if the patients were not counseled appropriately.

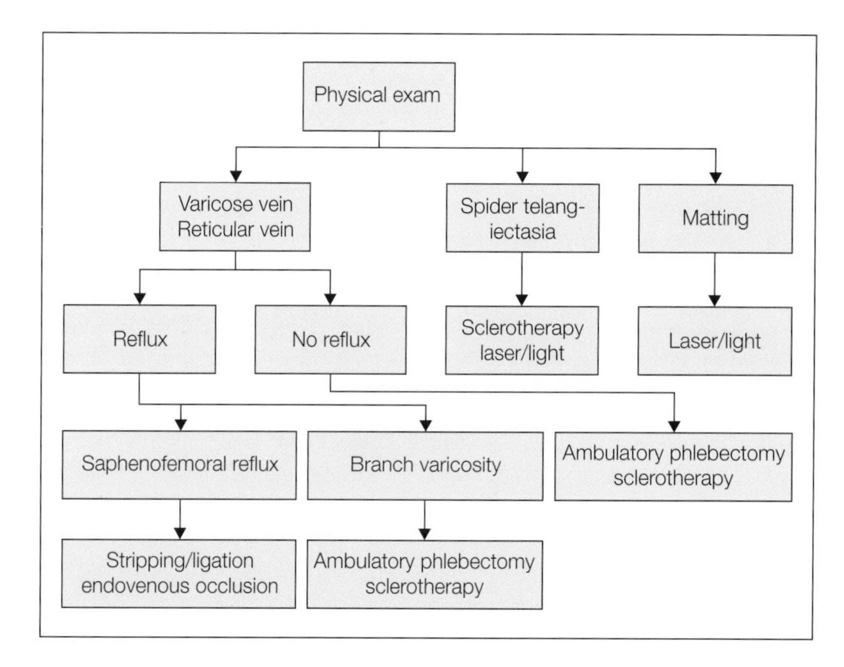

Fig. 3.6 Flowchart showing the appropriate treatment algorithm

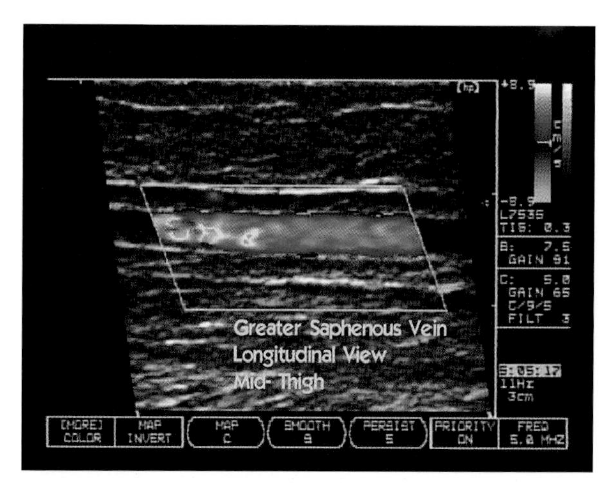

Fig. 3.7 Duplex ultrasound

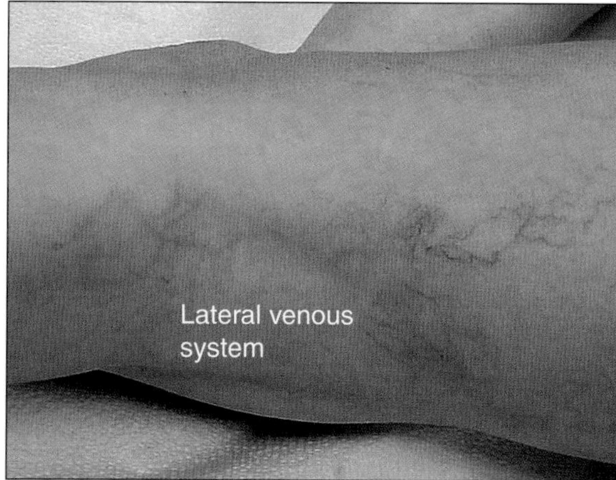

Fig. 3.8 Reticular veins

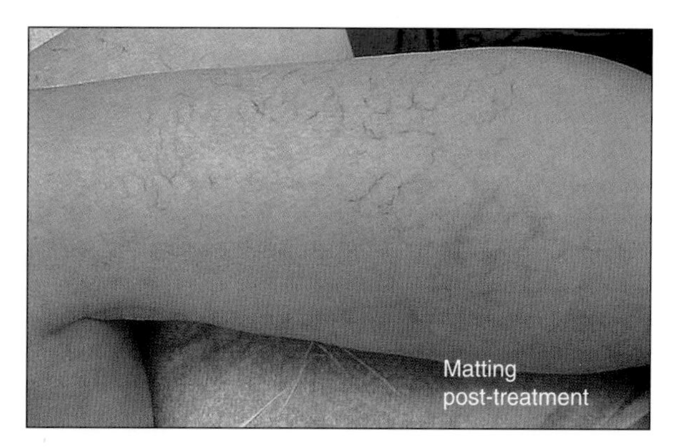

Fig. 3.9 Telangiectatic matting

Using needle gauge to estimate vein size	
Needle gauge	**Outer diameter (mm)**
12	2.77
18	1.25
20	0.91
25	0.50
26	0.45
28	0.38
30	0.32
32	0.26

Table 3.2 Using needle gauge to estimate vein size

Parameter selection

The challenge in laser treatment of leg veins is that the veins vary widely in size and depth in the skin. Furthermore, the superficial vessels are connected to deeper reticular veins, which often require adjunctive treatment such as sclerotherapy. The choice of wavelength and pulse duration is related to the type and size of the vessels treated. One may compare the target vessel to a needle of known gauge to estimate the vessel size (Table 3.2). In general, longer wavelengths allow for deeper penetration and longer pulse durations are needed to slowly heat vessels with larger diameters. Larger spot sizes penetrate deeper and optimize fluence delivery to the target. Another advantage of the longer wavelength laser is the dynamic nature of absorption peaks as a function of vessel size and depth. While hemoglobin absorption peaks in green (541 nm) are higher than red to infrared (800–1000 nm) for superficial small vessels, as the vessels approach 0.5 mm in size and 0.5 mm in depth, absorption by hemoglobin in the long visible and near infrared range becomes more important.

Laser selection

Potassium titanyl phosphate (KTP) lasers

The earliest successful treatment of leg veins came in the form of pulsed lasers and light sources. Pulsed KTP at 532 nm was initially chosen due to the favorable absorption by hemoglobin. The KTP crystals are reliable, convenient, and easily available to manufacturers (Box 3.1). Although these millisecond devices proved valuable in treating facial telangiectases, early experiences with small spot sizes and pulse durations of 10 ms or less were disappointing. The outcomes were much more favorable with larger spot sizes of 3–5 mm, and longer pulse durations of 10–50 ms at fluences of 12–20 J/cm^2.

> **KTP lasers**
>
> - Pulsed KTP (532 nm), 1–200 ms)
> - VersaPulse (Lumenis)
> - Illustra (Cynosure)
> - Diolite (Iriderm)
> - Aura (Laserscope)

Box 3.1 KTP lasers

The disadvantages of the KTP laser are the inadequate penetration and also heavy absorption by melanin, both properties of the 532 nm wavelength. Patients with darker or tanned skin experience a high risk of dyspigmentation. Cooling is especially important in these cases to protect the epidermis. Given these limitations, the pulsed KTP is best suited for small, superficial telangiectases in skin types I–III. Treatment is technique dependent. Multiple passes often are needed to achieve the clinical endpoints of vessel spasm or intravascular coagulation, which are associated with better results. However, pulse stacking should be avoided, as this may lead to 'grooving' or scarring.

Pulsed dye laser

The original pulsed dye laser (PDL) at 585 nm and 450 µs pulse duration was successful in treating port wine stains, which are composed of very superficial (average depth of 0.46 mm) and minute 100 µm vessels. However, they proved to be unsatisfactory in treating leg veins. The short pulse duration is effective only for superficial fine vessels of 0.1 mm or less. Based on the theory of selective photothermolysis, the ideal pulsed duration for destruction of leg veins 0.1 mm to several millimeters in diameter is in the 1–50 ms range. The high energy delivered in the short time frame lead to rupture of the vessels with purpura and hemosiderin deposit, seen clinically as long term hyperpigmentation. Polla et al used this laser to achieve 75% clearing in only 15% of telangiectases treated and found little if any improvement in 73% of the vessels. As expected, the vessels that responded were minute superficial telangiectases. Furthermore, 50% of the patients experienced dyspigmentation. However, when used appropriately, the results can be favorable. In another study, superficial red telangiectases of 0.2 mm or less and telangiectatic matting induced by sclerotherapy

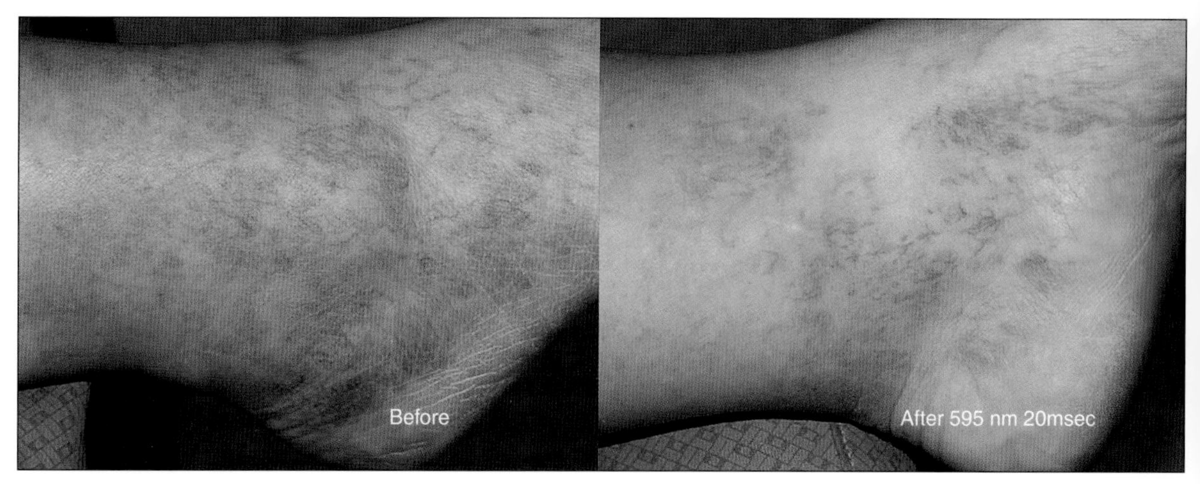

Fig. 3.10 Treatment with PDL

Pulsed dye lasers	
Pulsed dye (585, 590, 595, 600 nm)	**Pulse duration (ms)**
SPTL-1b (Candela)	0.45
LV (Cynosure)	0.45
ScleroPlus (Candela)	1.5
PhotoGenica LVS (Cynosure)	1.5
Vbeam (Candela)	0.5–40
PhotoGenica V-Star (Cynosure)	0.5–40

Table 3.3 Pulsed dye lasers

underwent treatment with the 450 nm PDL, using 5 mm spot and fluence of 6.5–8 J/cm^2, followed by compression for 72 hours. Seventy six per cent of linear telangiectases cleared completely within 4 months of a single treatment. Transient hyperpigmentation developed in 10% of the subjects.

The advent of long pulsed dye laser enabled treatment beyond superficial tiny telangiectases. Several devices using rhodamine dye are capable of pulse durations ranging from 1.5 to 40 ms (Table 3.3). The wavelengths range from 585 to 600 nm, which has better penetration to target deeper vessels. However, at these wavelengths, melanin absorption is still significant. The risk for dyspigmentation can be high without proper epidermal cooling.

Several studies with the 1.5 ms PDL revealed variable results. A single treatment with a 585 nm PDL on vessels up to 1 mm in size, using a 3 × 7 mm elliptical handpiece and up to 18 J/cm^2 in fluences, yielded 67% clearing. Another study using the 595 nm PDL showed slightly better results. Both studies reported side effects including crusting and dyspigmentation. Reichert showed more success when the areas treated were first cleared of refluxing reticular veins. In this study, telangiectases of 0.1–1 mm were treated with the 1.5 ms PDL at wavelengths of 585–600 nm. Total clearing was observed in vessels less than 0.5 mm in diameter after one or two treatments, while 80% clearing was achieved in vessels 0.5–1.0 mm after four treatments. Transient dyspigmentation was found in 50% of subjects. Although there are no published controlled studies on the efficacy of ultra-long pulsed dye laser (up to 40 ms), the authors have had predictable success in treating very small telangiectasias (<0.3 mm) using fluences of 15–20 J/cm^2 and pulse widths of 10–20 ms. Larger veins up to 1.5 mm may require a longer pulse duration (Fig. 3.10).

Long pulsed alexandrite laser

Several other pulsed lasers have successfully taken advantage of the small peak of hemoglobin absorption in the 700–900 nm range. They include long pulsed alexandrite, diode lasers, and long pulsed Nd : YAG lasers. The longer wavelengths afford deeper penetration to treat larger caliber veins and relative low absorption by melanin.

With wavelengths of 755 nm, alexandrite lasers are capable of penetrating 2–3 mm into the skin (Table 3.4). Coupled with a pulse duration up to 20 ms, these lasers have treated telangiectases with some success. McDaniel et al reported 63% overall clearing after three treatments. Medium sized vessels (0.4–1 mm) responded best, followed by

Alexandrite lasers	
Alexandrite laser (755 nm)	**Pulse duration (ms)**
EpiTouch (Lumenis)	2–40
GentleLaser (Candela)	3
LPIR/Apogee (Cynosure)	5–20

Table 3.4 Alexandrite lasers

Diode lasers	
Diode laser (800, 810 nm)	**Pulse duration (ms)**
FeatherLite (LaserLite)	50–250
LightSheer (Star Medical)	5–30

Table 3.5 Diode lasers

larger vessels (1–3 mm). Vessels smaller than 0.3 mm responded poorly, highlighting the need for shorter pulse durations to target these tiny vessels. The optimal parameter in the study was a pulse duration of 5 ms and a fluence of 20 J/cm^2. Another study showed up to 75% clearing of two thirds of all veins (0.3–2 mm) with a single treatment, using 8 mm spot, 3 ms pulse, at a fluence of 60–80 J/cm^2. Transient hyperpigmentation occurred in a third of the treatment sites.

Diode lasers

At 800–930 nm, the diode lasers are similar to alexandrite lasers in their ability to penetrate deeper and target larger reticular veins, and to match the tertiary hemoglobin absorption peak at approximately 900 nm with relatively less interference from melanin (Table 3.5). Using an 800 nm diode array laser, Dierickx saw more than 75% clearing in two thirds of veins after three treatments, with 5–30 ms pulses and 15–40 J/cm^2 in fluence. The 940 nm wavelength penetrates about 3 mm into the skin, which is capable of reaching most small veins up to 1 mm in diameter when coupled with fluences of 250–400 J/cm^2. Theoretically, red telangiectasias contain proportionally higher oxyhemoglobin and therefore should respond more favorably. Kaudewitz et al report short term results of more than 50% clearance of vessels less than 1 mm in 76% of patients and 75–100% clearance in 46% of patients after one laser pass. Interestingly, 1 year follow up demonstrated continued improvement, with 75% of the patients achieving 75–100% clearance. The mechanism of this process is yet undetermined. Based on this observation, the patients should be reassured that results may continue to improve over time, and that additional treatment may be unnecessary. Transient dyspigmentation and telangiectatic matting were observed in some patients, but cleared within 1 year.

Nd : YAG Lasers	
Nd : YAG laser (1064 nm)	**Pulse duration (ms)**
CoolGlide (Altus)	10–100
CoolTouch Varia (CoolTouch)	0.3–100
Lyra (Laserscope)	1–100
Vasculight (Lumenis)	2–16
VeinLaser (HGM Medical)	1–50

Table 3.6 Nd : YAG Lasers

Long pulsed Nd : YAG 1064 nm laser

The development of long pulsed Nd : YAG lasers was an exciting milestone in the treatment of leg veins (Table 3.6). The long wavelength affords even deeper penetration into the skin to target deep, relatively large caliber vessels. The Nd : YAG laser has maximum penetration of 3 mm, making it ideal for the destruction of large vessels in the mid-dermis. The scant absorption by melanin also decreases the potential for epidermal damage, even in darker skin types. However, a high fluence is needed for the deep penetration. This increases the risk for collateral damage as heat is dissipated to the tissue surrounding the target vessels. Furthermore, treatment with the long pulsed 1064 nm laser is relatively painful, requiring cooling and topical anesthesia. Whereas other lasers with lower fluences may require several passes to achieve this clinical response, multiple passes with the high fluence Nd : YAG laser should be performed with extreme caution.

Larger caliber vessels greater than 0.5 mm and up to 3 mm in diameter respond the best (Fig. 3.11). A recent study showed 75% clearing of vessels 0.5–3 mm in diameter after just one treatment,

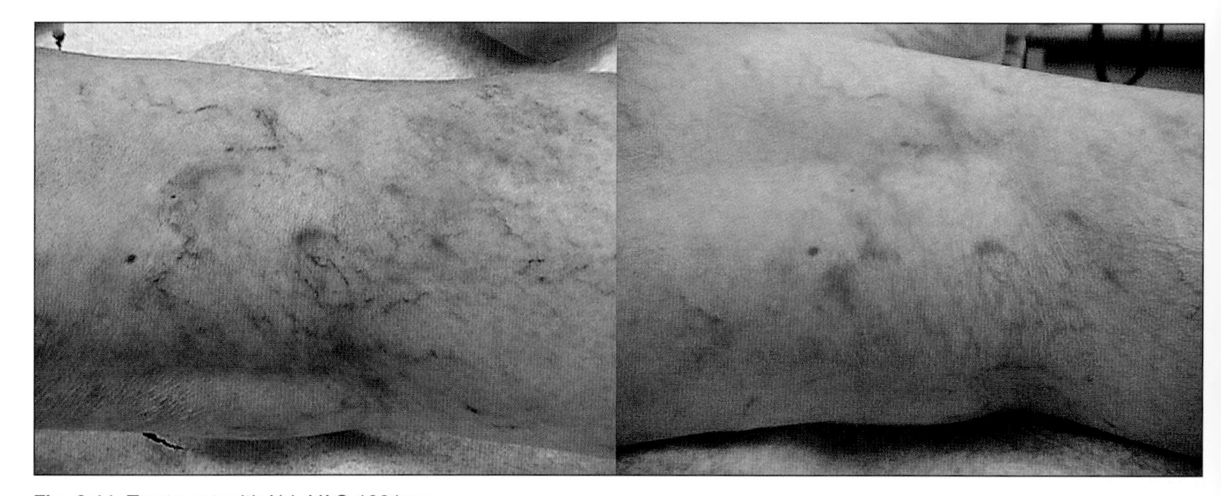

Fig. 3.11 Treatment with Nd : YAG 1064 nm

utilizing 16 ms pulse width and fluences of 130–140/cm^2. Unlike previous lasers, no epidermal injury was noted in any sites, even in Fitzpatrick skin types IV. Another study showed that greater than 85% of telangiectasias (0.3–1.5 mm) and reticular veins (1.5–3 mm) showed 75% improvement with just two treatments. In comparing the 1064 nm Nd : YAG to 810 nm diode and 755 nm alexandrite laser in treating veins up to 3 mm diameter, Eremia et al found a much better outcome with the Nd : YAG laser. Although the Nd : YAG laser appears to be very promising in treating veins, a comparison study still shows superior results with sclerotherapy, with earlier vessel clearing and more improvement overall. A recent effort has described ideal parameters using the 1064 nm Nd : YAG laser for various vessel sizes in a rat model. The applicability to the clinical situation is yet undetermined. Just as in other lasers, the treatment goal is to achieve blanching of the vessels without burning the skin.

Recent evidence has shown that methemoglobin formation leads to increase in the absorption of 1064 nm wavelength. Heating of hemoglobin causes oxidative reactions to form methemoglobin. Methemoglobin has three times the absorbance of oxyhemoglobin and 13 times that of deoxyhemoglobin. This information suggests that in theory it would be advantageous to deliver the energy in trains of pulses, rather than firing all the energy in one pulse with the risk of overheating the target and damaging the surrounding tissues. Each pulse would generate methemoglobin as a target for the subsequent pulse. The multipulse mode thereby increases efficacy while preserving the surrounding tissue and reducing the discomfort of treatment. Using a 1064 nm Nd : YAG laser with nonuniform pulse sequence mode, 2 mm spot, and 300–360 J/cm^2, 55% of 1–2 mm blue vessels were cleared after one session, 86% after two sessions, and 98% after three sessions.

Intense pulsed light

The intense pulsed light (IPL) device is a noncoherent, 515–1200 nm, flashlamp pumped light source that is capable of fluence up to 90 J/cm^2 and a pulse duration range of 2–100 ms, depending on the model. Unique to IPL is the ability to use filters that remove lower wavelengths in order to increase selectivity. Multiple filters are available, ranging from 560 to 755 nm. The filters most useful for vascular lesions are 550 and 570 nm filters that deliver primarily the yellow and red wavelengths with some infrared.

The broadband light of the IPL takes advantage of the dynamic optical properties of hemoglobin as the size and depth of the vessels change. As the size increases from 0.1 to 1 mm, and the depth increases from 0.3 to 1 mm, the peak absorption of hemoglobin shifts from 600 to approximately 900 nm. Therefore, having a broadband source of 515–1200 nm allows the physician to target the smaller, superficial vessels and the larger, deeper vessels simultaneously. Another practical advantage of the IPL is the relatively larger spot size that facilitates treatment.

Initial studies have shown success of up to 90% clearance in vessels less than 0.2 mm, 80% in vessels

0.2–0.5 mm, and 80% in vessels 0.5–1.0 mm in diameter. Later studies have also shown good results, but have not duplicated the dramatic results. All have reported few adverse events, with transient dyspigmentation occurring up to 3% of the patients. For vessels less than 0.2 mm, useful parameters include single 3 ms pulse of 22 J/cm^2 or double pulse of 35–40 J/cm^2 given in 2.4 and 4.0 ms with a 10 ms delay. Larger vessels 0.2–0.5 mm can be treated with 35–45 J/cm^2 with a 3–6 ms pulse and 20 ms delay time. Another protocol utilized the versatility of the IPL by combining long and short pulses in a single treatment for the best outcome. Using fluences up to 70 J/cm^2, the first pulse is given in 2.4 or 3 ms and the second pulse is given in 7 ms, separated by a 10–20 ms delay. Based on the theory of photoselectivity, the shorter pulse targets the smaller vessels while the longer pulse targets the underlying larger vessels. This protocol has allowed 74% clearing in two treatments with 8% incidence of dyspigmentation.

Advanced Topics: Treatment Tips for Experienced Practitioners

Sclerotherapy vs. lasers

While large varicosities are still best treated with surgical techniques or endovenous procedures, sclerotherapy remains the gold standard for the treatment of smaller leg veins. Recent comparison studies still show that most leg telangiectases respond better to sclerotherapy with fewer treatment sessions required. However, recent advances in laser technology have expanded the utility of lasers and light sources, such that the practitioner and the patient can now select laser as the treatment of choice in certain cases. In making this decision, the first consideration is the contraindications to sclerotherapy, such as patient predisposition to deep vein thrombosis, history of clotting disorders, hypersensitivity to sclerosants, and pregnancy. Patient bias must be considered as well. Many patients are 'needle phobic' and would much prefer the discomfort from laser treatments to the anxiety of undergoing multiple transcutaneous injections. Others expect treatments using the latest technology without regard to the clear advantage of sclerotherapy in certain cases. It is the physician's responsibility to counsel the patient appropriately, weighing the risk and benefit profile of the two approaches. One must recognize that as in all esthetic treatments, the treatment of unwanted leg veins can be an emotional and subjective process. As such, patients' perception of quality of treatment is paramount to their satisfaction. Another consideration is the physician's own preference. Success with sclerotherapy is heavily technique dependent; the novice may undergo a learning curve before becoming adept in sclerotherapy. One may choose instead to focus on lasers only and refer sclerotherapy to other physicians. The decision to offer laser treatment can be a financial decision as well as a technical decision. When it is considered that purchasing the latest laser requires an initial investment of tens of thousand of dollars in addition to costly maintenance, compared to a few dollars for sclerosants and needles, the practitioner may be limited to sclerotherapy.

The size of the vessels can be an important determinant. Very small vessels less than 0.3 mm, such as those in telangiectatic matting, are very difficult to cannulate. These can be excellent candidates for lasers. Vessels 0.3–1.5 mm still respond well to lasers, but can be treated just as effectively by an experienced sclerotherapist. Although medium size vessels between 1.5 and 3 mm respond moderately well to lasers, sclerotherapy is the first choice. Lasers have a very limited role in vessels larger than 3 mm. Patient skin type can also limit the use of lasers. Skin types IV–VI have a higher risk of dyspigmentation with light sources; these patients are better triaged to sclerotherapy.

Skin cooling

Skin cooling is an integral part of laser therapy both for cryoanesthesia and for protection. It is particularly crucial when treating darker skinned individuals. Epidermal melanin can absorb the light intended for the underlying targeted chromophores, such as oxyhemoglobin, leading to epidermal injury. One way to overcome this problem is to selectively cool the epidermis. Devices designed to cool the skin reduce epidermal damage and allow the use of higher fluences and the treatment of darker skin types. All forms of cooling entail putting a cold medium, usually cold air, cryogen spray, cold gel, or cold sapphire window, in contact with the skin. To ensure adequate cooling, several parameters must be considered regardless of the medium: duration of contact, temperature of the cooling source, and quality of contact. There are three basic modes of cooling: precooling, parallel cooling, and postcooling. Precooling lowers the skin temperature prior to the laser pulse. Because of the possibility of freeze injury to the epidermis, there is a limit on the degree of safe precooling. Protective precooling is best for pulse widths shorter than 5 ms, and best delivered by cryogen spray. Parallel cooling lowers the skin temperature concurrent with the laser pulse. With short pulse widths, the limited time of contact provided by parallel cooling tends to afford little epidermal protection. Parallel cooling becomes much more protective when it is coincident with pulses longer than 5–10 ms. A common parallel cooling medium is cold sapphire. Cryogen spray is less appropriate once the laser is firing since it may interfere with the laser beam. Postcooling is mainly used for minimizing pain and edema, and may serve to protect the skin by thermal quenching of the heat released from larger vessels following laser heating. The skin temperature can also be lowered with air chilled as low as –30°C. The cooling time for this medium can be longer than other methods, but this results in deeper penetration of the cooling effect. Consequently, the entire skin can be cooled ('bulk cooling') with little selectivity for the epidermis. On the other hand, there are certain advantages to air cooling. This medium does not disturb the laser light, can be used regardless of skin topography, and requires no compression of the skin, which can be important when treating vascular lesions.

Laser and radiofrequency treatment of varicose veins

The successful long term treatment of truncal varicose veins requires the elimination of the highest point of reflux and the elimination of the incompetent venous segment. Until recent years, the standard for the treatment of saphenous vein reflux has been ligation with or without stripping, despite little evidence of long term success. Recurrences occur due to reanastamoses of previously ligated tributaries or failure to ligate a functional tributary which subsequently becomes varicose. Furthermore, the traditional method of stripping involved significant scars and a long painful recovery period. With the work of Dr Oesch, the inversion perforate invagination (PIN) stripping method has dramatically improved the procedure. However, US surgeons are slow to adopt the newer technique, and instead continue to subject patients to unnecessary trauma. Sclerotherapy of truncal varicosities under ultrasound guidance is an alternative. But it remains imperfect, with 10–42% recanalization in a year. With foam sclerotherapy, the long term success rate may increase, but the safety of the procedure remains in doubt, as the sclerosant may flow into the deep venous system, although this is rare. When used correctly, foam sclerotherapy can even quickly eliminate smaller venulectases (Fig. 3.12).

A recent technological development involves endovenous occlusion with radiofrequency (RF). First, an entry point along the greater saphenous vein is selected, usually at or slightly below the level of the knee. Under duplex ultrasound guidance, a needle is inserted into the saphenous vein to gain access, followed by placement of a guide wire. The sheath is then guided over the wire into the access site. Finally, the RF catheter is inserted through the sheath into the greater saphenous vein and positioned at the base of the terminal valve under ultrasound visualization. Following the placement of the catheter, tumescent anesthesia is injected along the course of the vein. The tumescence serves as a heat sink to minimize heat damage to tissue surrounding the vein, and also helps to compress the vein, improving the contact between catheter tips and the vein wall. The RF is then applied while the catheter is slowly withdrawn. This enables shrinkage of the vein wall without electrocoagulation of blood. A continuous feedback mechanism allows the physician to monitor the impedance and the temperature at the treatment site. At the conclusion of the procedure there is no flow through the

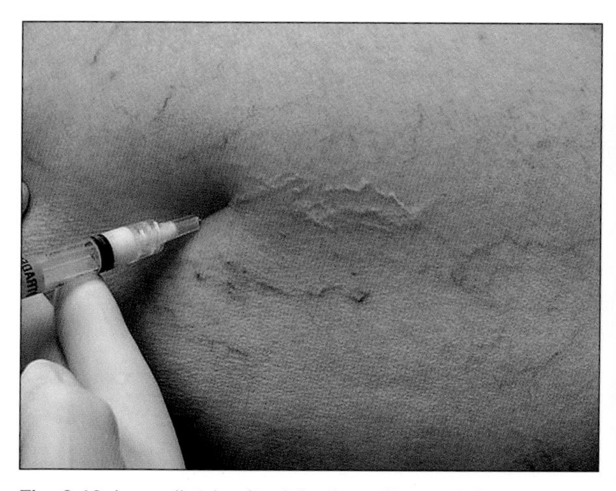

Fig. 3.12 Immediately after injection of foamed detergent solution

greater saphenous vein. After the application of a compression bandage, the patient is able to ambulate off the surgical table and resume normal activity. Duplex ultrasound is repeated within 72 hours to verify closure of the saphenous vein and absence of deep vein thrombosis. Over time, one observes the improvement of symptoms and shrinkage of distal varicosities (Fig. 3.13). Short term advantages of the RF procedure over traditional stripping and ligation have been documented in a prospective multicenter randomized comparison. The authors conclude that there are significant early advantages to endovascular obliteration of the GSV compared with conventional vein stripping, with less pain and a shorter recovery time. Long term results have been quite favorable also. Two year follow up shows elimination of GSV refluxing in greater than 90% of limbs, with symptom improvement in 95% of limbs.

Alternatively, endovenous ablation using laser sources has seen success as well. A laser fiber is inserted into the saphenous vein through a process similar to the insertion of a RF catheter. Tumescent anesthesia is also used. However, instead of using RF, a laser source is employed to generate heat.

Several lasers are capable of this task; the prototype model used an 810 nm diode laser. Over a 3 year period, 499 GSVs in 423 subjects with varicose veins were treated with 810 nm diode laser energy delivered into the GSV. Long term results available in 499 limbs treated with endovenous laser demonstrate a recurrence rate of less than 7% at 2 year follow up. However, a study using the animal model suggests that the 810 nm endovenous laser technique may be at a higher risk compared to the RF technique for vein perforations and failure to cause significant collagen shrinkage. Previous evidence indicates that coagulation of blood without shrinkage of the vein wall leads to early recanalization and recurrence.

Subsequently, other laser systems have been used for endovenous ablation. The 940 nm diode and the 980 nm diode lasers are equally successful in this role. Most recently the 1320 nm Nd : YAG laser has been outfitted with an automatic pullback mechanism for use in endovenous ablation with great success. There appears to be no difference in postoperative tenderness or bruising in comparison to RF.

Although the laser fiber with its aiming beam light affords easy visualization of the exact placement, no laser system thus far offers a safety feedback mechanism that allows the physician to monitor the treatment temperature. In expert hands, the side effect profile is similar. However, the laser fiber is more flexible and more maneuverable, and the treatment pullback time is significantly shorter than RF (4 min vs 15–20 min). But the greatest advantage of the laser system over the RF system may be financial, as the operating cost of the laser system is lower than the RF system.

Both the RF and the laser system eliminate the need for general anesthesia and extensive convalescence in comparison to the traditional stripping and ligation. The majority of patients resume normal activity immediately after the procedure. Three year data suggests high success rates, even higher than stripping surgery.

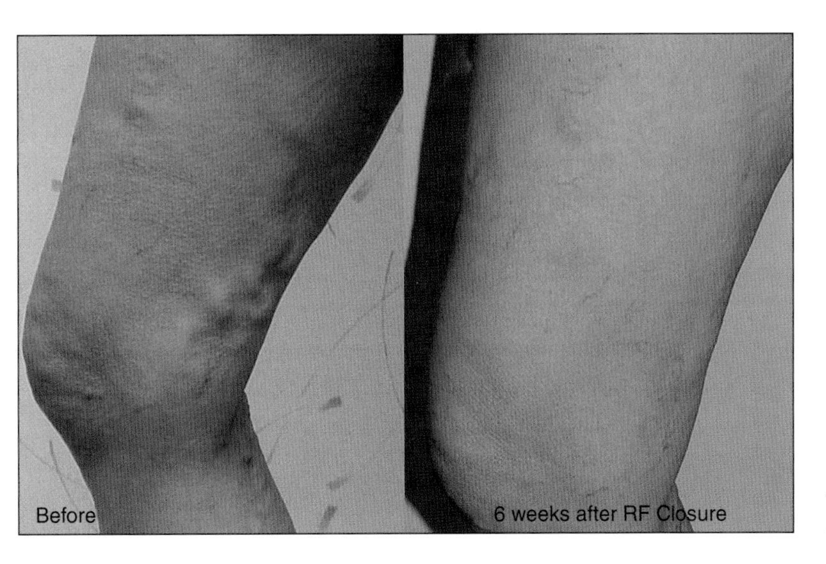

Fig. 3.13 Before and after treatment with endovenous radiofrequency ablation

Summary

Surgical interventions, endovenous ablative techniques, and sclerotherapy remain the primary choices for varicose veins and reticular veins 3 mm or larger. Lasers and light sources can be considered when telangiectases 3 mm or smaller are present. The current role for these devices are in (i) patients with medical contraindications to sclerosants, (ii) patients who are needle phobic, (iii) patients who have failed sclerotherapy, (iv) vessels too small for cannulation (less than 0.3 mm), and (v) foot or ankle vessels that are difficult to treat with sclerotherapy. Sclerotherapy is heavily technique dependent, however. Physicians who are unfamiliar with sclerotherapy may find more use for lasers. Nevertheless, all physicians interested in the treatment of leg veins, regardless of their expertise, must approach the issue with a solid foundation in venous anatomy and the physiology of reflux, and treat in a logical progression, starting with varicosities, incompetent perforators, reticular veins, and finally telangiectases.

Despite recent therapeutic advances, the ideal treatment for unwanted leg veins remains elusive due to their variable nature. Currently, the variety of methods and permutations in parameters underscores the lack of community standard in laser therapy of leg veins. However, as it represents one of the most common vascular lesions and most common cosmetic complaints, the drive to improve laser treatment of leg veins will continue.

Further Reading

Barton JK, Frangineas G, Pummer H, Black JF 2001 Cooperative phenomena in two-pulse, two-color laser photocoagulation of cutaneous blood vessels. Photochemistry and Photobiology 73:642–650

Davis LT, Duffy DM 1990 Determination of incidence and risk factors for postsclerotherapy telangiectatic matting of the lower extremity: a retrospective analysis. Journal of Dermatology and Surgical Oncology 16:327–330

Dierickx CC, Casparian JM, Venugopalan V, Farinelli WA, Anderson RR 1995 Thermal relaxation of port-wine stain vessels probed in vivo: the need for 1–10-millisecond laser pulse treatment. Journal of Investigative Dermatology 105:709–714

Eremia S, Li CY 2001 Treatment of leg and face veins with a cryogen spray variable pulse width 1064-nm Nd : YAG laser—a prospective study of 47 patients. Journal of Cosmetics and Laser Therapy 3:147–153

Garden JM, Backus AD 1996 Treatment of leg veins with high energy pulsed dye laser. Lasers in Surgery and Medicine 8(suppl):34

Goldman MP, Eckhouse S 1996 Photothermal sclerosis of leg veins. ESC Medical Systems, LTD Photoderm VL Cooperative Study Group. Dermatologic Surgery 22:323–330

Goldman MP, Fitzpatrick RE 1990 Pulsed-dye laser treatment of leg telangiectasia: with and without simultaneous sclerotherapy. Journal of Dermatologic and Surgical Oncology 16:338–344

Hoopman J, Ozturk S, Kenkel J 2004 An algorithm for determining ideal pulse width and energy settings vs. vessel diameter using 1064 nm Nd : YAG laser. Lasers in Surgery and Medicine 16(suppl):18

Hsia J, Lowery JA, Zelickson B. Treatment of leg telangiectasia using a long-pulse dye laser at 595 nm. Lasers in Surgery and Medicine 20:1–5

Kanter A 1998 Clinical determinants of ultrasound guided sclerotherapy outcome. Part I: The effects of age, gender, and vein size. Dermatologic Surgery 24:131–135

Kaudewitz P, Klovekorn W, Rother W 2002 Treatment of leg vein telangiectases: 1-year results with a new 940 nm diode laser. Dermatologic Surgery 28:1031–1034

Kauvar AN, Lou WW 2000 Pulsed alexandrite laser for the treatment of leg telangiectasia and reticular veins. Archives of Dermatology 136:1371–1375

Lupton JR, Alster TS, Romero P 2002 Clinical comparison of sclerotherapy versus long-pulsed Nd : YAG laser treatment for lower extremity telangiectases. Dermatologic Surgery 28:694–697

Lurie F, Creton D, Eklof B, et al 2003 Prospective randomized study of endovenous radiofrequency obliteration (closure procedure) versus ligation and stripping in a selected patient population (EVOLVeS Study). Journal of Vascular Surgery 38:207–214

Min RJ, Khilnani N, Zimmet SE 2003 Endovenous laser treatment of saphenous vein reflux: long-term results. Journal of Vascular and Interventional Radiology 14:991–996

Mordon S, Brisot D, Fournier N 2003 Using a 'non uniform pulse sequence' can improve selective coagulation with a Nd : YAG laser (1.06 micron) thanks to Met-hemoglobin absorption: a clinical study on blue leg veins. Lasers in Surgery and Medicine 32:160–170

Perrin MR, Guex JJ, Ruckley CV, et al 2000 Recurrent varices after surgery (REVAS), a consensus document. REVAS group. Cardiovascular Surgery 8:233–245

Politowski M, Zelazny T 1966 Complications and difficulties in electrocoagulation of varices of the lower extremities. Surgery 59:932–934

Polla LL, Tan OT, Garden JM, Parrish JA 1987 Tunable pulsed dye laser for the treatment of benign cutaneous vascular ectasia. Dermatologic 174:11–17

Reichert D 1998 Evaluation of the long-pulse dye laser for the treatment of leg telangiectasias. Dermatologic Surgery 24:737–740

Weiss RA 1993 Evaluation of the venous system by Doppler ultrasound and photoplethysmography or light reflection rheography before sclerotherapy. Seminars in Dermatology 12:78–87

Weiss RA 2001 Endovenous techniques for elimination of saphenous reflux: a valuable treatment modality. Dermatologic Surgery 27:902–905

Weiss RA 2002 Comparison of endovenous radiofrequency versus 810 nm diode laser occlusion of large veins in an animal model. Dermatologic Surgery 28:56–61

Weiss RA, Dover JS 2002 Leg vein management: sclerotherapy, ambulatory phlebectomy, and laser surgery. Seminars in Cutaneous Medicine and Surgery 21:76–103

Weiss RA, Weiss MA 1999 Early clinical results with a multiple synchronized pulse 1064 nm laser for leg telangiectasias and reticular veins. Dermatologic Surgery 25:399–402

4 Pigmented Lesions and Tattoos

Chrysalyne D. Schmults, Ronald G. Wheeland

Introduction

This chapter will cover laser treatment options for removing or lightening tattoos and benign pigmented lesions. These two topics are being covered together as many of the lasers used for treating both benign pigmented lesions and tattoos are the same. However, the approaches used to manage each problem can be quite different depending upon the nature of the specific lesion.

In tattoo removal, the target for the laser light consists of small particles of tattoo ink which are found either within macrophages or scattered extracellularly throughout the dermis. For treating benign pigmented lesions, the laser primarily targets melanin as its chromophore. However, unlike laser hair removal, in which the large melanin-laden unit of the hair follicle is the target, treatment of benign pigmented lesions relies upon targeting small particles of melanin found within melanocytes, keratinocytes or dermal macrophages. The targets in both tattoos and benign pigmented lesions are quite small in size. As a result, using the concept of thermal relaxation time to minimize collateral thermal injury to the normal surrounding tissue, the pulses of light required for effective treatment must be very short. Thus, Q-switched lasers with pulse durations in the nanosecond range are the mainstay of therapy for both benign pigmented lesions and tattoos. Most of these lasers have pre-set, nonvariable pulse durations that cannot be changed by the operator. The recent development of lasers, like the titanium:sapphire laser with shorter pulse durations than the Q-switched lasers (in the picosecond range), offer the potential for further reducing unwanted injury and simultaneously improving the results. Although this is still a current area of active research, these devices may ultimately prove superior to Q-switched lasers for treatment of some lesions.

The discussion of tattoo removal applies equally well to the treatment of decorative tattoos applied by professional and nonprofessional personnel, cosmetic tattoos for enhancing the lips, brows or areolae, and medical tattoos for radiation therapy of internal malignancies. [See the Advanced Topic section at the end of this chapter for a discussion of cosmetic and flesh-toned tattoos.] The discussion of treatment of benign pigmented lesions will be limited to solar lentigines, nevi of Ota and Ito, and café au lait macules (CALMs). This limitation on discussing laser treatment for other pigmented lesions, like melasma, nevocellular nevi and lentigo maligna, is warranted as the efficacy of laser therapy for these lesions has not yet been firmly established. Despite the fact that some of these lesions have been successfully treated with lasers, the small number of cases reported and the tremendous variability in the responses does not allow laser therapy to be considered as the standard of care for such lesions and consequently should only be attempted by experienced practitioners in carefully selected cases. (See the Further Reading section for articles on laser therapy for nevi.) It is also extremely important to state that laser therapy has no role in the treatment of invasive melanoma at this time.

Patient selection for tattoo removal

The recent growing trend of decorative tattooing among teens and young adults has led to an increase in the number of patients requesting tattoo removal. Most tattoos encountered today are professional tattoos. Professional tattoos are more difficult to remove than the amateur variety (Figs 4.1–4.4) due to the fact that they are often composed of multiple colors of inks placed at a variety of depths within the dermis that are often impossible to remove

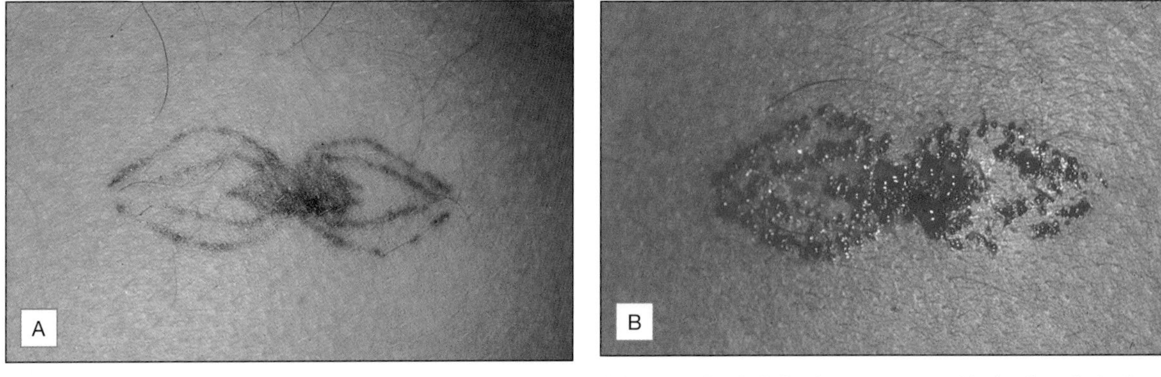

Fig. 4.1 Black amateur tattoo on the chest seen: pre-operatively (A), immediately following treatment with the Q-switched Nd:YAG laser showing punctuate bleeding (B)

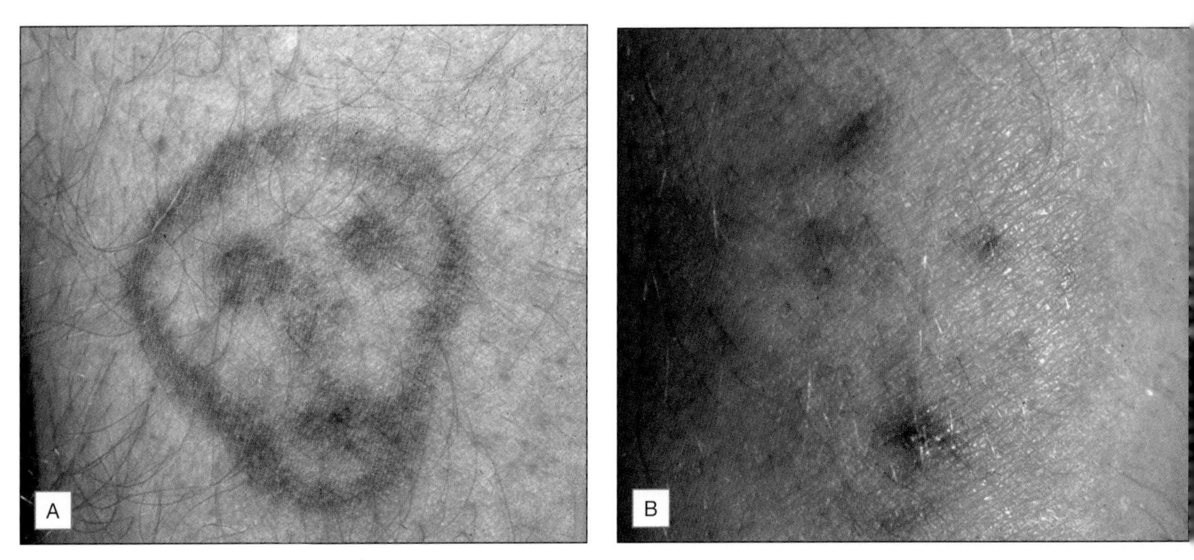

Fig. 4.2 Black amateur tattoo on the arm seen: pre-operatively (A) and 6 weeks later following a single treatment with the Q-switched ruby laser (B) with only small speckles of ink remaining

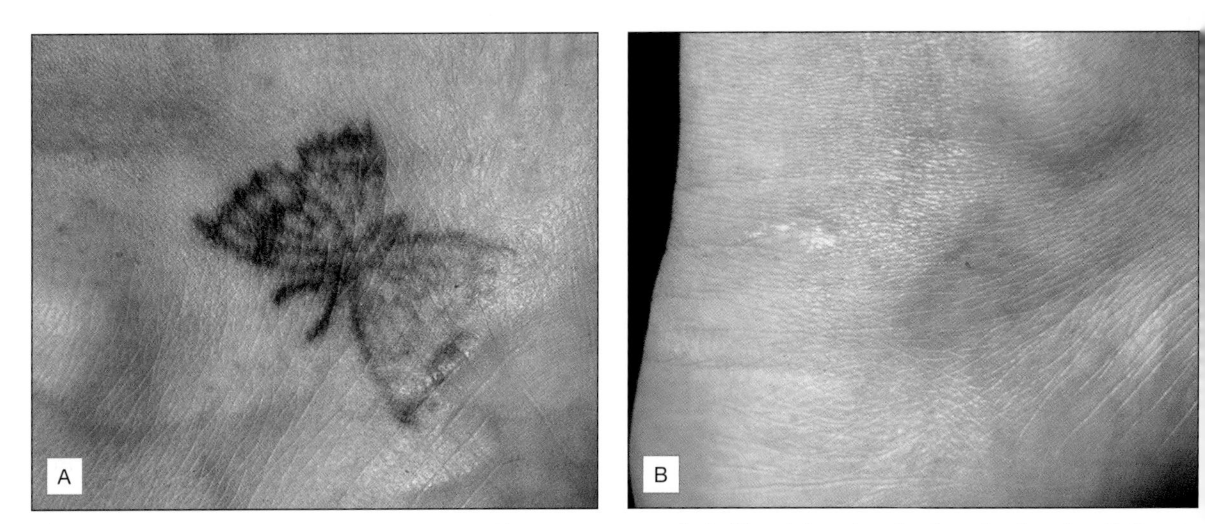

Fig. 4.3 Small, professional black tattoo on the ankle seen: pre-operatively (A) and 6 weeks after three treatments with the Q-switched ruby laser (B) with complete resolution

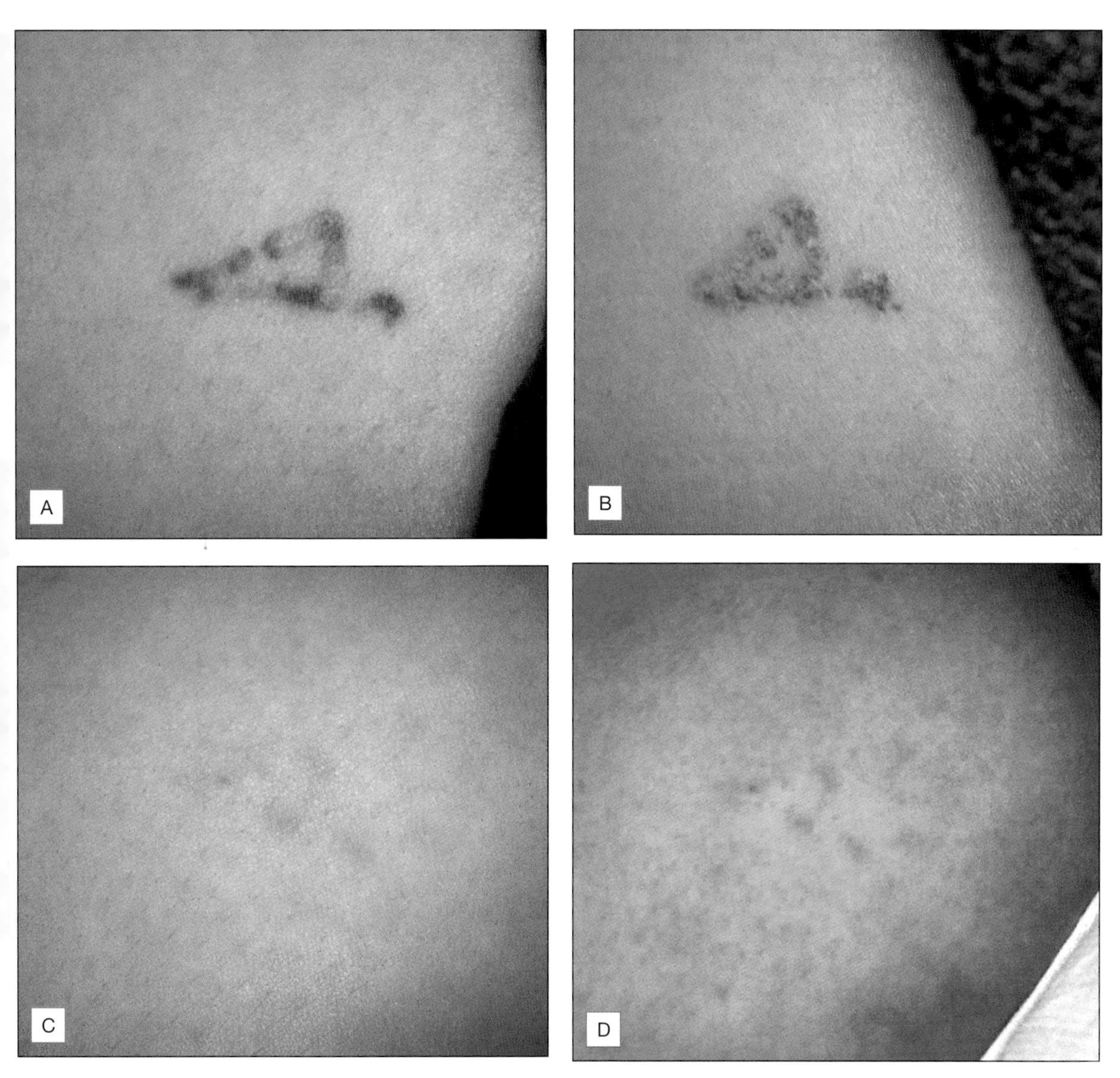

Fig. 4.4 Small, amateur black tattoo on the breast seen: pre-operatively (A), immediately following treatment with the Q-switched Nd:YAG laser showing punctuate bleeding (B), prior to third treatment with only speckles of pigment remaining (C), and 6 weeks after the third treatment showing complete resolution (D)

completely with current technology. Thus, establishing realistic expectations for every patient is paramount in achieving a result with which the patient will be satisfied. It must be emphasized that multiple treatments are normally required and may vary anywhere from five to as many as 20 in number. Furthermore, even after numerous treatments, some tattoo pigment may still remain (Fig. 4.5).

One must proceed with extreme caution in patients with darker skin (Fitzpatrick skin types IV–VI) or with tanned skin as temporary hypopigmentation (Fig. 4.6) or even permanent hyperpigmentation or hypopigmentation (Fig. 4.7) may be an adverse side effect of laser treatment in these patients due to competitive absorption of the laser light by melanin found within the epidermis. Because more light is

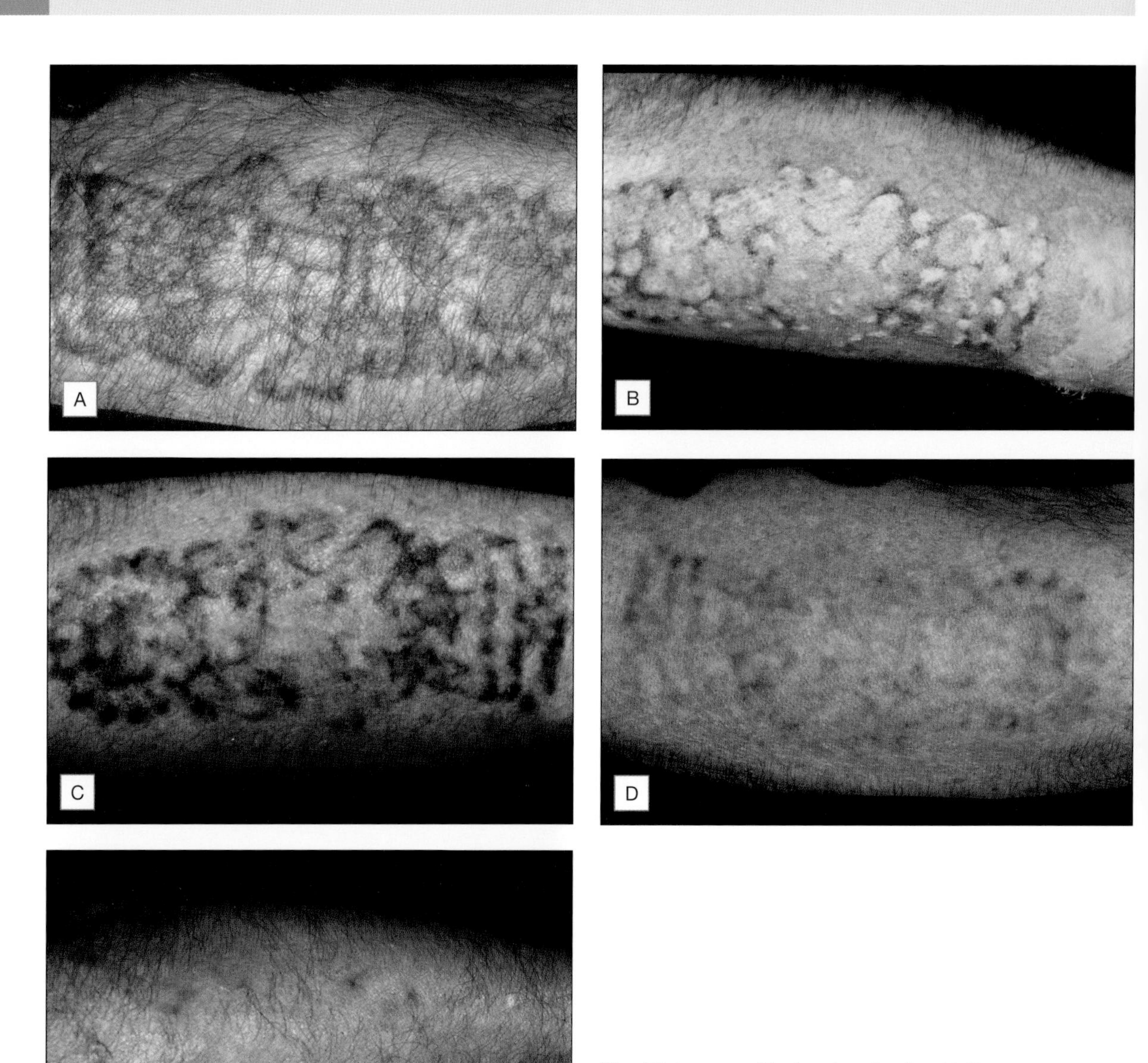

Fig. 4.5 Large multicolored professional tattoo seen: preoperatively (A), immediately following the first treatment with the Q-switched ruby laser showing the temporary whitening that occurs with the laser impacts (B), partially faded 6 weeks after the fourth treatment (C), additionally faded 6 weeks after the fifth treatment (D), and nearly completely resolved 6 months after the seventh treatment (E)

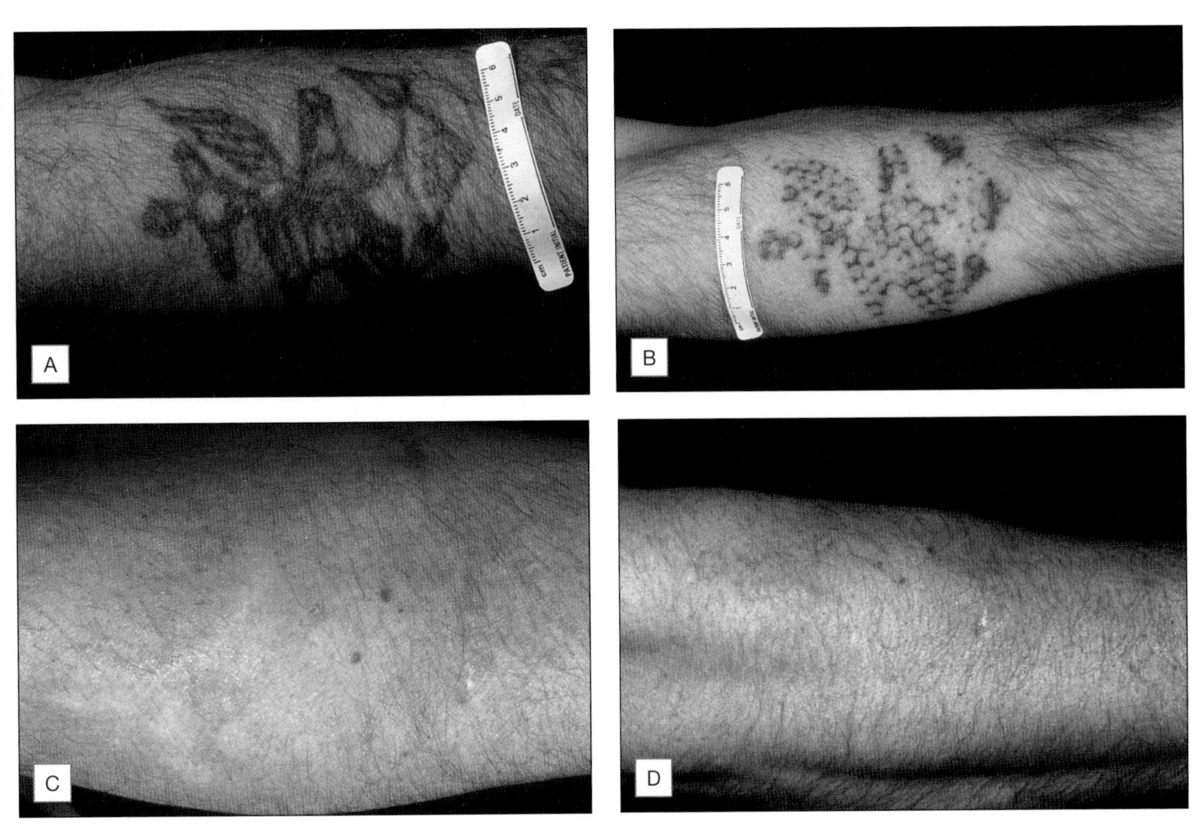

Fig. 4.6 Medium black professional tattoo seen: pre-operatively (A), following the first treatment with the Q-switched ruby laser showing breaking up of the ink focally throughout the tattoo (B), completely removed 6 weeks after the fourth treatment but with residual temporary hypopigmentation (C), 12 months after the last treatment with completely normal skin color and loss of the tattoo (D)

absorbed by the epidermis there is more potential injury to the melanocytes and this may also increase the risk of scarring. In addition, because more light is absorbed by the epidermal pigment, less light reaches the dermal target (tattoo ink) so more treatments than usual may be necessary.

The ideal patient for tattoo removal is a fair-skinned, untanned patient with type I or II skin and a dark blue or black tattoo that has been present for at least a year. The older the tattoo, the better the response to laser treatment as macrophages are already present in the skin and are actively trying to phagocytose the foreign pigment particles and remove them from the skin. This natural attempt by the body to remove the foreign tattoo ink pigment is the reason why older tattoos are often illegible and have blurry or indistinct margins. When a tattoo is treated with light from a Q-switched laser, the tattoo particles shatter into smaller fragments, facilitating more rapid removal by macrophages, and in some cases may allow complete removal of the tattoo. Conversely, recently applied, multicolored tattoos in darker-skinned patients can be very difficult to remove completely and treatment should be attempted only by experienced laser surgeons in order to reduce the potential for scarring and pigmentary alterations described above.

Patient selection for benign pigmented lesion removal

A primary consideration in treatment of benign pigmented lesions is establishing the correct diagnosis prior to initiating treatment. A biopsy must be per-

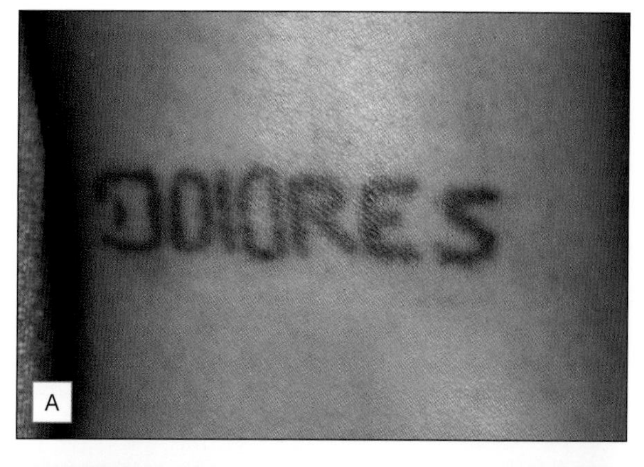

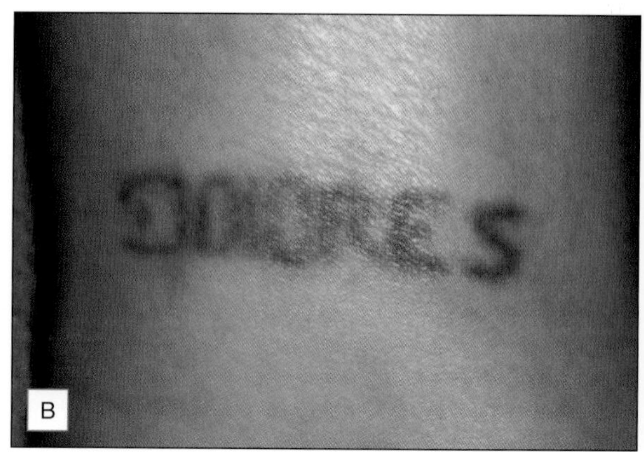

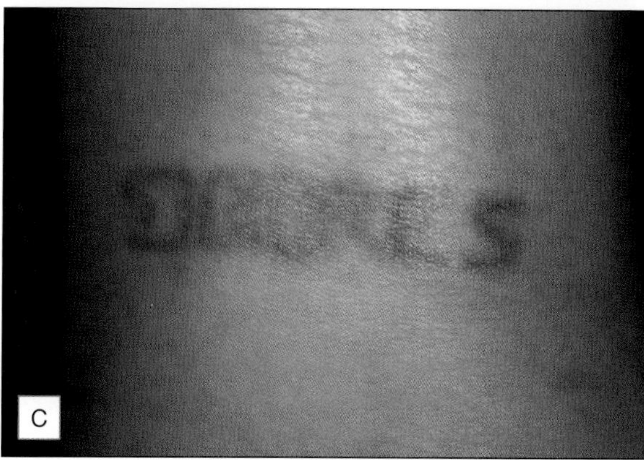

Fig. 4.7 Small black amateur tattoo seen: pre-operatively (A), following the first treatment with the Q-switched Nd:YAG laser showing approximately 80% loss of the tattoo ink but with post-inflammatory hyperpigmentation (B), nearly completely removed 6 weeks after the third treatment but with residual hyperpigmentation (C)

formed if melanoma or any other malignancy is in the differential diagnosis.

As with tattoo removal, there is a significant risk of pigmentary alteration and scarring in darker-skinned patients (Fitzpatrick skin types IV–VI) undergoing benign pigmented lesion removal. Care must be taken to avoid such risk of complications in these patients.

Expected benefits of pigmented lesion treatment

Lentigines can usually be removed completely in one to three treatments (Figs 4.8–4.10). However, CALMs (Fig. 4.11), post-inflammatory hyperpigmentation (Fig. 4.12), and nevi of Ota (Fig. 4.13) and Ito may require multiple treatments, perhaps as many as five to 10 in number, and some cannot be completely removed with any number of treatments. Nevus of Ota patients should be made aware that the scleral component of the lesion is not treatable with current technology.

The results of laser treatment of benign pigmented lesions are generally permanent. However, due to the relationship between chronic ultraviolet light (UVL) exposure and the later development of lentigines, patients should be told that in spite of an excellent response new lesions may develop over a period of 3–4 years after the treatment has been successful. This is especially true if the patient is not compulsive about protecting their skin by using sunscreens or clothing when outside. [See Tables 4.1 and 4.2 for information on clearance and improvement rates for pigmented lesions treated with laser and IPL therapy.] The treatment of the lentigines found on the mucosal surfaces in Peutz–Jeghers syn-

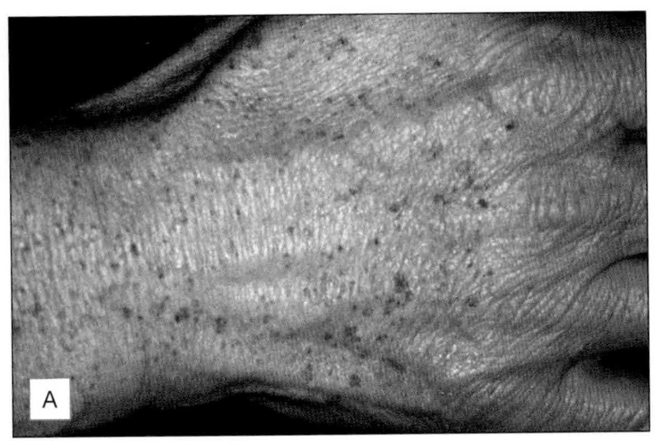

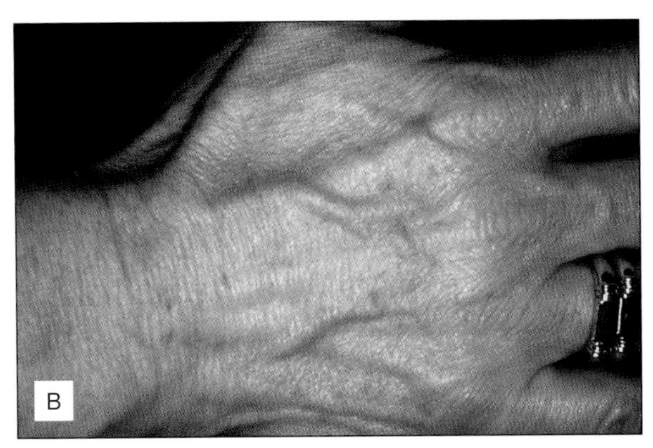

Fig. 4.8 Multiple small brown lentigines on the back of the hand seen: pre-operatively (A), with nearly complete resolution 6 weeks after a single treatment with the Q-switched Nd:YAG laser (B)

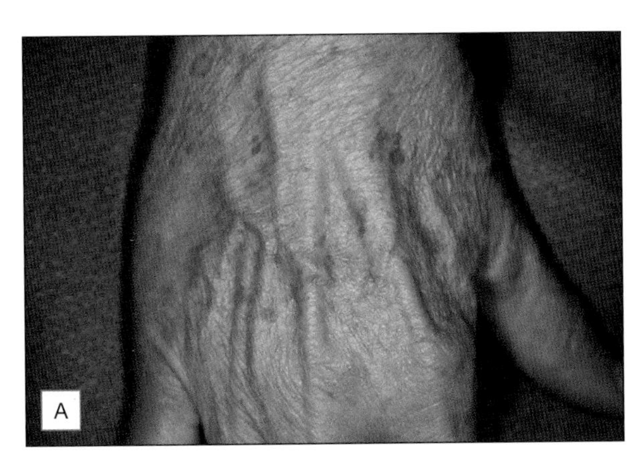

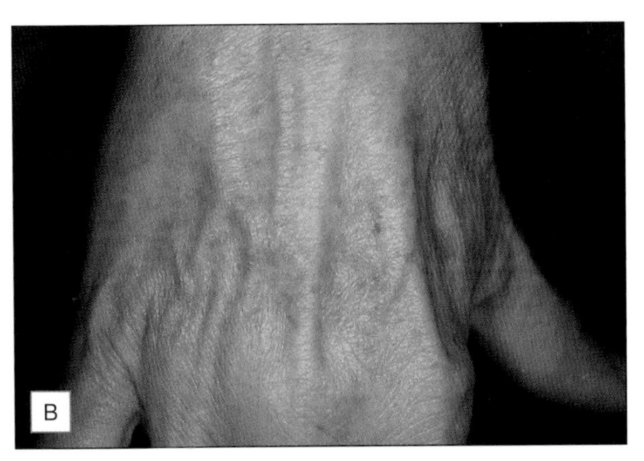

Fig. 4.9 Multiple small brown lentigines on the back of the hand seen: pre-operatively (A), with complete resolution 6 weeks after a single treatment with the Q-switched Nd:YAG laser (B)

drome may produce equally good results (Fig. 4.14) as those found on the skin surface.

Costs: Before initiating laser treatment of benign pigmented lesions, it is very important to discuss with the patient the cost of treatment, as the removal of lentigines is generally not covered by health insurance while some insurance plans will cover laser treatment of CALMs, nevi of Ota and, and nevus of Ito. Individual practitioners vary greatly in what they charge for benign pigmented lesion treatment, primarily as a reflection of the purchase price of the equipment they use (IPL, Q-switched ruby, Q-switched Alexandrite, or Q-switched Nd:YAG lasers), the number of lesions being treated, and the time it takes to perform that treatment.

Expected benefits of tattoo treatment

As mentioned above, often five to 20 treatments will be required to substantially fade or remove tattoos, and even after numerous treatments some tattoos cannot be completely removed with current laser technology. Even when removal is complete or nearly complete, there is still often a slight 'ghost-like' variation in color that may resemble the original shape of the former tattoo.

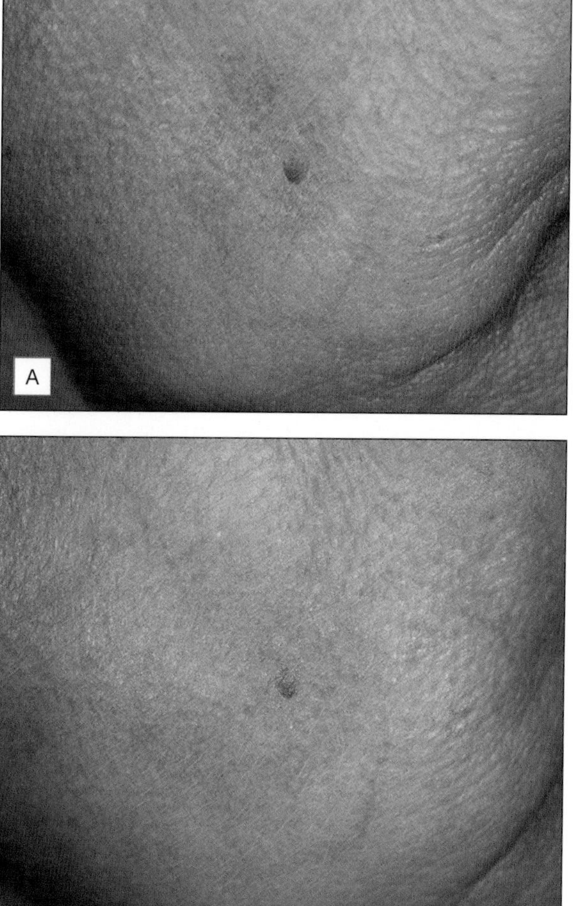

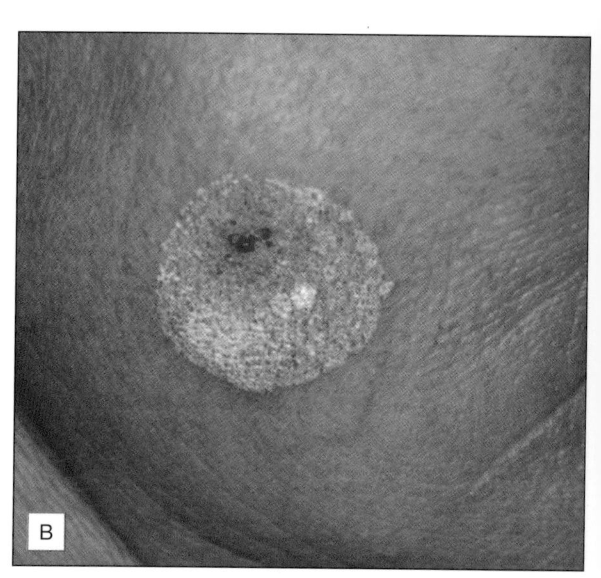

Fig. 4.10 Solitary medium-sized brown lentigo with one central black macule on the right lower cheek seen: pre-operatively (A), immediately following the first treatment with the Q-switched Nd:YAG laser showing the typical temporary whitening of the skin (B), and 6 weeks later showing resolution of the larger lentigo but persistence of the central dark macule which should be biospied to rule out a more serious problem (C)

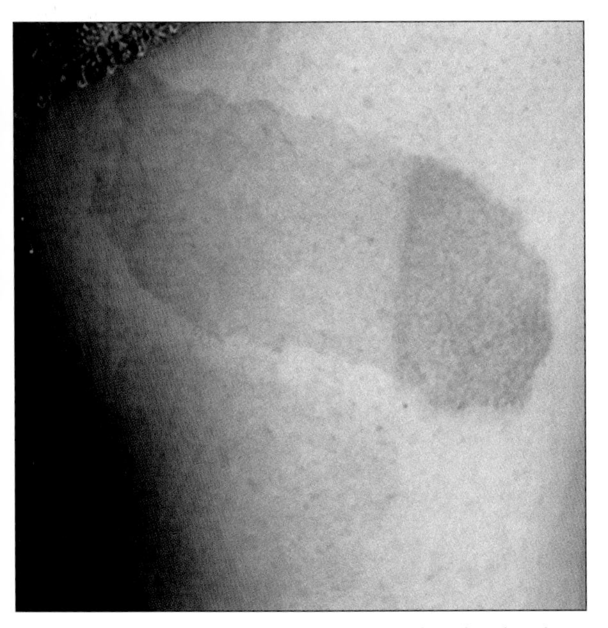

Fig. 4.11 Solitary café-au-lait patch on the leg showing the complication of hyperpigmentation of the lateral portion of the lesion twelve weeks after testing with the Q-switched Nd:YAG laser

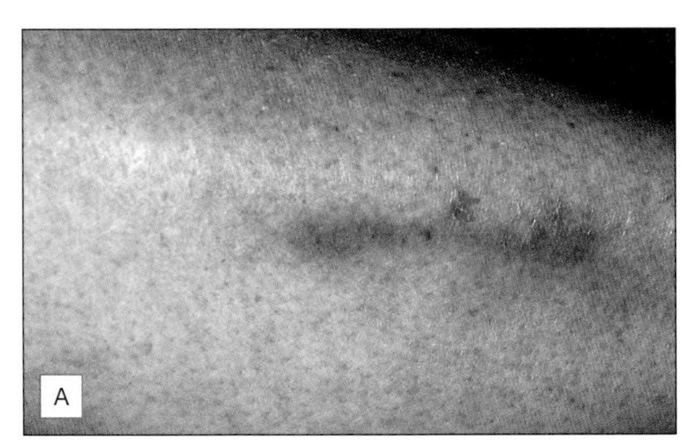

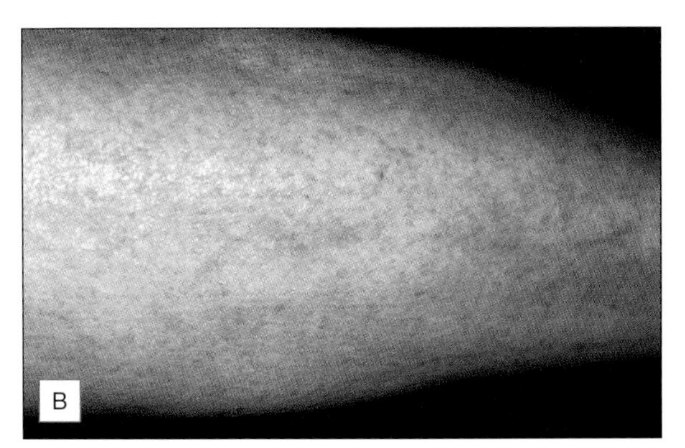

Fig. 4.12 Area of post-inflammatory hyperpigmentation following sclerotherapy for small leg veins seen: pre-operatively (A), and 6 weeks after multiple treatments with the Q-switched ruby laser (B)

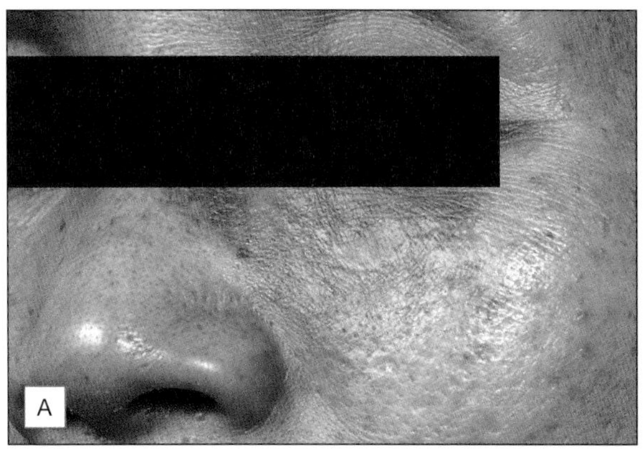

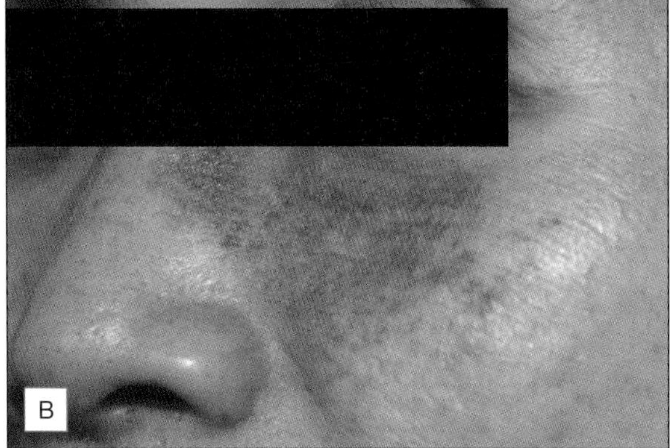

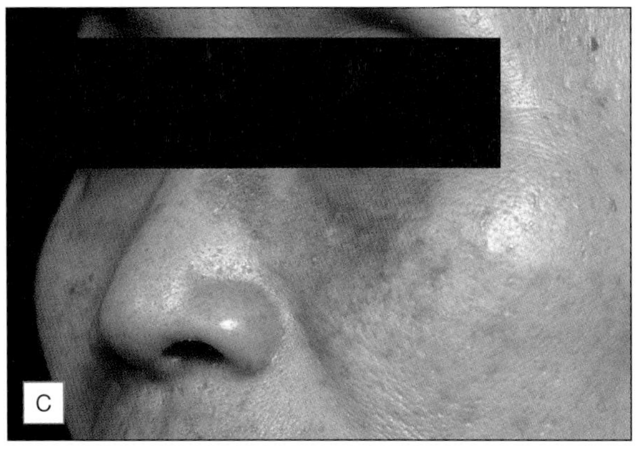

Fig. 4.13 Small nevus of Ota is seen: pre-operatively (A), 6 weeks after two treatments with the Q-switched ruby laser showing some fading (B), and with nearly complete fading 6 weeks after the fourth treatment (C)

Laser and IPL removal of lentigines: a summary of studies		
Reference	**Study design**	**Results**
Todd MM, Hata TR et al. A comparison of three lasers and liquid nitrogen in the treatment of solar lentigines: A randomized, controlled, comparative trial. Archives of Dermatology 2000;136:841–846	27 patients treated once for dorsal hand lentigines	>45% of patients were cleared and >35% had lightening of 76-90% with Q-s 532 nm Nd:YAG treatment. This was superior to liquid nitrogen, krypton laser and a 532 nm diode-pumped vanadate laser
Rashid T, Haroon TS et al. Laser therapy of freckles and lentigines with quasi-continuous, frequency-doubled, Nd:YAG (532 nm) laser in Fitzpatrick skin type IV: a 24-month follow-up. Journal of Cosmetic Laser Therapy 2002;4:81–85	6 lentigo patients and 14 freckle patients with type V skin received three to eight treatments	80% of patients had >50% improvement. 25% had hypopigmentation and 10% had hyperpigmentation
Li YT, Yang KC. Comparison of frequency-doubled Q-switched Nd:YAG laser and 35% trichloroacetic acid for the treatment of face lentigines. Dermatological Surgery 1999;25:202–204	20 patients with 37 facial lentigos and skin types III–IV underwent a single treatment. Half of each lentigo was treated with 35% TCA and the other half with Q-s Nd:YAG	Mean clearance score was 4.2 (76–95% clearance) for Q-s Nd:YAG. Mean TCA score was 3.7 (statistically significant difference but only small clinical difference)
Tse Y, Ashinoff R et al. The removal of cutaneous pigmented lesions with the Q-switched ruby laser and the Q-switched Nd:YAG laser: a comparative study. Journal of Dermatologic Surgery and Oncology 1994;20:795–800	20 patients were treated once	100% of patients had >30% lightening. Ruby was superior to 532 nm Q-s Nd:YAG
Kilmer SL, Wheeland RG, Goldber DJ, Anderson RR. Treatment of epidermal pigmented lesions with the frequency-doubled Q-switched (532 nm) Nd:YAG laser: a controlled single-impact, dose-response multicenter trial. Archives of Dermatology 1994;130:1515–1519	37 patients with lentigines were treated once at 2, 3, 4 or 5 J/cm^2	Higher fluences produced better clearance with >75% clearance in 60% of patients at higher fluences. Hyper- and hypopigmentation resolved within 3 months
Kawanda A, Tezuka T et al. Clinical improvement of solar lentigines and ephelides with an intense pulsed light source. Dermatologic Surgery 2002; 28:504–508	60 patients with facial lesions were treated three to five times	48% of patients had >50% improvement and 20% had > 75% improvement. Ephelides responded slightly better than lentigines
Bjerring P, Christiansen K. Intense pulsed light source for treatment of small melanocytic nevi and solar lentigines. Journal of Cutaneous Laser Therapy 2000;2:177–181	18 patients with lentigines were treated once	Average lentigo clearance was 74%
Kopera D, Landthaler M et al. Q-switched ruby laser application is safe and effective for the management of actinic lentigo. Acta Dermatologica Venereologica 1996; 76:461–463	10 patients with lentigines of arms and hands were treated once. One arm was treated with Q-s ruby laser and the other with glycolic acid peel	Q-s ruby laser treatment resulted in complete clearance of lesions. Glycolic acid peel showed little to no improvement

Table 4.1 Laser and IPL removal of lentigines: a summary of studies

Laser removal of CALMs and Nevi of Ota and Ito: a summary of studies		
Reference	**Study design**	**Results**
Laser Removal of Café au Lait Macules (CALMs)		
Alster TS. Complete elimination of large café au lait birthmarks by the 510 nm pulsed dye laser. Plastic and Reconstructive Surgery 1995; 96:1660–1664	34 patients were treated multiple times at 2–4 J/cm^2	An average of 8.4 treatments were required for complete removal. No recurrences were seen at 1 year
Grossman MC, Grevelink JM et al. Treatment of café au lait macules with lasers: a clinicopathologic correlation. Archives of Dermatology 1995; 131:1416–1420	9 CALMs in 10 patients were treated once, half of each lesion with Q-s Nd:YAG (532 nm) and half with Q-s ruby	No lesions were cleared after this single treatment. Responses varied and included lightening, clearance with rapid recurrence, transient darkening, and no change
Laser Removal of Nevi of Ota and Ito		
Chan HH, Ho WS et al. A retrospective analysis of complications in the treatment of nevus of Ota with the Q-switched alexandrite and Q-switched Nd:YAG lasers. Dermatologic Surgery 2000;26:1000–1006	171 patients with 211 lesions were evaluated. 58 were treated with alexandrite alone, 105 with Nd:YAG (1064 nm) alone and 48 with both lasers	13/171 patients had recurrences. 15% had hypopigmentaion, 3% hyperpigmentation, 3% textural changes, 2% scarring. Using both lasers in a given patient increased the risk of side effects. It took more treatments to achieve a 50% clearance with the Nd:YAG as compared to ruby
Chan HH, King WW et al. An in vivo trial comparing the efficacy and complications of Q-switched 755 nm alexandrite and Q-switched 1064 nm Nd:YAG lasers in the treatment of nevus of Ota. Dermatologic Surgery 2000;26:919–922	45 patients were treated three or more times. Half of each lesion was treated with each laser	The Q-s Nd:YAG (1064 nm) was found to be more effective than the Q-s alexandrite
Kono T, Nozaki M et al. Use of Q-switched ruby laser in the treatment of nevus of Ota in different age groups. Lasers in Surgery and Medicine 2003;32:391–395	46 children and 107 adults who had >75% clearance were studied	A mean of 3.5 treatments resulted in complete clearing in children versus six treatments for adults. A 5% complication rate was seen in children versus 22.4% in adults
Kono T, Mikashima Y et al. A retrospective study looking at the long-term complications of Q-switched ruby laser in the treatment of nevus of Ota. Lasers in Surgery and Medicine 2001;29:156–159	101 patients were evaluated at least 1 year after treatment completion	One patient had a recurrence. 17% had hypopigmentation, 6% had hyperpigmentation
Alster TS, Williams CM. Treatment of nevus of Ota by the Q-switched alexandrite laser. Dermatologic Surgery 1995;21:592–596	7 patients were treated	2 treatments resulted in average of 50% clearance. 5 of the patients had 100% clearance after five treatments. No recurrences had occurred after 1 year. No pigmentation alteration or scarring occurred

Table 4.2 Laser removal of CALMs and Nevi of Ota and Ito: a summary of studies

Continued

Laser removal of CALMs and Nevi of Ota and Ito: a summary of studies—cont'd		
Reference	**Study design**	**Results**
Laser Removal of Nevi of Ota and Ito—cont'd		
Watanabe S, Takahashi H. Treatment of nevus of Ota with Q-switched ruby laser. New England Journal of Medicine 1994; 331:1745–1750	114 patients underwent multiple treatments	After 4–5 treatments: 33/35 patients had >70% lightening. 2/35 had 40–69% lightening. After three treatments: 26/31 had 40–69% clearance, 4/31 had >70% clearance. After two treatments: 2/25 had >70% clearance, 16/25 had 40–69% clearance. After a single treatment: 3/23 had >70% clearance, 13/23 had 40–69% clearance. Only eight patients had hyperpigmentation that resolved in 2 months
Geronemus RG. Q-switched ruby laser therapy of nevus of Ota. Archives of Dermatology 1992;128:1618–1622	15 patients were treated one to seven times	4/15 patients had 100% clearance. >50% clearance occurred in 11/15. The higher fluences studied produced a greater effect

Table 4.2, cont'd Laser removal of CALMs and Nevi of Ota and Ito: a summary of studies

Dark blue and black tattoos respond best to laser therapy, while yellow, red, and green (Figs 4.15 & 4.16) pigments may respond poorly or only incompletely to treatment. Treatment of white and cosmetic flesh-toned tattoos should be avoided by inexperienced practitioners as they may change to a permanent darker black or gray color immediately following Q-switched laser therapy and be impossible to remove.

When a tattoo is completely removed by laser therapy, it is generally permanent. [See Table 4.3 for clearance and improvement rates for tattoos treated with lasers.]

Costs: As with laser removal of benign pigmented lesions, there is wide variation in the cost of removing a tattoo with a laser. Not only is the purchase price for the Q-switched ruby, Nd:YAG, and alexandrite lasers variable, but the size of the tattoos

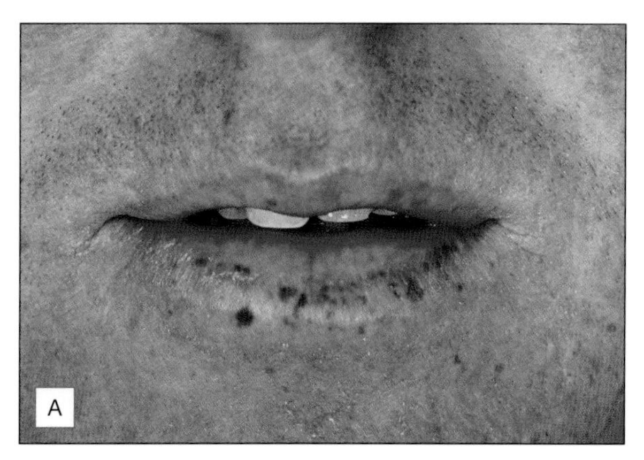

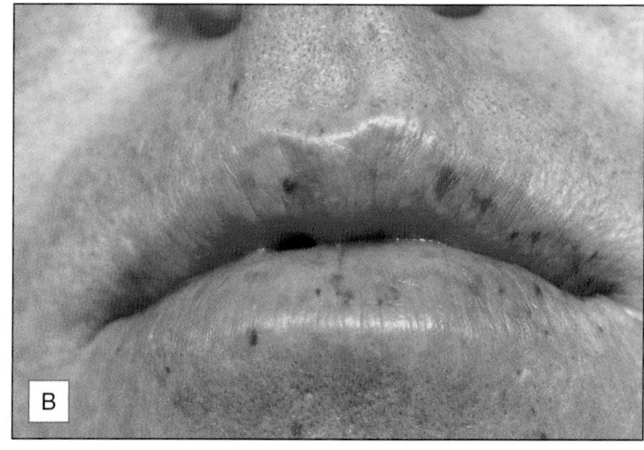

Fig. 4.14 Multiple small lentigines of the oral mucosa seen with Peutz–Jeghers syndrome seen: pre-operatively (A), 6 weeks after three treatments with the Q-switched ruby laser showing excellent fading without scarring (B)

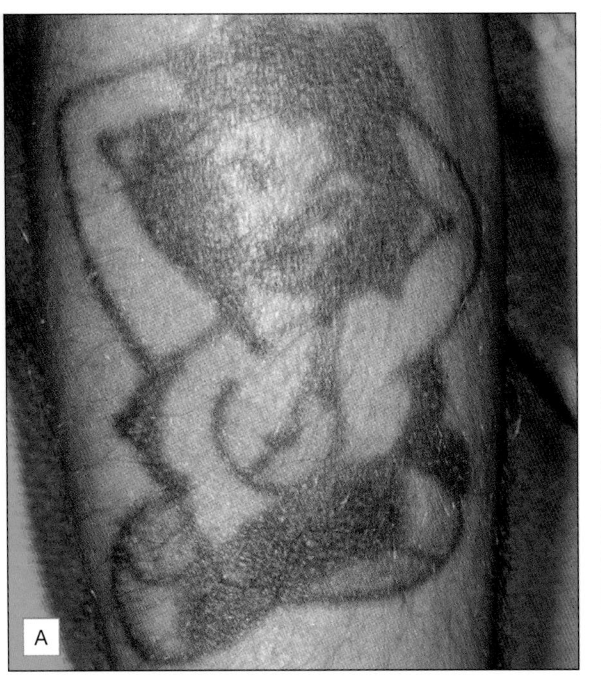

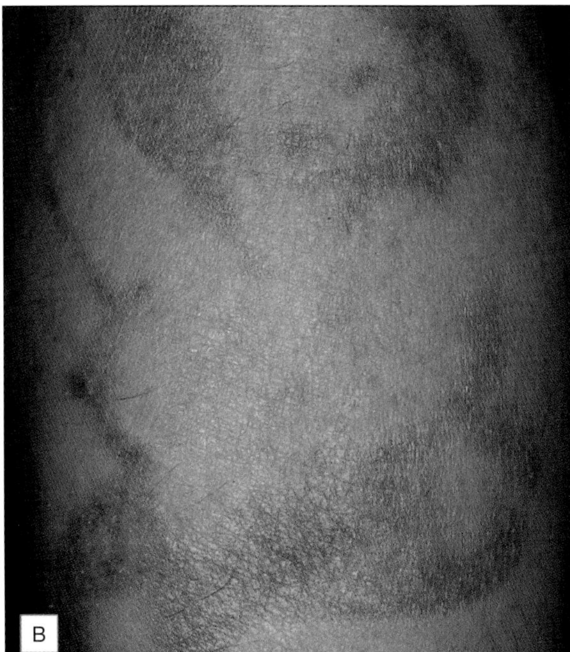

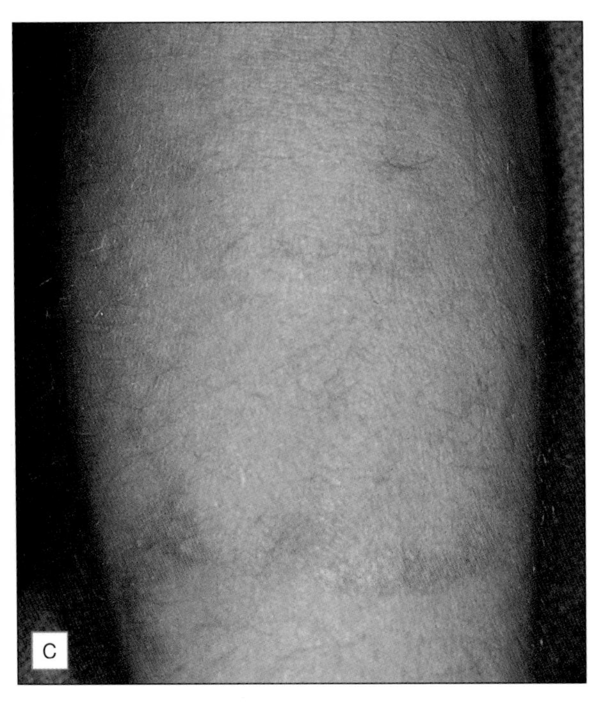

Fig. 4.15 Medium-sized, multicolored professional tattoo seen: pre-operatively (A), 6 weeks following the second treatment with the Q-switched Nd:YAG laser showing significant fading of the black tattoo ink but with nearly complete persistence of the green tattoo ink (B), and 6 weeks after the fifth treatment showing fading, but persistence, of much of the green tattoo ink (C)

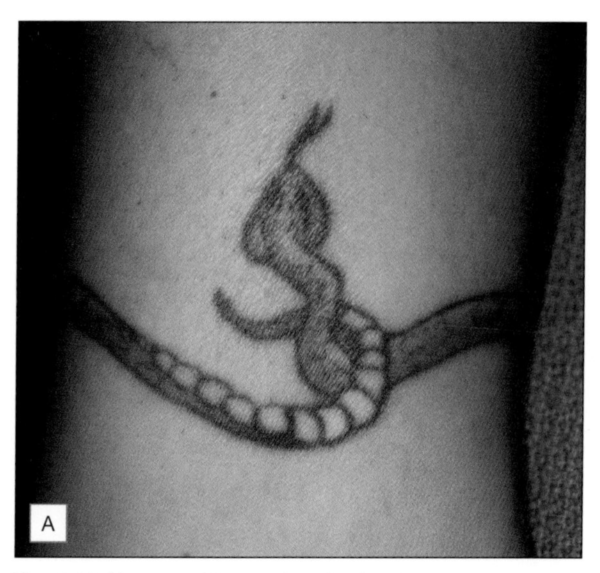

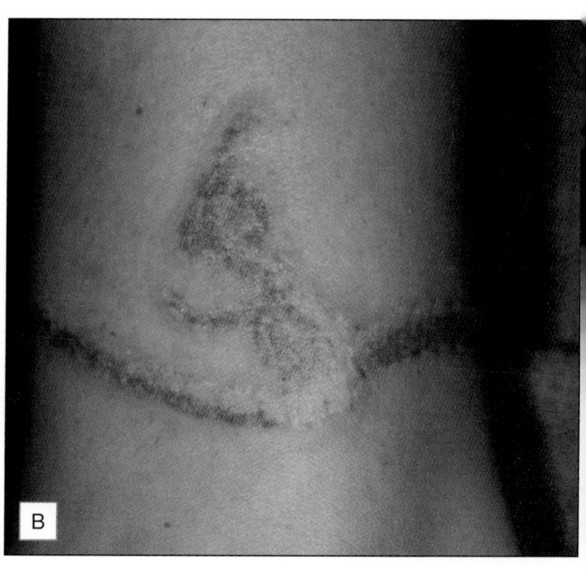

Fig. 4.16 Linear, multicolored professional tattoo seen: pre-operatively (A) and 6 weeks following the third treatment with the Q-switched Nd:YAG laser showing significant fading of the black tattoo ink but only mild fading of the green tattoo ink (B)

Laser removal of tattoos: a summary of studies		
Reference	**Study design**	**Results**
Laser Removal of Tattoos Kilmer SL, Anderson RR et al. The Q-switched Nd:YAG laser (1064 nm) effectively treats tattoos: a controlled dose–response study. Archives of Dermatology 1993;129:971–978	25 patients with 39 tattoos were treated four times	>75% clearance occurred in 77% of lesions. >95% clearance was achieved in 28% of lesions. 10–12 J/cm^2 was superior to 6–8 J/cm^2
Alster T. Q-switched alexandrite laser (755 nm) treatment of professional and amateur tattoos. Journal of American Academy of Dermatology 1995;33:69–73	24 multicolored and 18 blue-black tattoos were treated with Q-s alexandrite. Red tattoos were treated with a 510 nm, 300 nsec laser.	Professional tattoos required an average of 8.5 treatments for complete clearance versus 4.6 treatments for amateur tattoos. An average of two treatments with the 510 nm laser cleared red ink
Jones A, Rosen T et al. The Q-switched Nd:YAG laser effectively treats tattoos in darkly pigmented skin. Dermatologic Surgery 1996;22:999–1001	15 patients with amateur tattoos and type VI skin were treated two to four times.	75–95% clearance occurred in 8/15 patients. 5/15 were 50% cleared. 2/15 had 25% clearance but this was with only two treatments. 2/15 patients had slight hypopigmentation
Grevelink JM, Anderson RR et al. Laser treatment of tattoos in darkly pigmented patients: efficacy and side effects. Journal of American Academy of Dermatology 1996;34:653–656	5 patients with skin types V and VI were treated three to eight times. 4 patients had amateur tattoos and 1 had a professional tattoo. Q-s ruby and (1064nm) Nd:YAG lasers were used	All tattoos were cleared. No scarring or permanent pigment changes occurred

Table 4.3 Laser removal of tattoos: a summary of studies

Continued

Reference	Study design	Results
Laser Removal of Tattoos—cont'd		
Levine VJ, Geronemus RG. Tattoo removal with the Q-switched ruby laser and the Q-switched Nd:YAG laser: a comparative study. Cutis 1995;55:291–296	48 amateur and professional tattoos were treated once; half of each lesion with Q-s ruby and half with Q-s Nd:YAG.	532 nm Nd:YAG was superior for removal of red pigment. Ruby was superior to 1064 nm Nd:YAG for black and green. Ruby and 1064 nm Nd:YAG were equivalent for other colors. One hypertrophic scar occurred
Stafford TJ, Tan OT et al. Removal of colored tattoos with the Q-switched alexandrite laser. Plastic and Reconstructive Surgery 1995;95:313–320	7 patients were treated	9–10 treatments were required for removal of green, red and mauve colors. Orange and yellow showed no improvement
Fitzpatrick RE, Goldman MP. Tattoo removal using the alexandrite laser Archives of Dermatology 1994; 130:1508–1514	17 patients with professional tattoos and eight patients with amateur tattoos were treated	9 treatments yielded >95% clearance of blue-black and black tattoos. Only transient side effects were seen
Goyal S, Dover JS et al. Laser treatment of tattoos: a prospective paired comparison study of the Q-switched Nd:YAG (1064 nm), frequency-doubled Q-switched Nd:YAG (532 nm), and Q-switched ruby lasers. Journal of American Academy of Dermatology 1997;36:122–125	12 black and 8 multicolored tattoos were divided into thirds and treated once with each of the three lasers	Ruby was best for black blue yellow and green. 532 nm YAG was best for red. 1032 nm YAG and ruby were equally effective for brown and purple
Scheibner A, Wheeland RG et al. A superior method of tattoo removal using the Q-switched ruby laser. Journal of Dermatologic Surgery and Oncology 1990;16:1091–1098	101 amateur and 62 professional tattoos were treated	For amateur tattoos, nearly complete or complete removal was achieved in 88/101 lesions after an average of three treatments. Professional tattoos were refractory with only 7/62 achieving complete or near-complete removal. Red yellow and green pigments were especially difficult. No permanent side effects occurred
Lauenberger ML, Grevelink JM et al. Comparison of the Q-switched alexandrite, Nd:YAG, and ruby lasers in treating blue-black tattoos. Dermatologic Surgery 1999;25:10–14	42 blue-black tattoos were divided into three and treated with the three different lasers three to six times	The Q-switched ruby was statistically significantly superior to the Nd:YAG and alexandrite. All three lasers had increased clearance rates with increased number of treatments

Table 4.3, cont'd Laser removal of tattoos: a summary of studies

and the number of treatments required to obtain maximal clearing of the pigment are also highly variable. Tattoo removal is generally not covered by health insurance except on rare occasions. Coverage may be provided for the laser removal of medical tattoos placed for radiation therapy, traumatic tattoos resulting from explosions or motor vehicle (Figs 4.17–4.19) accidents ('road rash'), and tattoo granulomas, which require use of the ablative carbon dioxide laser for effective treatment (Fig. 4.20). Suffice it to say that some larger, resistant, multicolored tattoos may require many expensive treatments to produce sufficient fading or lightening to satisfy the patient.

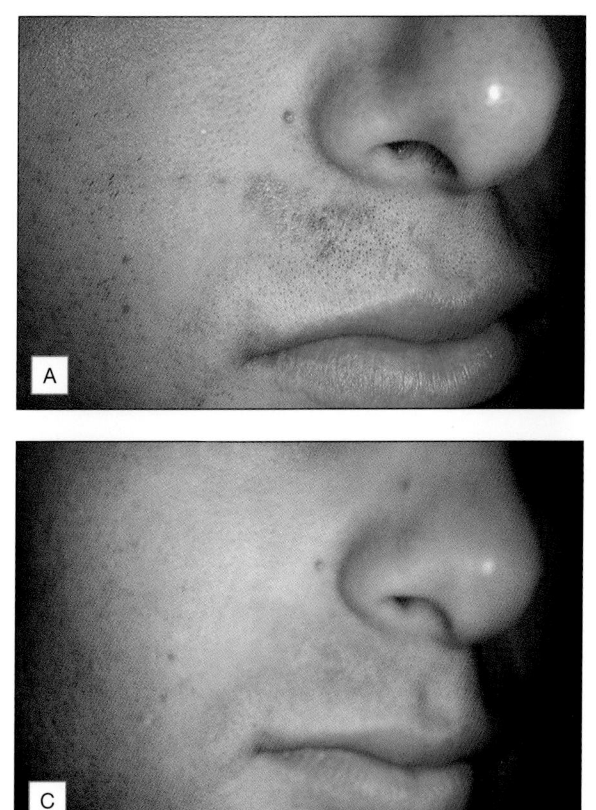

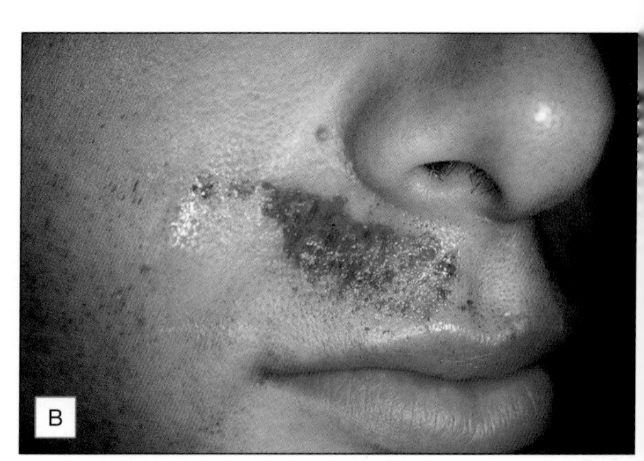

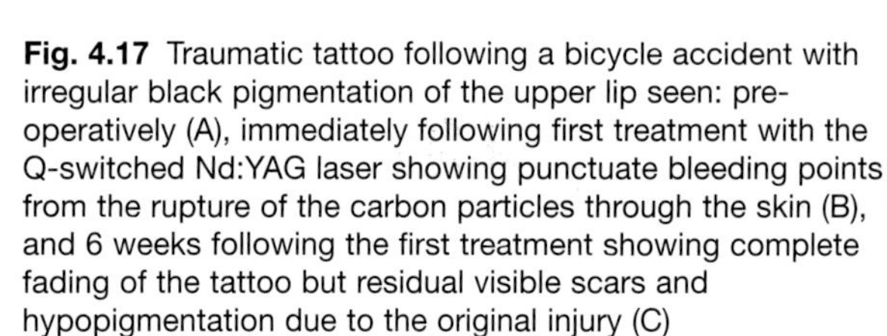

Fig. 4.17 Traumatic tattoo following a bicycle accident with irregular black pigmentation of the upper lip seen: pre-operatively (A), immediately following first treatment with the Q-switched Nd:YAG laser showing punctuate bleeding points from the rupture of the carbon particles through the skin (B), and 6 weeks following the first treatment showing complete fading of the tattoo but residual visible scars and hypopigmentation due to the original injury (C)

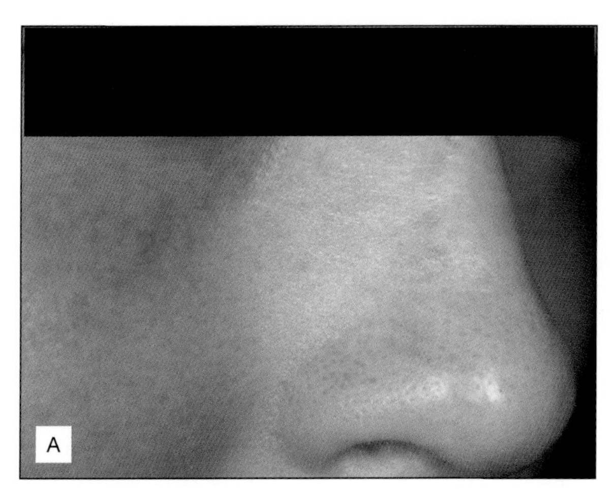

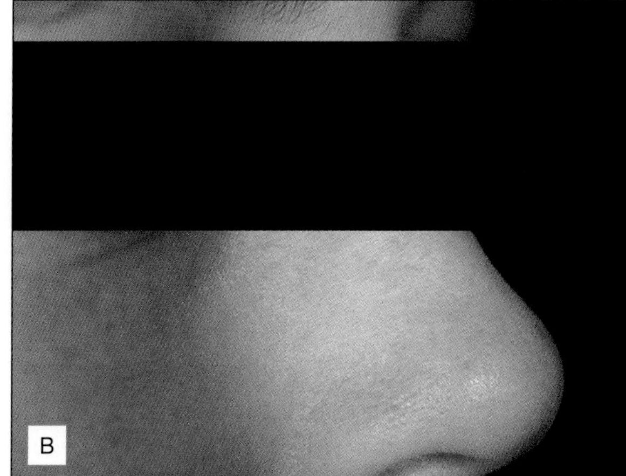

Fig. 4.18 Traumatic tattoo following a motor vehicle accident with irregular linear black pigmentation of the right nasal bridge seen: pre-operatively (A) and 6 weeks after the first treatment with the Q-switched Nd:YAG laser showing complete fading of the tattoo but with residual visible scars from the original injury (B)

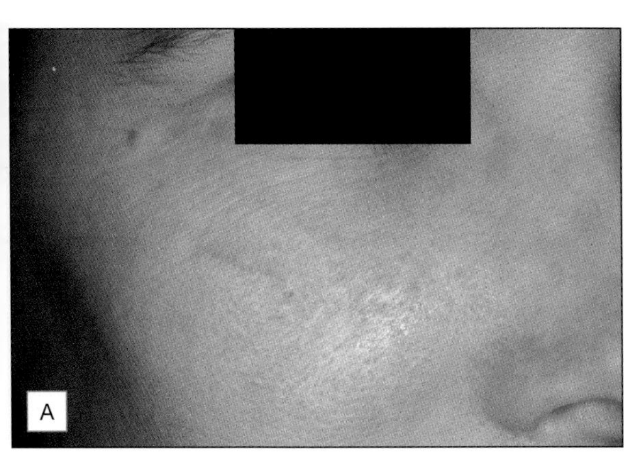

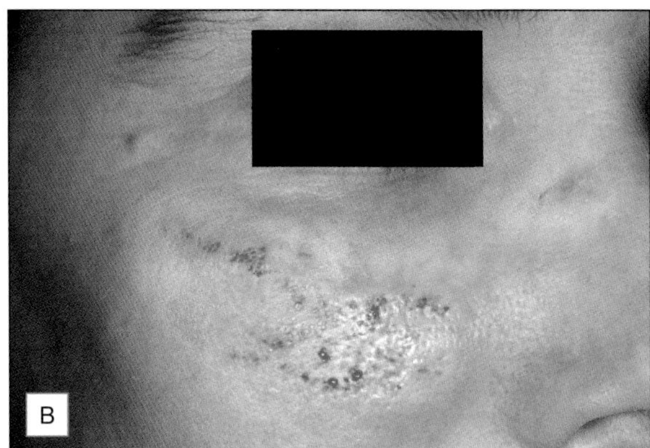

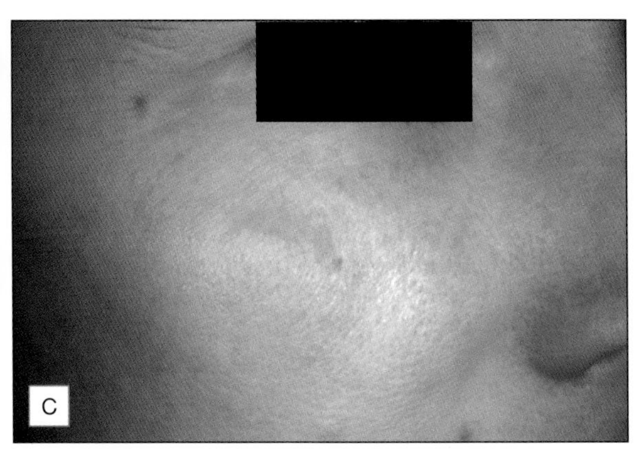

Fig. 4.19 Traumatic tattoo following a motor vehicle accident with irregular linear black pigmentation of the right superior cheek seen: pre-operatively (A), immediately after the first treatment with the Q-switched Nd:YAG laser showing punctuate bleeding points from the rupture of the foreign carbon particles back through the skin (B), and 6 weeks after the first treatment with the Q-switched Nd:YAG laser showing complete fading of the tattoo but with slight residual post-inflammatory hyperpigmentation (C)

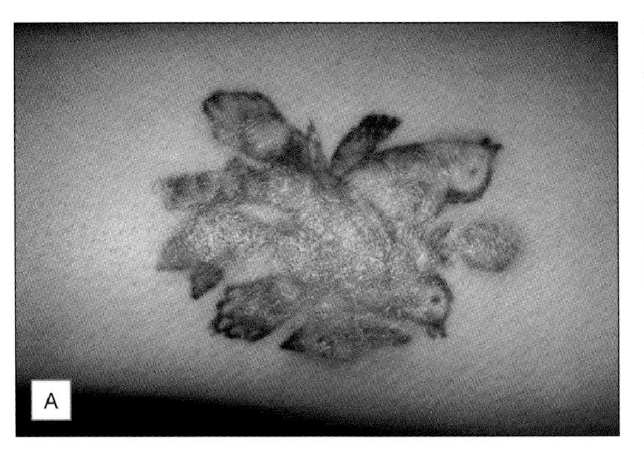

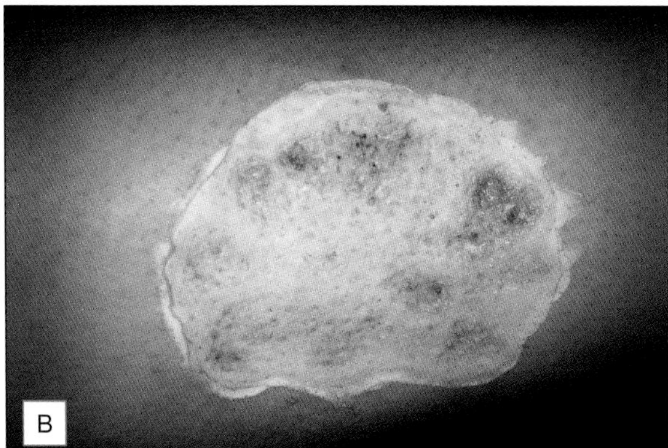

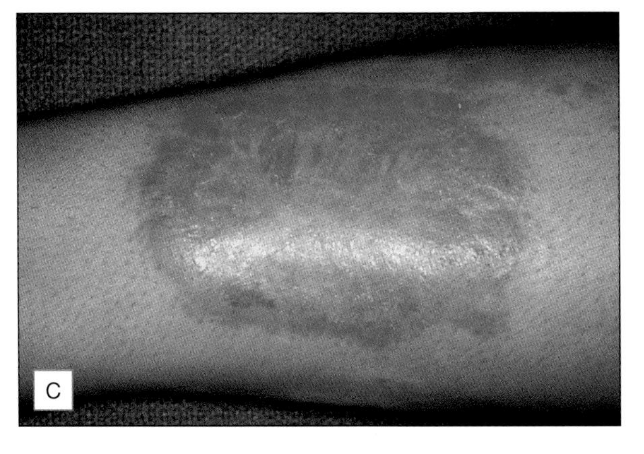

Fig. 4.20 Tattoo granulomas from an allergic reaction to the red (cinnabar or mercury tattoo ink) color in a multicolored tattoo, seen: pre-operatively (A), immediately after removal of the tattoo and all granulomas with the vaporizational mode of the carbon dioxide laser (B), and 3 months later showing the residual erythematous permanent scar (C)

Overview of Treatment Strategy

Major determinants

The natural, untanned color of the patient's skin is a major determinant in appropriately selecting the proper laser for treating benign pigmented lesions and tattoos. In tattoo removal, the size, age, anatomic location, and color of the tattoo are other major determinants (see Figs 4.21 & 4.22 and Treatment Techniques below).

Patients with lighter skin types have less risk of pigment alteration following laser therapy compared to darker skinned patients. Fitzpatrick skin types are helpful but only approximate a patient's risk of permanent pigment disturbance following laser therapy. Thus, the performance of small representative test spots prior to initiating full treatment may be useful. **It is advisable for all beginning practitioners to perform laser test spots (Figs 4.23 & 4.24) in all patients prior to treating an entire lesion.** Many seasoned experts continue to perform small test spots since skin type and color do not always perfectly predict the response to treatment.

It is very important to ensure that the patient is not tanned. This is important because epidermal melanin produced by UVL exposure may interfere with laser treatment and increase the risks of scarring, hypopigmentation, or hyperpigmentation. To ensure a tan is not present, it is wise to compare the color of exposed skin at the potential treatment site to that of a nonexposed skin site, like the buttock or axilla. If a tan is present (due to natural sunlight, tanning beds, or even topically applied bronzers), treatment should be delayed until the tan has faded as much as possible in the treatment area. Use of sun protection, protective clothing or bleaching creams can be useful in expediting fading.

Many practitioners do not treat patients who have been on oral retinoids within the previous 12 months due to reports of increased risks of scar formation and poor healing. Oral anti-viral prophylaxis should be always be considered for patients with a history of herpes simplex (HSV) infections in or near the planned treatment site. If active HSV infection is present on the day of planned laser treatment, the appointment should be cancelled and delayed until the area has healed completely and the patient can be placed on appropriate pre-operative prophylactic antiviral therapy prior to the initiation of treatment.

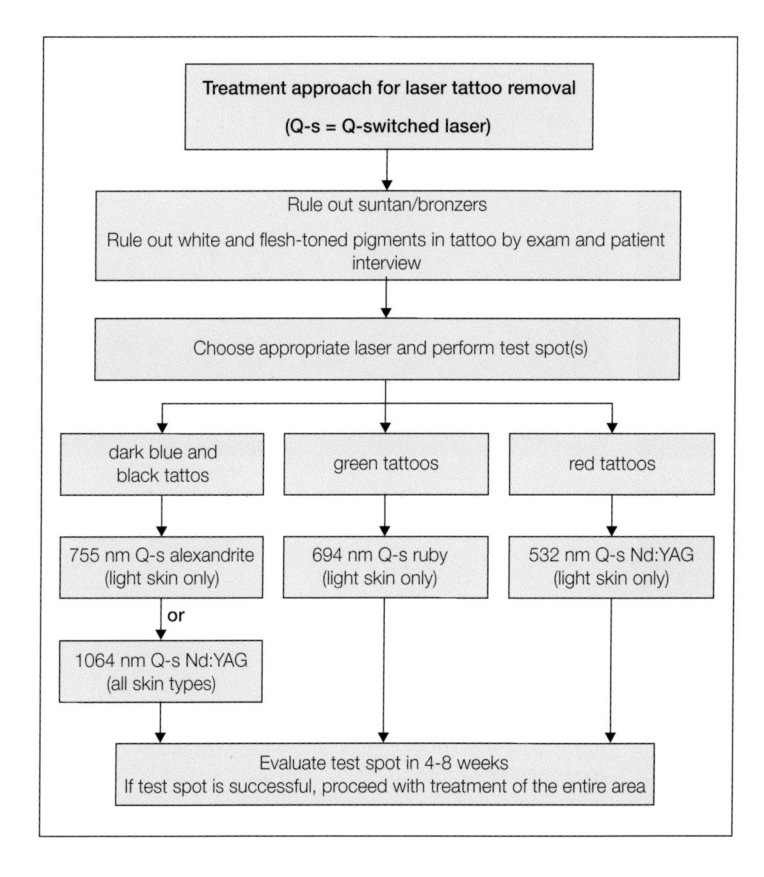

Fig. 4.21 Treatment approach for laser tattoo removal

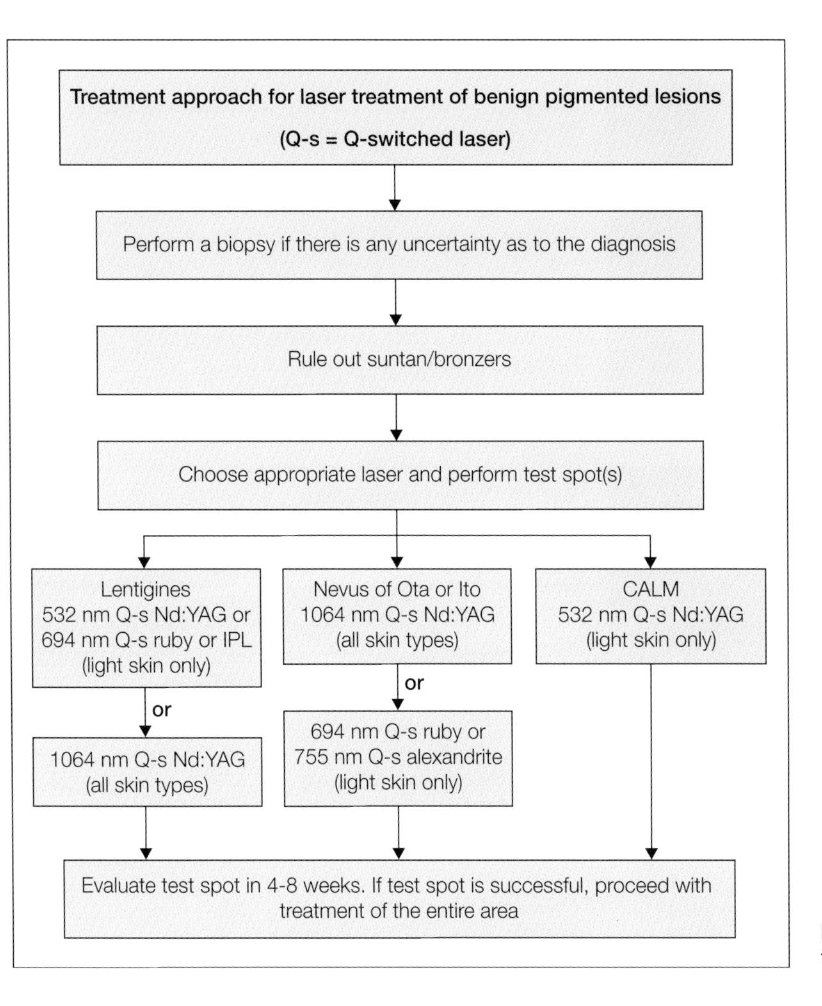

Fig. 4.22 Treatment approach for laser treatment of benign pigmented lesions

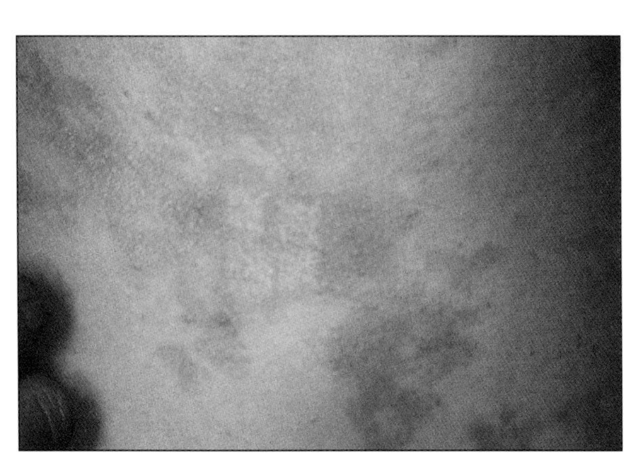

Fig. 4.23 Four distinct lighter test spots within a larger hyperpigmented patch on the right anterior neck 6 weeks after testing with the Q-switched Nd:YAG laser

Patient interviews

The questions to ask a tattooed patient and one with a pigmented lesion are shown in Boxes 4.1 and 4.2, respectively.

Treatment Techniques

Patients and equipment for dark blue or black tattoo treatment in lighter-skinned patients (Fitzpatrick skin types I–III)

In lighter-skinned patients (in the absence of a tan or bronzer), the Q-switched alexandrite laser operated at a wavelength of 755 nm, the Q-switched ruby laser operated at a wavelength of 694 nm or the Q-switched Nd:YAG laser operated at a wavelength of 1064 nm are the preferred devices for treatment for dark blue and black tattoos.

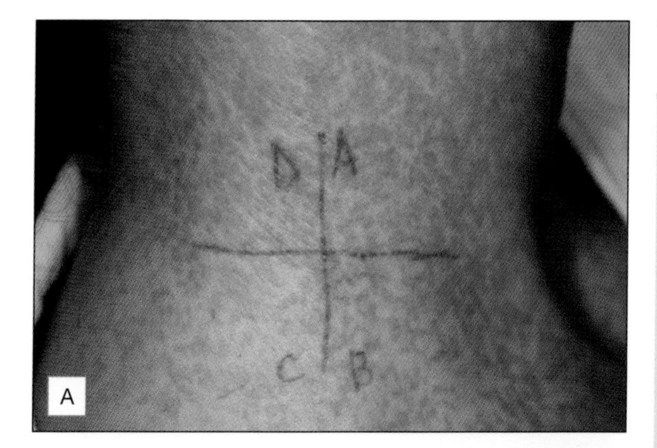

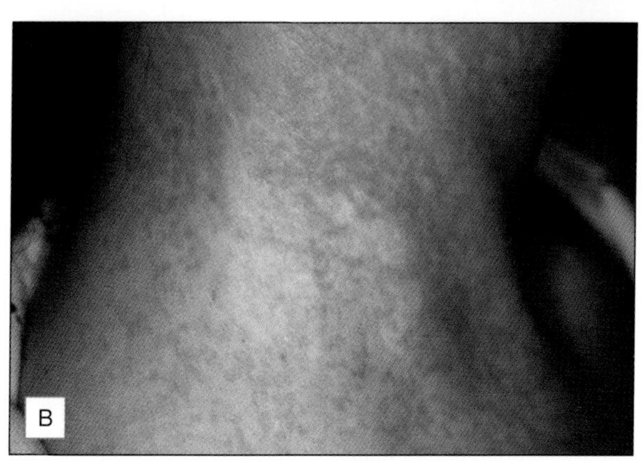

Fig. 4.24 Four different areas within a large hyperpigmented patch on the right anterior neck are seen: pre-operatively (A) and 6 weeks after testing with the Q-switched Nd:YAG laser showing better fading of the pigment at some of the test sites than others (B) which represent different energy fluences; the best results are now used to initiate treatment at the proper dosage

Tattoo patient history

Amateur, professional, cosmetic, or medical tattoo?
When was it placed?
What inks/dyes were used?
Were inks mixed together to make the colors?
Is there any white ink in the tattoo to the patient's knowledge?
Has the patient attempted to remove or alter the tattoo previously? If so, how?
Has patient used oral retinoids within the past year? (These can increase risk of scarring)
History of herpes infection or cold sores?
History of keloid formation or easy scarring?
Current suntan, tanning bed or bronzer use?
Fitzpatrick skin type?

Box 4.1 Tattoo patient history

Pigmented lesion patient history

How long has the lesion(s) been present?
Has a biopsy of the lesion ever been performed?
Has it grown, changed color, or changed in any other way?
Does patient or any blood relative have a history of melanoma?
Has the patient attempted to remove or alter the lesion previously? If so, how?
Has patient used oral retinoids within the past year? (These can increase risk of scarring)
History of herpes infection or cold sores?
History of keloid formation or easy scarring?
Current suntan, tanning bed or bronzer use?
Fitzpatrick skin type?

Box 4.2 Pigmented lesion patient history

Patients and equipment for dark blue or black tattoo treatment in darker-skinned patients (Fitzpatrick skin types IV–VI)

In darker-skinned patients, lasers having longer wavelengths are generally safer as they spare injury to the epidermis to a greater degree than shorter wavelength lasers. Thus, the Q-switched Nd:YAG laser operated at a wavelength of 1064 nm is the treatment of choice for dark blue and black tattoos in darker-skinned patients.

Patients and equipment for red tattoo treatment

The optimal laser wavelength for removing red tattoo ink is 532 nm. Thus, the Q-switched, frequency-doubled Nd:YAG laser operated at a wavelength of 532 nm is the best laser for red tattoo ink removal. This wavelength can cause both hyperpigmentation (Fig. 4.25) and hypopigmentation in darker-skinned patients so treatment should be limited to light-skinned (type I–III) patients. [See Advanced Topics section for treatment options for darker-skinned patients.]

Patients and equipment for green tattoo treatment

The optimal laser wavelength for removing green tattoo ink is 694 nm. Thus, the Q-switched ruby laser operated at a wavelength of 694 nm is the best laser for green tattoo ink removal. Like the 532 nm Nd:YAG, this wavelength can cause pigmentary alterations in darker-skinned patients which may

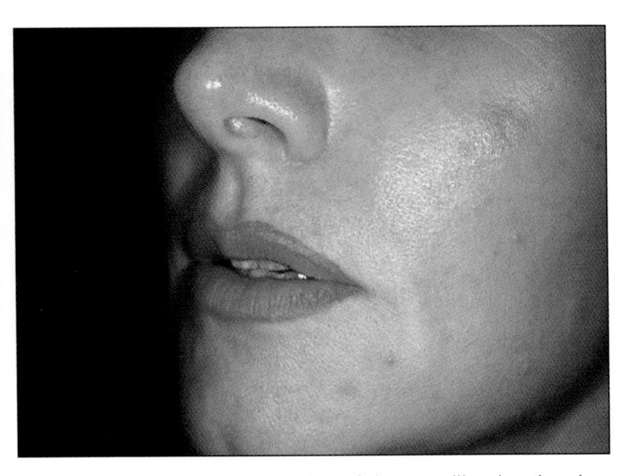

Fig. 4.25 Red cosmetic tattooing of the vermilion borders is present and should represent danger since hyperpigmentation or even blackening of this tattoo can occur following treatment with any of the Q-switched lasers [Note: This patient was not treated after having been consulted on the risks and complications.]

make green tattoos difficult to treat (Figs 4.15 & 4.16) in dark-skinned patients. [See Advanced Topics section.]

Patients and equipment for lentigo treatment

For light-skinned patients, the Q-switched, frequency-doubled Nd:YAG laser operated at a wavelength of 532 nm is usually the safest and most effective choice available. However, the ruby laser operated at a wavelength of 694 nm can also be very effective for treating lentigines. Intense pulsed light (IPL) systems can also be effective but somewhat less predictable than the Q-switched lasers due to the wider range of wavelengths being used. Most often the removal of lentigines by the IPL is an added benefit that occurs during full face photorejuvenation to correct rhytides and poor skin turgor from chronic sunlight exposure. Because the light from the IPL must traverse the epidermis in order to stimulate the dermal fibroblasts in photorejuvenation, the focal melanin deposits that account clinically for the appearance of lentigines are inadvertently treated as well. These lesions generally immediately turn a slightly darker chocolate brown color and then peel off in 7–10 days. Because the rejuvenation aspects of IPL treatments generally take 6–8 weeks to be seen, much of the early patient enthusiasm seen with these treatments is the eradication of the lentigines and not the reduction in rhytides. In darker-skinned patients, the Q-switched Nd:YAG laser operated at 1064 nm laser is usually the safest choice and also very effective.

Patients and equipment for nevus of Ota and Ito treatment

In darker-skinned (type IV–VI) patients, the Q-switched Nd:YAG laser at 1064 nm is usually the safest laser to lighten a nevus of Ota or a nevus of Ito. In lighter-skinned patients, Q-switched ruby laser at 694 nm and Q-switched alexandrite laser at 755 nm can also be used. It is important to inform patients that there is currently no effective treatment for the scleral pigmentation of nevus of Ota and that a corneal protective eye shield must be placed on the surface of the cornea using topical anesthesia to protect the globe if the periorbital area or eyelids are being treated.

Patients and equipment for café au lait macule (CALM) treatment

Green light from the Q-switched Nd:YAG laser at 532 nm is often the best choice for treating CALMs. Darker-skinned patients are at risk for the complications of hyperpigmentation and hypopigmentation. Light-skinned patients are the ideal candidates for CALM removal, but it should be remembered that recurrences, residual hyperpigmentation (Fig. 4.11) and incomplete pigment removal are common.

Treatment algorithm

1. **Anesthesia:** Each laser pulse causes a brief, sharp, hot pain whose intensity is variable depending on the individual patient and the anatomic location being treated. Lentigines can usually be treated without anesthesia. However, topical or intradermal local anesthesia is often required for tattoo removal and for larger pigmented lesions such as CALMs and nevi of Ota and Ito. For small tattoos and test spots, local anesthesia using an intradermal injection of lidocaine may be helpful. However, most tattoos, nevi of Ota and Ito, and CALMs are too large for local anesthesia to be considered practical. In these cases, treatment is generally well tolerated after application of a topical anesthetic such as EMLA or Ela-Max under plastic wrap occlusion for 1 hour prior to therapy.

Excess anesthetic cream should be wiped away prior to beginning the laser treatment.

2. **Eye protection:** Q-switched laser light can cause permanent retinal damage and vision loss. The light from the IPL can also cause eye damage with repeated exposure. Thus, eye protection in the form of optically coated glasses or goggles for the specific laser being used is required. All persons present in the room during laser treatment must also wear appropriate eye protection. The door to the treatment room must be kept closed and locked during laser firing to protect innocent intruders or passers-by from possible injury.

   Eye protection must block the particular wavelength being used. Because many laser goggles look alike, it is important to read the label on the goggles or glasses each time before putting them on or giving them to a patient. Always ensure that the eyewear blocks the wavelength being used and the lenses provide an optical density (OD) of at least 4. If the goggles obstruct the treatment area in the periorbital area, use of an anodized external metal eye cup can be used to protect the patient's eyes. If the eyelids are to be treated, a metal corneal eye shield should be placed on the eye using topical anesthesia to protect the globe.
3. **Determine treatment parameters** with the aid of a test spot. The test spot should be evaluated 4–8 weeks after having been performed. Parameters will vary depending upon the laser being used. To establish initial treatment parameters, read the users' manual and consult experienced laser surgeons who have been working with the laser being used.

   Because the spot size may be fixed or adjustable depending upon the laser, it is important to adjust the spot size to best match the size of the lesion. **Begin with the lowest energy fluence (J/cm^2) that produces a visible response.** If using a Q-switched laser, the desired response is when the skin turns white in the treatment area. If using an IPL system for lentigo treatment, it may be difficult to gauge the effect during the treatment. Again, consult persons familiar with the particular device you are using for ideal treatment endpoints.
4. **Position the laser handpiece** at a 90 degree angle perpendicular to the skin surface.
5. **Ensure that the handpiece is held at the appropriate distance from the patient.** Some lasers have a removable stylus that can be used to deliver laser light at the correct focal length depending upon the spot size being used. **Holding the laser too close or too far from the patient or using the wrong stylus can result in an improper energy fluence being delivered to the skin and can cause unwanted thermal injury and scarring.**
6. **Once the parameters and focal length have been verified,** begin delivering light pulses across the treatment area, ensuring that a 90 degree angle to the treatment area is maintained. Try to place the pulses close to one another without significant overlap. While a small amount of overlap will generally not have an adverse effect, **repeatedly delivering multiple pulses to the same area can result in unwanted thermal injury and scarring.** Continue delivering pulses of light until the entire treatment area has been covered once. If using a Q-switched laser, a popping sound will be heard with each light pulse as pigment particles and the cells that contain melanin are heated and explode. Pinpoint bleeding may occur if there is a great deal of pigment or tattoo ink present in the epidermis or upper papillary dermis.
7. **Post-operative care:** If a Q-switched laser was used for treatment, the area will appear somewhat abraded after treatment. Apply a layer of polysporin ointment, petrolatum, or bacitracin, beneath a dressing of nonstick gauze and paper tape. Instruct the patient to change the dressing twice daily after first gently cleansing the area with soap and water. This should be continued until the area has completely re-epithelialized. The area should be kept moist with petrolatum or antibiotic ointment at all times and a dry crust should never be allowed to form. The treatment area should heal within 5–14 days. If an IPL system was used for treatment, typically only erythema is seen postoperatively and dressings are not generally required.
8. **Follow-up and additional treatments:** Treatments should be at least 6–8 weeks apart. At subsequent treatments, the energy fluence (J/cm^2) can be increased by small increments of 1–2 joules to a maximum that will vary according to the laser and the nature of the patient's lesion. **Remember, using too high an energy fluence can result in thermal injury and scarring.**

Troubleshooting for tattoo removal

When evaluating a tattoo patient prior to initiating therapy, carefully palpate and examine the site to be sure that no scarring, hypopigmentation or induration is present. Many patients may not realize that the actual tattooing procedure can cause both scars and loss of normal pigmentation. If laser tattoo removal treatments 'unmask' either of these complications (Figs 4.17 & 4.18), the patient may unjustly blame the physician for causing them when, in fact, they were present prior to laser treatment. Preoperative photography is another excellent way to document the appearance of the tattoo both prior to, as well as during, the course of treatment. Many patients may become discouraged by their seeming lack of improvement with multiple treatments, but photographs taken prior to treatment and at intervals during treatment can be shown to the patient and demonstrate how effective the treatments have been.

Incomplete removal of the tattoo is a common problem following laser treatment. Despite numerous treatments being required to obtain the best results, complete ink removal may not possible. Still, effectiveness can be improved by optimizing laser treatment parameters. If treatment is ineffective, an increase in energy fluence may be necessary but care must always be taken to stay within safe treatment parameters to avoid scarring or pigmentary alterations. In some cases, switching to a different laser may be worthwhile due to the intrinsic differences in wavelengths, pulse durations and spot sizes.

Troubleshooting for pigmented lesion removal

As with tattoos, incomplete removal is the chief problem with laser treatment of benign pigmented lesions. However, unlike tattoos, additional treatments usually lead to total or near total removal of CALMs, lentigines, and nevi of Ota and Ito. Increasing the energy fluence is often beneficial for resistant lesions. Again, care should always be taken to ensure that the safe treatment parameters are not exceeded. Appropriate eye protection must always be of paramount concern when treating nevus of Ota or nevus of Ito because of the proximity to the eyes. When treating lentigines, if the patient has lesions on both their hands and face, it is always best to treat the hand lesions first so that if an untoward reaction results it will be the cause of less patient unhappiness than if the same problem were to have developed on the face. It is important to recognize that the value of treating congenital or large pigmented nevocellular nevi with any laser has not been substantiated as both residual pigment and regrowth of the nevi can be anticipated in some cases (Figs 4.26 & 4.27).

Side effects and complications

Alterations in pigmentation

Even when all the precautions have been taken, hyperpigmentation or hypopigmentation can still occur after laser treatment of tattoos or benign pigmented lesions. Hyperpigmentation usually improves with the passage of time or the application of topical bleaching creams, such as 4–5% hydroquinone compounded with 1–2% hydrocortisone and 0.05–0.1% tretinoin. Hypopigmentation is more difficult to treat, but the use of the excimer laser or narrow band ultraviolet light (UVB) light can produce improvement. Still, multiple treatments are often required and incomplete resolution is common. While many cases of pigmentary alteration will resolve spontaneously over time, some cases are permanent.

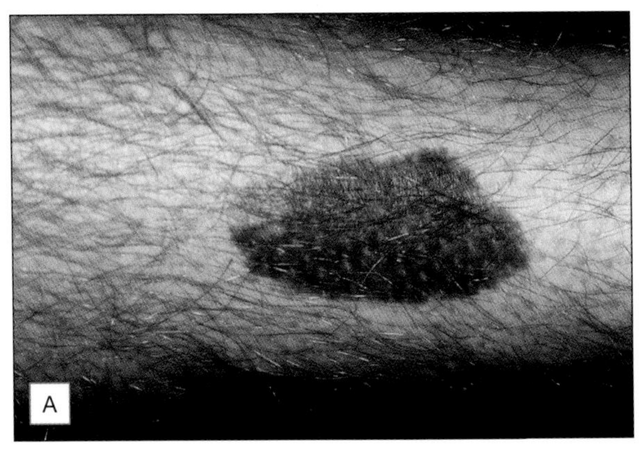

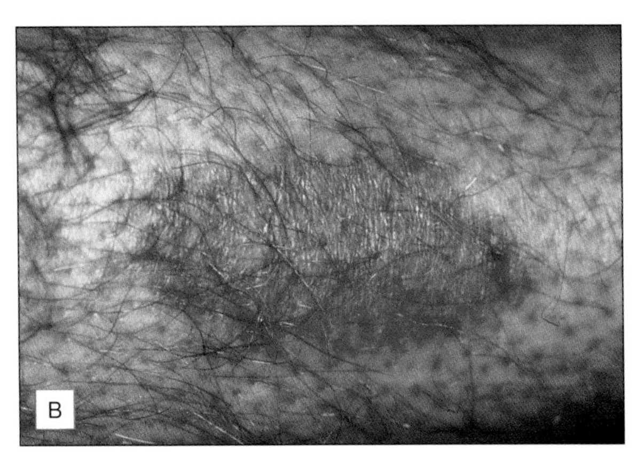

Fig. 4.26 Small, slightly raised compound nevus on the leg of a young adult seen: pre-operatively (A) and 6 weeks after two treatments with the Q-switched ruby laser showing residual, but faded, light brown color (B)

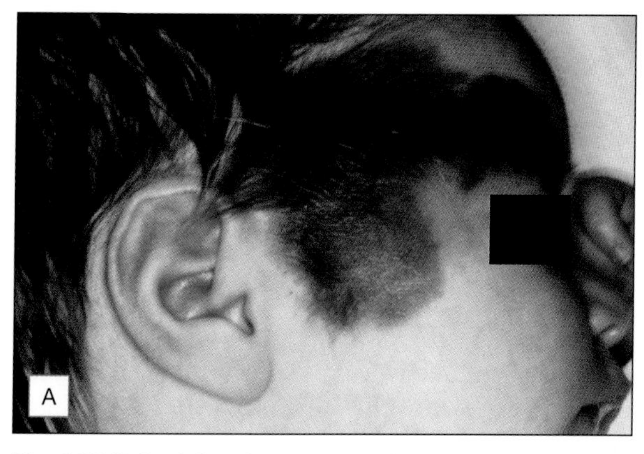

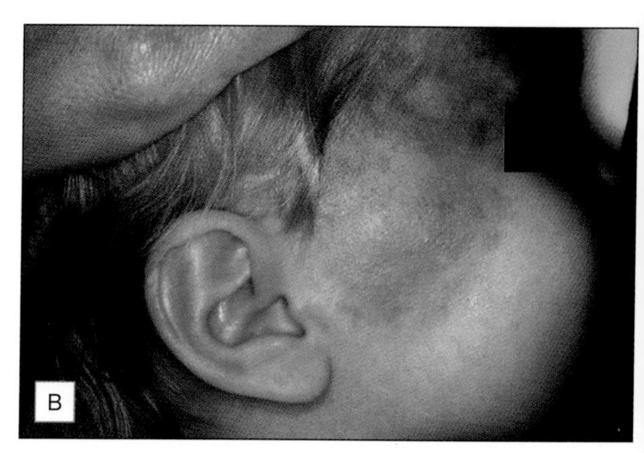

Fig. 4.27 Raised deep brown congenital nevus on the face of a newborn seen: pre-operatively (A) and after multiple treatments with the Q-switched ruby laser showing residual, but faded, light brown color (B) [Note: These Figs are courtesy of Dr David Goldberg.]

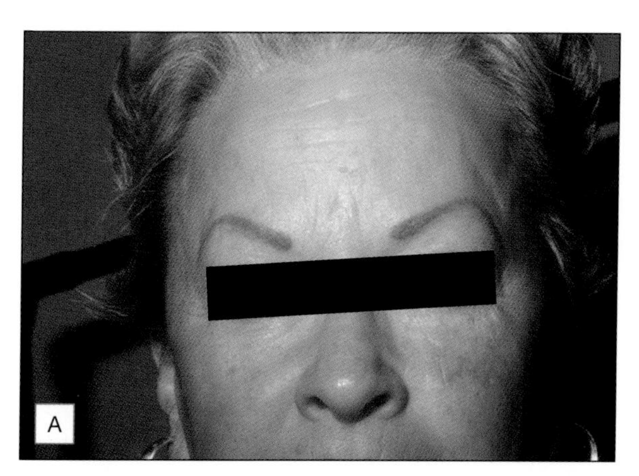

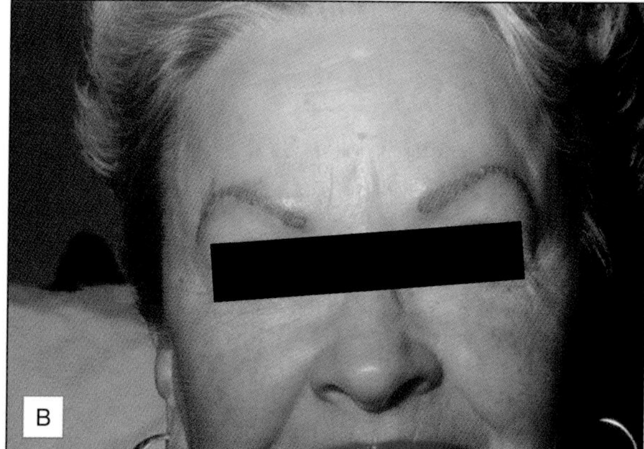

Fig. 4.28 Cosmetic tattoos of the brows are seen: pre-operatively (A) and immediately after treatment with the Q-switched ruby laser showing instantaneous darkening of the tattoo color (B) [Note: This patient slowly responded to multiple retreatments with the laser and the dark color finally faded. Photographs courtesy of Dr Lynn Roberts.]

Darkening of tattoo pigment

White, skin-colored or even red cosmetic tattoos (Fig. 4.28) used for enhancing the borders of the lip or reconstructing the areola after breast cancer surgery may contain white pigment to lighten the ink. Pastels such as light blue, turquoise, yellow, light green, lavender, and pink may also contain white pigment. This white material may turn black with laser therapy. White tattoos should not be treated with lasers unless the patient is informed of the potential risk and a very small, inconspicuous test site is first performed to ensure that this complication does not result. [See the Advanced Topics section for information on treating cosmetic tattoos.] Test spots can help to determine if a pastel-colored tattoo that contains white dye may turn black with laser therapy. If pigment darkening does occur, it may be improved with subsequent treatment with the Q-switched Nd:YAG laser operated at 1064 nm. However, this type of ink darkening may be refractory to treatment and can be permanent.

Thermal injury and scarring

Thermal injury and subsequent scarring is very rare when the proper laser treatment guidelines are followed and the appropriate treatment parameters are used. However, if a thermal injury does occur, ideal wound care with normal saline cleansing and application of petrolatum or polysporin ointment with a nonstick gauze dressing may prevent infection and help to minimize scarring. In spite of these efforts, if scarring does occur subsequent treatment with the pulsed dye laser, intradermal injection of low dose triamcinolone acetonide, and topical application of silicone gel sheeting or Mederma cream may improve the appearance of the scar.

Alternative approaches

Tattoo granulomas

When a patient develops an allergic granuloma to one of the tattoo inks, most commonly those that produce a red color in the skin, the use of the Q-switched Nd:YAG, ruby or alexandrite lasers is contraindicated as it may worsen the allergic reaction beyond the original site. In these cases, use of a destructive laser, such as the carbon dioxide laser, can be employed to remove the offending agent and also destroy the granulomas at the same time (Fig. 4.20).

Treating multicolored tattoos

When treating a tattoo of multiple colors, especially black, red or green, more than one laser wavelength can be employed during a single visit to maximize the degree of improvement. In these situations, the black outline of the tattoo is usually first treated with infrared light from the Nd:YAG laser operated at 1064 nm. Once that portion of the treatment has been completed, then green light from the frequency-doubled Nd:YAG laser operated at 532 nm is used on a limited basis to just treat the red portions of the tattoo. Once that second portion of the treatment has been completed, red light from the Q-switched ruby or alexandrite lasers is used to treat just the green portions of the tattoo. Care should be taken to avoid overlapping the treatment pulses as much as possible by adjusting the spot size being used to most closely match the size of the color being treated. In this way, all of the tattoo is treated at one time and resolution of the three different inks should occur in an orderly fashion simultaneously over time.

Advanced Topics: Treatment Tips for Experienced Practitioners

Cosmetic tattoo removal

When tattoos are used to enhance the shape of the upper or lower lips, reconstruct or augment the appearance of the eyebrow (Fig. 4.28), or to reconstruct the appearance of the areola following mastectomy, the technique is known as cosmetic tattooing. The tattoo inks are usually a mixture of white (titanium) and red (ferric oxide) pigments, the relative concentration of each is determined by the location and the natural pigmentation of the affected area. On occasion these tattoos are applied inexpertly, or the cosmetic style has changed making the appearance of the tattoo look 'old fashioned' or obsolete, or the patient may just not like the appearance. In any event, some patients will request removal of these cosmetic tattoos. Care must always be taken in these situations due to the phenomenon of pigment darkening, which has now been seen with all of the Q-switched lasers used for tattoo removal and also the dye laser that was specifically designed for treating tattoos and benign pigmented lesions. A chemical reaction occurs in the skin almost immediately following laser light treatment which changes the original white or red color into a gray or black color. This color is not only cosmetically unacceptable, it is also extremely difficult to remove with subsequent laser treatments. For that reason, extreme caution must be taken by first performing a very small test site on the least noticeable portion of the tattoo using the smallest spot size possible. Typically, the color change is immediate. To use maximum safety, it is wise to perform the test and then wait 6–8 weeks before seeing the patient in follow-up to determine if further treatment is indicated. If there has been no darkening of the tattoo, and the color has faded, it would be reasonable to proceed with actual treatment but only with the patient's written consent that darkening may still occur during future treatments and this darkening may be permanent.

Tattoo removal in darker skin types (Fitzpatrick IV–VI)

Decorative tattoos in skin types IV–VI present a difficult problem for the laser surgeon as all the current devices used to treat tattoos are also used to treat benign pigmented lesions. As a consequence, complications such as epidermal blistering, hypopigmentation and incomplete tattoo removal can be anticipated. In these situations, it is prudent to always perform a small test treatment to an inconspicuous portion of the tattoo, after first warning the patient about the potential complications, then wait 6–8 weeks to determine whether the results from the test support the initiation of actual treatment to the remainder of the tattoo.

Carbon dioxide laser

Initially, there was great enthusiasm for using the carbon dioxide laser operated in the infrared portion of the electromagnetic spectrum at a wavelength of 10,600 nm. This was largely a result of the fact that the carbon dioxide laser could be used to treat all of the different colors of tattoos, that extraordinary precision was possible with laser light compared to the longstanding use of the imprecise dermabrasion technique, and also the fact that complete removal of tattoo pigment could be accomplished in a single treatment session. However, the down side of carbon dioxide laser ablation of tattoos was multiple: long healing times of up to 2–3 months, permanent textural changes (Fig. 4.20), permanent scarring, sometimes keloid formation, and hypopigmentation. As a result, today the carbon dioxide laser is largely reserved for the removal of tattoo granulomas while the Q-switched lasers are utilized for all other types of tattoos.

Further Reading

Adrian RM, Griffin L. Laser tattoo removal. Clinics in Plastic Surgery 2000; 27: 181–192.

Carpo BG, Grevelink JM, Grevelink SV. Laser treatment of pigmented lesions in children. Seminars in Cutaneous Medicine and Surgery 1999; 18: 233–243.

Chan HH, Fung WK, Ying SY, Kono T. An in vivo trial comparing the use of different types of 532 nm Nd:YAG lasers in the treatment of facial lentigines in Oriental patients. Dermatologic Surgery 2000; 26: 743–749.

Chan HH, Ying SY, Ho WS, Kono T, King WW. An in vivo trial comparing the clinical efficacy and complications of Q-switched 755 nm alexandrite and Q-switched 1064 nm Nd:YAG lasers in the treatment of nevus of Ota. Dermatologic Surgery 2000; 26: 919–922.

Duke D, Byers HR, Sober AJ, Anderson RR, Grevelink JM. Treatment of benign and atypical nevi with the normal-mode ruby laser and the Q-switched ruby laser: clinical improvement but failure to completely eliminate nevomelanocytes. Archives of Dermatology 1999; 135: 290–296.

Grevelink JM, Van Leeuwen RL, Anderson RR, Byers HR. Clinical and histological responses of congenital melanocytic nevi after single treatment with Q-switched lasers. Archives of Dermatology 1997; 133: 349–353.

Herd RM, Alora MB, Smoller B, Arndt KA, Dover JS. A clinical and histologic prospective controlled comparative study of the picosecond titanium:sapphire (795 nm) laser versus the Q-switched alexandrite (752 nm) laser for removing tattoo pigment. Journal of American Academy of Dermatology 1999; 40: 603–606.

Kilmer SL. Laser eradication of pigmented lesions and tattoos. Dermatology Clinics 2002; 20: 37–53.

Lu Z, Fang L, Jiao S, Huang W, Chen J, Wang X. Treatment of 522 patients with nevus of Ota with Q-switched alexandrite laser. Chinese Medical Journal 2003; 116: 226–230.

Michel JL. Laser therapy of giant congenital melanocytic nevi. European Journal of Dermatology 2003; 13: 57–64.

Peach AH, Thomas K, Kenealy J. Colour shift following tattoo removal with Q-switched Nd:YAG laser (1064/532). British Journal of Plastic Surgery 1999; 52: 482–487.

Rosenbach A, Williams CM, Alster TS. Comparison of the Q-switched alexandrite (755 nm) and Q-switched Nd:YAG (1064 nm) lasers in the treatment of benign melanocytic nevi. Dermatologic Surgery 1997; 23: 239–244.

Todd MM, Rallis TM, Gerwels JW, Hata TR. A comparison of three lasers and liquid nitrogen in the treatment of solar lentigines: a randomized, controlled comparative trial. Archives of Dermatology 2000; 136: 841–846.

5 Laser Treatment for Scars

Keyyan Nouri, Sean W. Lanigan, Maria Patricia Rivas

Introduction

The problem being treated

Scars are ubiquitous and may be caused by surgical procedures, burns, trauma, or inflammation. Epithelial disruption unleashes a cascade of wound healing mechanisms that ultimately result in wound closure and scarring. A flat, flexible scar is the product of a normal wound healing process.

The wound healing process may be divided into three stages: inflammation, proliferation, and remodeling. The inflammation phase starts once the injury has occurred along with activation of the clotting and complement cascade. The release of chemotactic factors (i.e. prostaglandins, complement factors, interleukin 1 (IL-1), etc.) stimulate the migration of inflammatory cells such as neutrophils and macrophages. These cells initiate the debridement of the wound, and macrophages release cytokines and growth factors such as transforming growth factors (TGF-β) and platelet derived growth factors (PDGF), among others, leading to the formation of the provisional wound matrix. The proliferation stage is characterized by the migration of fibroblasts, endothelial cells, and keratinocytes to the wound site. Fibroblasts play a major role in the formation of the extracellular matrix composed of collagen III and I, fibronectin, elastin, and proteoglycans. The keratinocytes start the re-epithelialization of the wound with reconstitution of the basement membrane. The presence of endothelial cells in the wound bed, stimulated by hypoxia and angiogenic factors such as fibroblast growth factor (FGF), results in the formation of new blood vessels. During the maturation phase the collagen network and proteoglycans are remodeled. In the course of this process hyaluronic acid is gradually replaced by glycosaminoglycans, such as chondroitine-sulfate and dermatan-sulfate. Both collagen types I and III increase during the wound healing process; however, as the scar continues to mature and remodeling takes place, the proportion of collagen type III decreases.

The precise mechanism that leads to the development of hypertrophic scars and keloids has not been established, thus multiple disturbances in the wound healing process have been implicated. The development of excessive scar tissue may result from excessive matrix deposition, reduced degradation, or both. Fibroblasts from keloids show an abnormal response to stimulation, producing high levels of collagen, specially type I. Fibroblasts in hypertrophic scars, on the other hand, usually exhibit a normal response when exposed to growth factors, with a moderate increase in collagen synthesis. TGF-β linkage to increased collagen and fibronectin deposition has also been involved in the pathogenesis of excessive scarring. Furthermore, collagen fibers in these types of scars are found to be arranged as whorled, hyalinized bundles. Angiogenesis usually regresses during the maturation phase of the normal scarring process; however, keloids and scars are characterized by persistent hyperemia due to the constant presence of new vessels in the area. Other factors implicated in the development of hypertrophic scars and keloids are hyaluronic acid, proteoglycans, and mast cells, among others.

The estimated incidence has been reported to be between 4.5 and 16%, with African-Americans and hispanics showing the highest rates. Patients in their second decade of life are more commonly affected, with the same prevalence in both sexes.

Hypertrophic scars usually arise within 1 month of injury and are consistently confined to the original injury site. They appear as red, raised, and firm scars. Hypertrophic scars may arise anywhere in the body; however, those areas under constant pressure

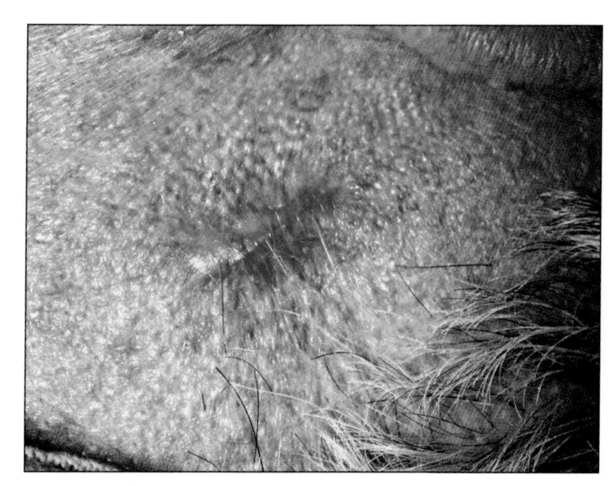

Fig. 5.1 White male with a hypertrophic scar. Red, raised, firm scar limited to incision site on the right side of his forehead

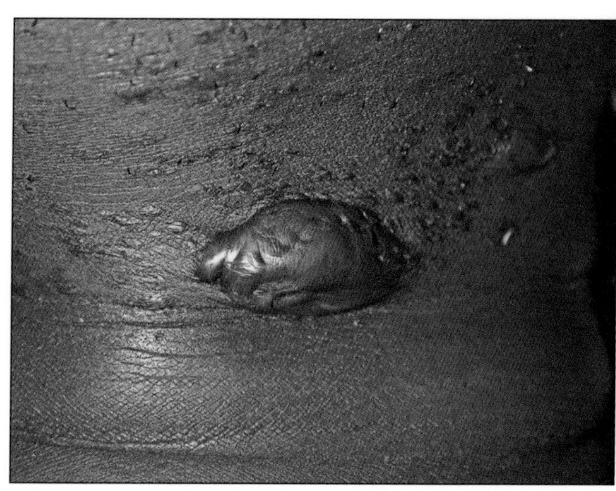

Fig. 5.2 African-American female with a keloid located on her lower, anterior neck

and movement stretching are more commonly affected (Fig. 5.1).

Keloids, on the other hand, are purple/red nodules that extend beyond the original injury site and are frequently disfiguring. These lesions may appear within weeks or years from the original cutaneous insult. The most common locations for keloids are the earlobes, anterior chest, shoulders, and upper back. In addition to the usual cutaneous injuries that result in scarring, keloids may also result from ear piercing, abrasions, tattooing, and vaccinations, among others (Fig. 5.2).

Keloids usually persist indefinitely, whereas hypertrophic scars may involute with time. However, whether a hypertrophic scar will ultimately regress or not cannot be predicted. Furthermore, besides obvious esthetic concerns, symptoms such as pruritus and dysesthesias may be associated with these abnormal scars, driving the patient to seek treatment alternatives.

Over the years several treatment options have been proposed, including surgery, cryotherapy, electrocautery and dessication, dermabrasion, intralesional corticosteroids, 5-fluorouracil, and radiation. Later on the Nd : Yag and CO_2 lasers were also included as therapeutic alternatives; however, the high recurrence incidence and side effects lead to its discontinued use for the treatment of hypertrophic scars. Overall, treatment of hypertrophic scars is consistently much more successful than treatment of keloids.

Currently, the pulsed dye laser is widely used and accepted as the laser of choice for the improvement and management of hypertrophic scars. Its benefits, indications, and technique will be discussed in this chapter. The treatment of acne scars is described in Chapter 7 of this volume.

Mechanism of action

Under the principle of selective photothermolysis, the pulsed dye laser (PDL) targets blood vessels, with the 585 nm wavelength selectively absorbed by hemoglobin. The precise mechanism by which the PDL improves scarring has not yet been established. Theories such as microvascular destruction with consequent ischemia, leading to deprivation of nutrients to the scar and interference in collagen deposition, have been proposed. Other hypotheses include increment of mast cells, disulfide bond disruption, and collagenolysis.

Patient selection

Patients with hypertrophic scars usually seek treatment because of cosmetic issues or associated symptoms. Therefore, hypertrophic scars are usually treated when they are functionally impairing, patients consider the lesions to be cosmetically unfavorable, or when associated symptoms such as pruritus and dysesthesias are present.

Patient-specific (skin type) and lesion-specific (age of scar and color) factors need to be considered when assessing therapeutic alternatives, such as lasers, for the treatment of hypertrophic scars.

The majority of the research studies on laser treatment of hypertrophic scars involve patients with skin types I–III. Skin tone is the main patient-specific characteristic to be taken into account when evaluating potential candidates for scar revision with lasers. Skin tone has a great influence on the outcome of the treatment, with fair skinned individuals having an overall better response, with fewer side effects such as pigmentation changes. Assessment of the patient's skin type is also used to establish the most appropriate laser parameters. In patients with Fitzpatrick skin types IV–VI, there is a high risk of laser light absorption by epidermal melanin, therefore less effective targeting of the skin and increased risk of postoperative pigment alteration along with reduced treatment outcome. Patients should be specifically warned about the high risk of pigmentation alterations that may result from laser treatment. Some authors suggest that laser fluences should be adjusted and lowered in dark skinned individuals. Due to the adjustment of the laser parameters, more sessions are usually required when treating these individuals. In general we do not recommend laser treatment of dark skinned individuals; however, when treating these patients we suggest doing a 'test spot' in an effort to foresee any side effects and help determine the most appropriate parameters to be used.

In summary, the ideal patients for scar revision with lasers are light skinned individuals, with relatively new (less than 1 year), red, raised scars.

Expected benefits

In general, most authors agree that laser treatment reduces the redness and height of the scar, improves the pliability, and usually provides relief from symptoms such as pruritus.

Alster and her coworkers noted that the PDL was able to alter argon laser induced scars, which are often erythematous and hypertrophic. By using optical profilometry measurements, she demonstrated a trend toward more normal skin texture as well as a reduction in observed erythema. This work was extended to the treatment of erythematous and hypertrophic scars using objective measurements; clinical appearance (color and height), surface texture, skin pliability, and pruritus could all be improved. Alster's work has been confirmed by that of Dierickx et al, who treated 15 patients with erythematous/hypertrophic scars and obtained an average improvement of 77% after an average of 1.8 treatments. Goldman and Fitzpatrick also treated 48 patients with similar laser parameters. Scars less than 1 year old did better than those more than 1 year old and facial scars did better; they obtained an 88% average improvement, with total resolution in 20% after 4.4 treatments.

The laser procedure is usually well tolerated. It may cause some discomfort that is consistently compared to a 'rubber band snapping'. When doing pain assessment in the laser clinic, most of our patients report a score of 1 or 2. After the procedure patients experience a burning or itching sensation in the treated area, which usually subsides within a couple of days. Purpura is the most commonly expected side effect, which usually appears immediately after the procedure and may persist 7–10 days.

Initial improvement in scar erythema and symptoms are usually seen within the first month after the first laser procedure. Multiple sessions are needed depending on the parameters being used, and the degree or severity of scarring. An average of three to five sessions is usually done to achieve satisfactory results. Newly formed scars that are red have a better response and require the least number of treatment sessions. The cost of the treatment varies according to the length and number of scars to be treated. The fact that multiple sessions are required and that insurance companies do not usually cover these expenses is an issue to be considered by the patients.

Overview of Treatment Strategy

Treatment approach

Currently, the pulse dye is the recommended laser for the treatment of hypertrophic scars. As stated before, the Nd : Yag and CO_2 lasers were also used; however, the high recurrence incidence and side effects have lead to their discontinued use over the years.

Although established hypertrophic scars can respond to treatment, the early treatment of scars within the first months might prevent hypertrophy in individuals who are keloid prone. We have found that the PDL 585 nm is effective and safe in improving the quality and cosmetic appearance of surgical scars starting on the day of suture removal (Fig. 5.3).

Other treatment modalities have been used alone or in combination with PDL, including intralesional corticosteroids or intralesional 5-fluoruouracil (5-FU). Two studies have compared the effects of PDL treatment with other treatment modalities, particularly intralesional steroids. Alster compared PDL treatment alone with laser therapy combined with intralesional corticosteroid treatment. Both

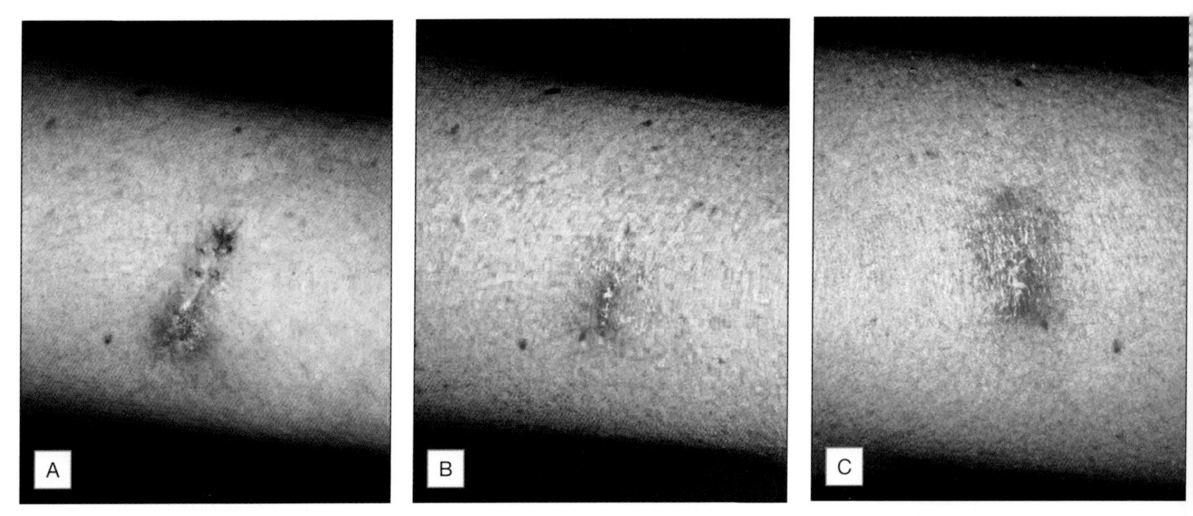

Fig. 5.3 (**A**) Female patient with a 3 cm surgical linear scar on anterior forearm. Patient received treatment of the inferior half of the scar. Superior half remained as control. (**B**) One month after the first PDL treatment. (**C**) One month after the second PDL treatment. Notice the difference in height and color between treated and control sites

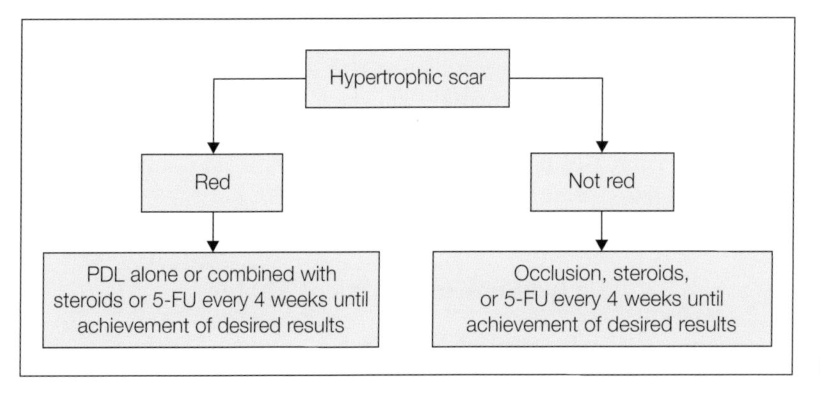

Fig. 5.4 Overview of treatment strategy

treatment arms produced improvement in scars and there was no significant difference between the two treatments. Manuskiatti and Fitzpatrick compared scar treatment with intralesional corticosteroids alone or combined with 5-FU or 5-FU alone or the PDL using fluences of 5 J/cm^2. All treatment areas were improved compared to baseline, and there was no significant difference in treatment outcome compared to method of treatment. The highest risk of adverse sequelae occurred in the intralesional corticosteroid group, and it was concluded that treatment with intralesional corticosteroid alone or in combination with 5-FU or 5-FU alone and PDL treatment are comparable.

When using intralesional corticosteroids or 5-FU in combination with PDL, certain considerations should be taken into account. If using intralesional steroids, it should be done following the laser procedure. You do not inject steroids in the scar before the laser treatment because it blanches the area, resulting in the risk of losing the laser target (vessel). An average of 10–40 mg/mL immediately after laser treatment can be used after the laser procedure (Fig. 5.4).

Laser therapy for keloids is mainly used to improve pliability, height, redness, and symptoms such as pruritus. Excision of keloids, as atraumatically as possible, with the least dessication is the main procedure that will achieve removal of the mass. On a recent study, Berman et al showed a decrease in the recurrence rate of excised keloids using topical imiquimod starting on the same day of

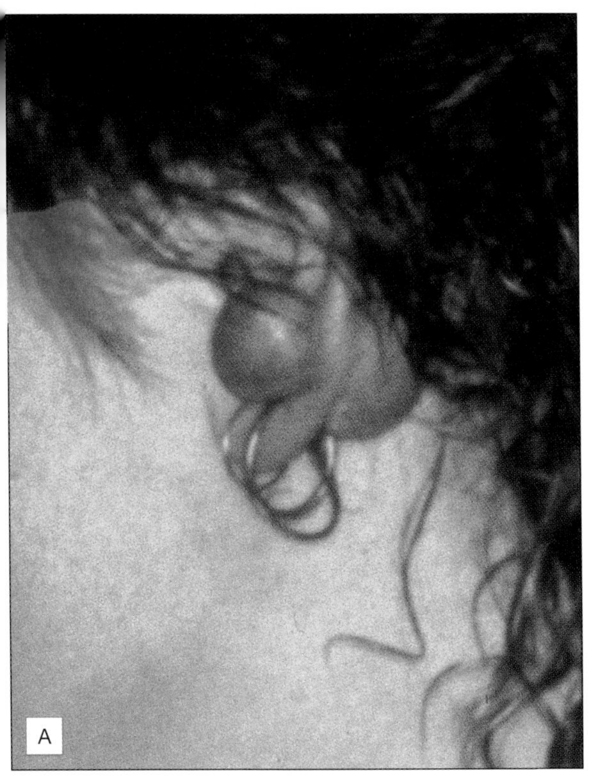

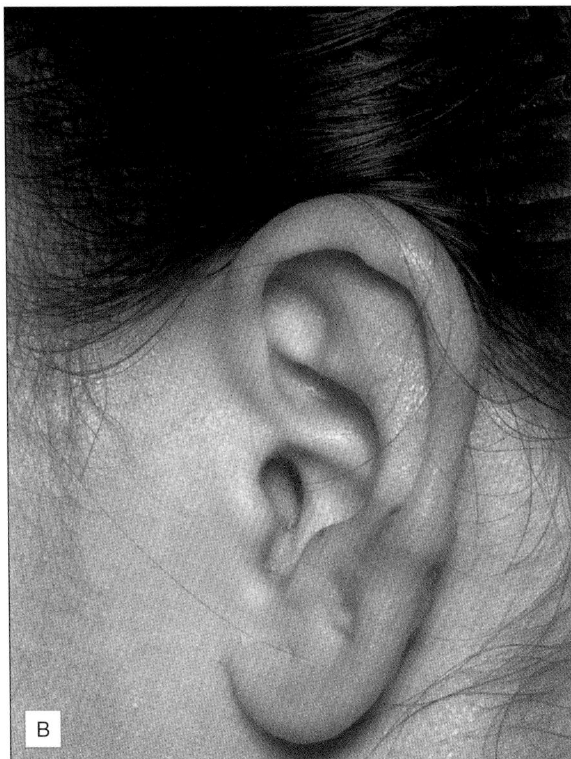

Fig. 5.5 (**A**) Three times recurring keloid scar of the ear lobe. (**B**) Appearance 3 months after initial excision and three subsequent PDL sessions

surgery. Lanigan et al, in unpublished observations, have seen benefits in early PDL treatment of excised recurrent keloids. In a group of 11 patients treated in this way, none had a recurrent keloidal scar (Fig. 5.5). Treatment at 6.5–7.5 J/cm^2 with a 5 mm spot or 6–6.75 J/cm^2 with a 7 mm spot is usually used. Treatment is repeated at 6 to 8 weekly intervals depending on clinical response. Keloidal scars require multiple treatments and the response is unpredictable. Similar to hypertrophic scars, laser treatment of keloids may also be combined with intralesional steroids (Fig. 5.4).

Patient interviews

Even though PDL for the treatment of hypertrophic scars and keloids renders very good results with a low side effect profile, certain information must be elicited prior to the procedure.

History of the scar or keloid

The history of the scar or keloid in terms of age, evolution, and previous treatments should be determined. As previously stated, the sooner you treat the scar the better the results that will be achieved. Hypertrophic scars that have been present for less than 1 year are considered optimal for PDL treatment. Newly formed scars that are only red may not need further treatment due to the likelihood of clearance with time. However, newly formed scars that are red and start becoming hypertrophic with time may greatly benefit with early laser treatment intervention. Patients may present with a history of previous failed intents to improve the appearance of their scars. Previous treatments such as cryotherapy may cause increased fibrosis of the scarring tissue; therefore, adjustments of the laser parameters and number of sessions may be necessary when treating patients with this type of history.

Determination of the patient's skin type

The skin type should be determined according to the Fitzpatrick classification. The best outcome has consistently been seen in fair skinned individuals. The majority of patients suffering from hypertrophic scars and keloids belong to the Fitzpatrick skin types IV–VI. As explained before, although these patients may benefit from laser treatment of their hypertrophic scars, there is a high risk of pigmentation alteration as a side effect. It is important for the treating physician to warn the patient of the high probability of hyperpigmentation. Nevertheless, it is likely that the patient will decide to continue with the procedure regardless of this risk. They usually consider that the cosmetic burden caused by their pathologic scars is much greater than the discomfort they may get from the resulting hyperpigmentation.

Treatment Techniques

Patients

Patients requesting therapy for the improvement of their hypertrophic scars or keloids may be eligible for laser treatment with the pulsed dye laser.

Equipment

In addition to the PDL, protective eyewear must be used. In order to protect from retinal damage, the protective eyewear must be capable of filtering the laser's specific wavelength. It must be worn by the patient and all personnel present in the room during the entire length of the laser procedure.

Treatment algorithm

The PDL treatment for hypertrophic scars and keloids is an outpatient procedure. A step by step explanation of the entire process follows:

1. The laser procedure is usually well tolerated, and usually does not require the use of anesthesia. However, if the patient requests it, topical anesthetic cream could be used. It must be applied 30–60 minutes before the procedure.
2. Make-up and any residual anesthetic creams (if used) must be removed (with soap and water) from the area to be treated so it does not interfere with light absorption.
3. Assessment of the lesion to be treated must be carried out. Include size, color, height, and pliability. It is recommended for the assessment always to be done by the same person and with the same parameters or scale. For this purpose you may use the Vancouver Scar Scale, or any other scar-related scale. The presence and degree of any symptoms associated must also be recorded.
4. Prelaser pictures of the lesion should be taken before the procedure in every session. Here, we also recommend the pictures always to be taken with the same camera, lightening, and distance, in order to maintain a standardized image.
5. Provide the patient and all personnel present with appropriate eyewear protection.
6. Calibrate the laser and set parameters to be used. In general, the following are the parameters that we most commonly use at our clinic: wavelength 585 nm, pulse duration 450 μs, spot size of 10 mm, and fluences ranging from 3 to 4 J/cm^2. When using smaller spot sizes the energy must be increased. Initial treatment visits should be started with low fluences, which can be adjusted according to the response in subsequent sessions. Energy densities are also adjusted according to the patient's and scar's characteristics (i.e. reduce fluence in dark skinned individuals).
7. Inform the patient that you are about to start the procedure. Remind him that he will experience a 'rubber band snapping' discomfort during the treatment.
8. Place the handpiece over one end of the scar and start applying laser pulses over the entire scar surface in a continuous pattern until reaching the opposite end. Overlapping of 10% is generally accepted.
9. Postoperative care instructions should include strict sun avoidance to avoid pigmentation alterations. The treated area may be normally cleansed with soap and water. Trauma to the site should be avoided.
10. The next treatment session can be done within 4–6 weeks.

Side effects, complications, and alternative approaches

Immediately after the laser treatment the patient will experience a pruritic or burning sensation, which usually persists from a few hours up to 2 days. The most commonly expected side effect after the procedure is purpura localized over the treated area. This side effect usually persists for up to 10 days. Hyperpigmentation of the treated area may also occur. If this happens, consider treating the area with a bleaching cream, or defer the following treatment session to avoid light absorption by epidermal melanin and assure effective laser targeting of the scar.

Crusting, oozing, and vesiculation are rare complications that sometimes occur. In such cases, the area should be kept moist with ointment and may be covered with nonstick occlusive dressing to avoid touching of the area. The following treatment session must be postponed until complete healing of the treated site has been achieved. Furthermore, laser energy should be lowered during the following treatment sessions.

Advanced topics

As previously stated, the use of intralesional steroids or 5-FU in addition to laser treatment is considered an alternative approach for hypertrophic scars and keloids.

When treating relatively new, red, hypertrophic scars, some dermatologists like to use intralesional steroids or 5-FU after the laser procedure has been done. When treatment of old, not red, scars is to take place the PDL is usually not as effective and occlusion plus intralesional steroids and/or 5-FU is one common approach. (Fig. 5.4). Flattening of the scar, as well as improved pliability and associated symptoms, could be achieved with this approach.

We recommend injection of the intralesional drugs to be done after the laser procedure, otherwise blanching of the area may occur with subsequent loss of the laser target, specifically the vessel. Triamcinolone (TAC) is one of the most commonly used steroids for intralesional injection of keloids and hypertrophic scars (10–40 mg/mL). Intralesional TAC can be administered every 4–6 weeks until the desired effect is achieved. 5-FU at concentrations of 45–50 mg/mL may be injected at different intervals ranging from three times per week to once per month depending on the degree of induration and inflammation.

The effects of corticosteroids on the scarring process include inhibition of the migration of inflammatory cells, vasoconstriction, and inhibition of fibroblasts and keratinocytes proliferation. The main mechanism implicated in 5-FU's effectiveness in the treatment of hypertrophic scars is inhibition of fibroblast proliferation.

Both intralesional 5-FU and steroids cause pain at the injection site. Other side effects such as purpura at the injection site, atrophy, and pigmentation changes have been associated with intralesional TAC injections.

Further Reading

Alster TS 1994 Improvement of erythematous and hypertrophic scars by the 585-nm flashlamp-pumped pulsed dye laser. Annals of Plastic Surgery 32:186–190

Alster TS 2003 Laser scar revision: comparison study of 585 nm pulsed dye laser with and without intralesional corticosteroids. Dermatologic Surgery 29:25–29

Alster TS, Tanzi EL 2003 Hypertrophic scars and keloids: etiology and management. American Journal of Clinical Dermatology 4:235–243

Alster TS, Williams CM 1995 Treatment of keloid sternotomy scars with 585 nm flashlamp-pumped pulsed dye laser. Lancet 345:1198–1200

Berman B, Kaufman J 2002 Pilot study of the effect of postoperative imiquimod 5% cream on the recurrence rate of excised keloids. Journal of the American Academy of Dermatology 47(4 suppl): S209–211

Dierickx C, Goldman MP, Fitzpatrick RE 1995 Laser treatment of erythematous/hypertrophic and pigmented scars in 26 patients. Plastic and Reconstructive Surgery 95:84–90

English RS, Shenefelt PD 1999 Keloids and hypertrophic scars. Dermatologic Surgery 25:631–638

Fitzpatrick RE 1999 Treatment of inflamed hypertrophic scars using intralesional 5-FU. Dermatologic Surgery 25:224–232

Goldman MP, Fitzpatrick RE 1995 Laser treatment of scars. Dermatologic Surgery 21:685–687

Lupton JR, Alster TS 2002 Laser scar revision. Dermatologic Clinics 20:55–65

Manuskiatti W, Fitzpatrick RE 2002 Treatment response of keloidal and hypertrophic sternotomy scars: comparison among intralesional corticosteroid, 5-fluorouracil, and 585-nm flashlamp-pumped pulsed-dye laser treatment. Archives of Dermatology 138:1149–1155

Niessen FB, Spauwen PH, Schalkwijk J, et al 1999 On the nature of hypertrophic scars and keloids: a review. Plastic and Reconstructive Surgery 140:1435–1458

Nouri K, Jimenez GP, Harrison-Balestra C, et al 2003 585 nm pulsed dye laser in the treatment of surgical scars starting on the suture removal day. Dermatologic Surgery 29:65–73

6 Treatment of Actinic Keratoses and Nonmelanoma Skin Cancer

Ramsey F. Markus, Janna Nunez-Gussman, Paul Martinelli

Introduction

The problem being treated

Physicians often encounter malignant and pre-cancerous skin conditions in daily practice. This chapter will cover the most common conditions: actinic keratoses, actinic cheilitis, basal cell carcinoma, squamous cell carcinoma. A proper diagnosis is essential in selection of the proper treatment (Box 6.1). Traditionally, such lesions were managed with destruction or excision of the targeted lesion. Surgical removal (i.e. electrodessication and curettage, excision with margins, or Mohs surgery) remains the standard approach to most common cutaneous malignancies. This chapter will focus on laser and other light-based therapies, an evolving and rapidly growing part of our arsenal. One focus will be the treatment of lesions by combining light and a light-activated medication, termed photodynamic therapy (PDT). Of note, the most dangerous skin cancer, melanoma (Fig. 6.1), is not covered in this chapter and should be treated according to the most updated melanoma treatment guidelines, which can be found on the American Cancer Society website, www.cancer.org.

Actinic keratoses (AK) are pink, scaly, thin papules often less than 1 cm in size and distributed in areas with extensive sun damage (Fig. 6.2). According to Gupta et al, AKs are clinically diagnosed in 14% of office visits with US dermatologists and accounted for 47 million office visits in the 1990s. AKs are of concern as a small number will progress to squamous cell carcinoma (SCC). A review of the literature by Glogau concluded that the risk of progression of AK to SCC was 0.025–16%. Cockerell argues that AKs are essentially very early squamous cell carcinomas. AKs can be differentiated from other non-malignant epidermal growths by their rough texture, their presence in usually sun-exposed areas, and lack of the greasy, stuck-on appearance of a seborrheic keratosis, although biopsy is the only way to know with certainty.

Chronic scaling and blurring of the vermillion border of the lower lip is a sign of actinic cheilitis. Similar to actinic keratoses, there is a risk of malignant progression to SCC. Once SCC develops in the mucocutaneous area of the lip, the potential for spread to the regional lymph nodes is greater than in glabrous skin.

Diagnostic methods
Actinic keratosis – clinical suspicion
Actinic cheilitis – clinical suspicion or biopsy (shave, punch, excision)
Basal cell cancer – biopsy (shave, punch, excision)
Squamous cell cancer – biopsy (shave, punch, excision)

Box 6.1 Diagnostic methods

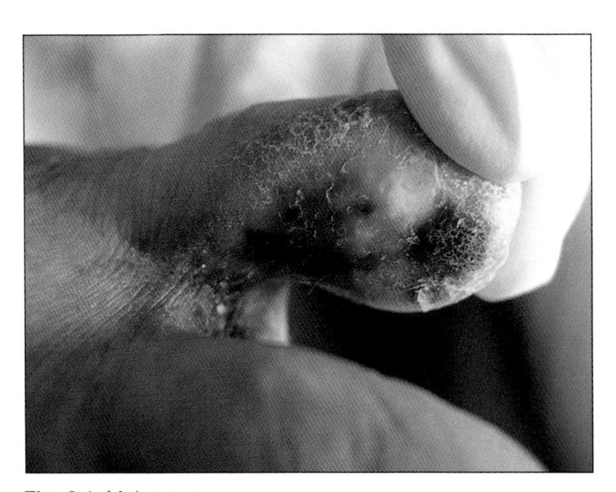

Fig. 6.1 Melanoma

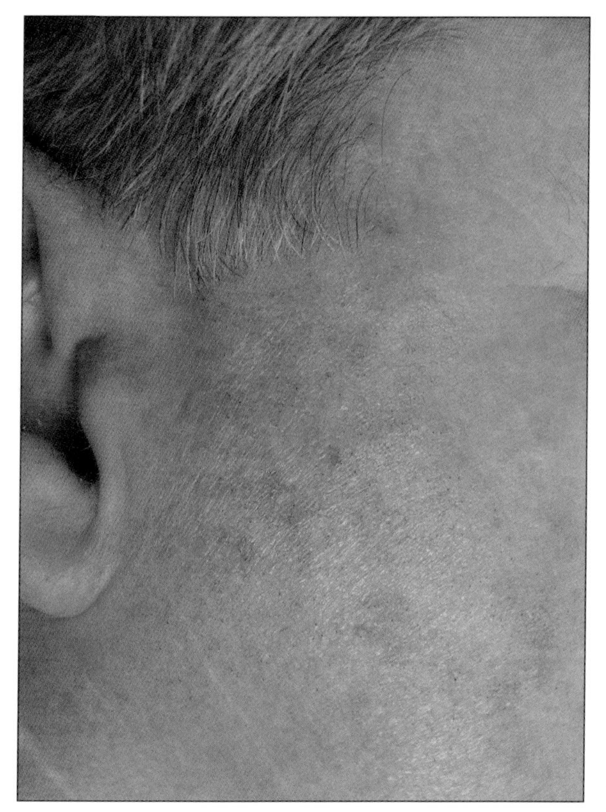

Fig. 6.2 Multiple actinic keratoses visible as thin, red, scaly lesions

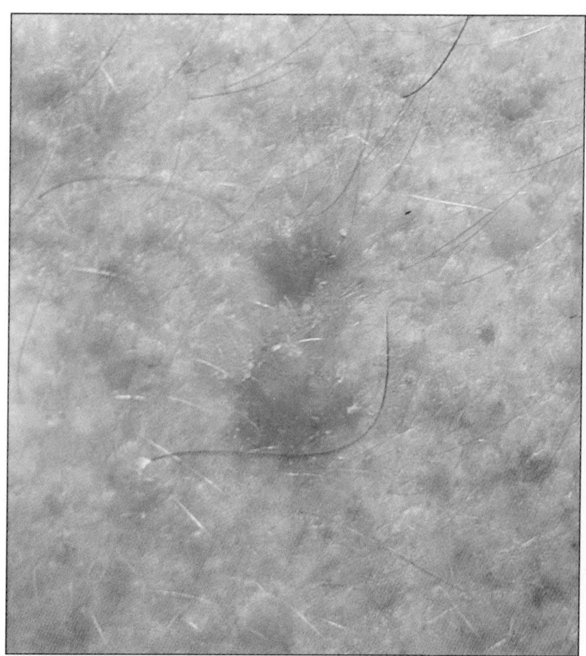

Fig. 6.3 Basal cell carcinoma with characteristic pearly appearance and telangiectasis

Basal cell carcinoma (BCC) is the most common cutaneous malignancy and often appears on sun-exposed areas as a pink, irregular plaque often with a rolled border, telangiectasis, and central erosion or crust (Fig. 6.3). Clues that a lesion is a basal cell rather than a benign growth such as an intradermal nevus, sebaceous hyperplasia, or seborrheic keratosis include frequent pinpoint bleeding, a shiny surface, and arborizing telangiectasis visible clinically and with a dermatoscope. Diagnosis is confirmed by skin biopsy. Several sub-types exist (nodular, superficial, morpheaform, infiltrating) and are classified based on morphologic and histologic grounds. Fortunately, BCCs usually produce only local tissue destruction. Metastasis, an extraordinarily rare event, has been reported.

Squamous cell carcinoma is the second most common cutaneous malignancy in the USA. The appearance can be similar to BCC, though often more scaly (Fig. 6.4). Diagnosis is confirmed by skin biopsy. SCC can metastasize, especially in the head and neck region. Patients with iatrogenic immune suppression after organ transplantation are at higher risk of cutaneous malignancy, especially SCC. Due to the metastatic potential, some clinicians prefer surgical excision or Mohs micrographic surgery instead of destructive modalities to ensure clear margins.

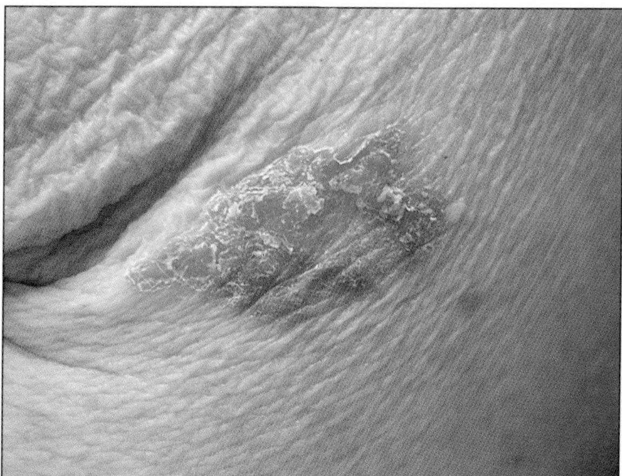

Fig. 6.4 Squamous cell carcinoma with overlying scale

Patient selection

Actinic keratoses and nonmelanoma skin cancer should be treated with light-based therapies in certain situations. There are many therapeutic choices for each type of lesion (Boxes 6.2–6.5). Major issues in determining the proper treatment include: cost, cosmetic concern, time constraints, compliance, effectiveness, and concurrent medical problems (Table 6.1). The cost of these new technologies may be prohibitive, especially if not covered by insurance. Topical creams and light-based therapy generally offer effective treatment with better cosmesis. Some patients may not be concerned by the hypopigmentation possible with liquid nitrogen or scarring with surgery. Light therapies avoid the difficulty in patient compliance that may be seen with the duration of therapy needed with topical treatment. Some types of light-based treatment may be more time-consuming for the physician than liquid nitrogen or surgery from start to finish. However, benefits of laser and photodynamic therapy (PDT) include quickness of the actual procedure [noted to be three times faster than surgery and more acceptable cosmesis]. In some instances, electrocautery is

Therapeutic options for actinic keratoses

Ablative therapies (physical tissue destruction)
Cryotherapy (LN2)
- Curettage and desiccation
- Medium depth to deep chemical peels (TCA or phenol)
- Ablative laser resurfacing (CO_2 or Erbium)
- Dermabrasion

Topical chemotherapy (patient-applied medication)
- 5-Fluorouracil
- Imiquimod
- Diclofenac

Photodynamic therapy (light + light-activated medicine)

Box 6.2 Therapeutic options for actinic keratoses

Therapeutic options for basal cell carcinoma

Imiquimod cream
Fluorouracil cream
Liquid nitrogen with thermocouple
Electrodessication and curettage
Surgical excision
Mohs micrographic surgery
Photodynamic therapy (PDT)
Laser vaporization (CO_2 or Erbium)
Radiation therapy

Box 6.4 Therapeutic options for basal cell carcinoma

Therapeutic options for actinic cheilitis

Cryosurgery
Electrosurgery
Chemical peeling
Vermillionectomy with mucosal advancement
Carbon dioxide laser ablation
Topical chemotherapy
- 5-Fluorouracil
- Imiquimod

Box 6.3 Therapeutic options for actinic cheilitis

Therapeutic options for cutaneous squamous cell carcinoma

Imiquimod cream
Fluorouracil cream
Electrodessication and curettage
Surgical excision
Mohs micrographic surgery
Photodynamic therapy
Laser vaporization (CO_2 or Erbium)
Radiation therapy

Box 6.5 Therapeutic options for cutaneous squamous cell carcinoma

Comparison of main treatment options

	Topical creams	Surgery/Liquid nitrogen	Laser/PDT
Cost to insured patient	$$	$	$$$
Cosmetic outcome	+++	+ or ++	+++
Patient compliance	+	+++	+++
Physician treatment time	Minimal	Moderate	Moderate to extensive
Effectiveness	Variable	Gold standard	Variable
Concurrent medical problems	Minimal	Important with surgery	Minimal

Table 6.1 Comparison of main treatment options

contraindicated (certain implanted electrical devices such as pacemakers), and surgery avoided. Any co-morbid conditions that complicate surgery may make PDT treatment more desirable: severe arrhythmia precluded by lidocaine or epinephrine, uncontrolled severe hypertension, severe dementia making a long procedure difficult, or anticoagulation. Multiple large lesions that would require a dangerously high amount of total local anesthetic could also benefit from PDT treatment. An ideal patient for PDT treatment of a nonmelanoma skin cancer would be a person with superficial actinic keratoses, SCC in situ, or BCCs with multiple lesions, including large lesions, who is concerned about cosmesis. Other reasons PDT or laser ablation of skin cancer might be preferable are listed in Box 6.6.

Expected benefits

Overview

Treatment of actinic keratoses and nonmelanoma skin cancer has been the subject of much research. Initially, laser therapy was mainly with the carbon dioxide (CO_2) or erbium laser. These lasers vaporize tissue resulting in lesion ablation. More recently, PDT has gained popularity as a more precise method in targeting abnormal cells. Of note, the varied study results are due to many factors: lesion type, study design, treatment technique, length of follow-up, number of study subjects, etc. As the data in Table 6.2 demonstrates for PDT efficacy, clearance and recurrence rates fall within a relatively large range when multiple studies are included.

Patient considerations for PDT and/or laser treatment of a nonmelanoma skin cancer

- Thin, nonaggressive cancers (superficial BCC, SCC in situ) or actinic keratoses
- Elderly or frail patient
- Multiple co-morbidities, including pacemaker or bleeding diathesis
- Multiple lesions (e.g. transplant patient or basal cell nevus syndrome)
- Large superficial lesions
- Lesions covering a cosmetic unit
- Lesions involving an important anatomic structure (genitals, digits)
- Lesions on slow-healing or poorly vascularized skin such as lower legs
- High patient concern for cosmesis
- Patients with low pain threshold, fear of needles, allergy to multiple anesthetics

Box 6.6 Patient considerations for PDT and/or laser treatment of a nonmelanoma skin cancer

Basics of photodynamic therapy

Photodynamic therapy, using an exogenous photosensitizer and a light source to illuminate the skin surface, has been shown to be highly selective for tumor cells. (Fig. 6.5) The mechanism of PDT uses the biosynthetic pathway for heme where precursor compounds are metabolized into phototoxic compounds such as protoporphyrin IX (PpIX), which in the presence of oxygen, produces reactive oxygen species, promoting tumor destruction. Preferential accumulation of PpIX in neoplastic tissue is thought to occur through increased penetration of ALA

PDT efficacy			
	Clearance	**Recurrence**	**Comments**
Actinic keratoses	44–91%	10%	Better for facial than acral sites; only PDT indication FDA-approved in USA
Superficial BCC	81–96%	4–44%	Higher clearance and lower recurrence with two or more treatments
Nodular BCC	50–91%	24%	Methyl ALA
SCC in situ	75–93%	0–40%, average 12%	Higher clearance with red than green light
SCC (invasive, not in-situ)	40–100%, average 69%	21–69%	Higher cure/clearance in thin lesions; PDT to be used cautiously in SCC

Table 6.2 PDT efficacy

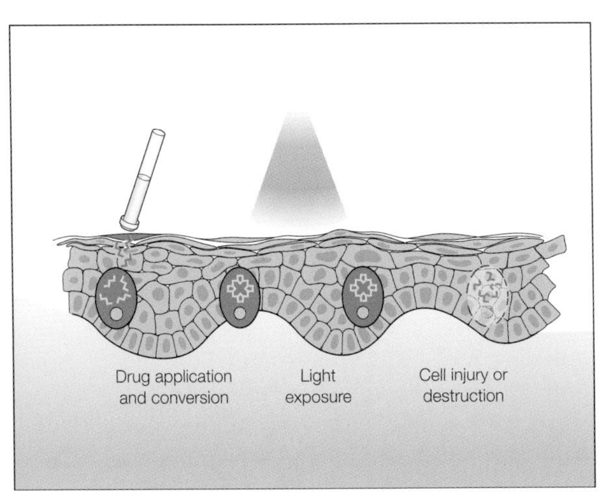

Fig. 6.5 Graphic depiction of photodynamic therapy. Courtesy of DUSA Pharmaceuticals, Inc.

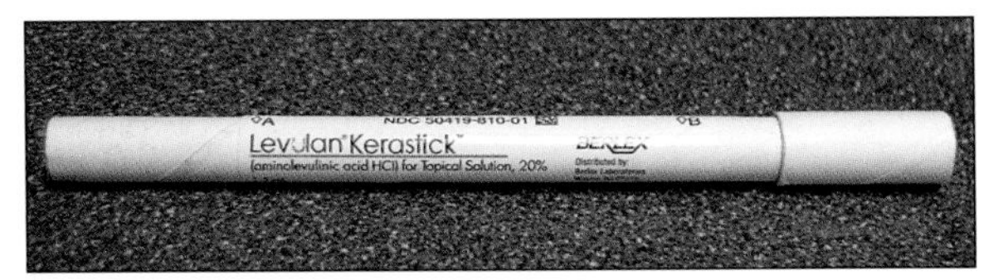

Fig. 6.6 Levulan® Kerastick™ applicator for ALA

Light sources used in PDT
Lamps (BLU-U, other fluorescent, halogen, tungsten, xenon arc)
Light-emitting diodes
Intense pulsed light
Laser (pulsed dye, argon, copper vapor, frequency doubled Nd : YAG)

Box 6.7 Light sources used in PDT

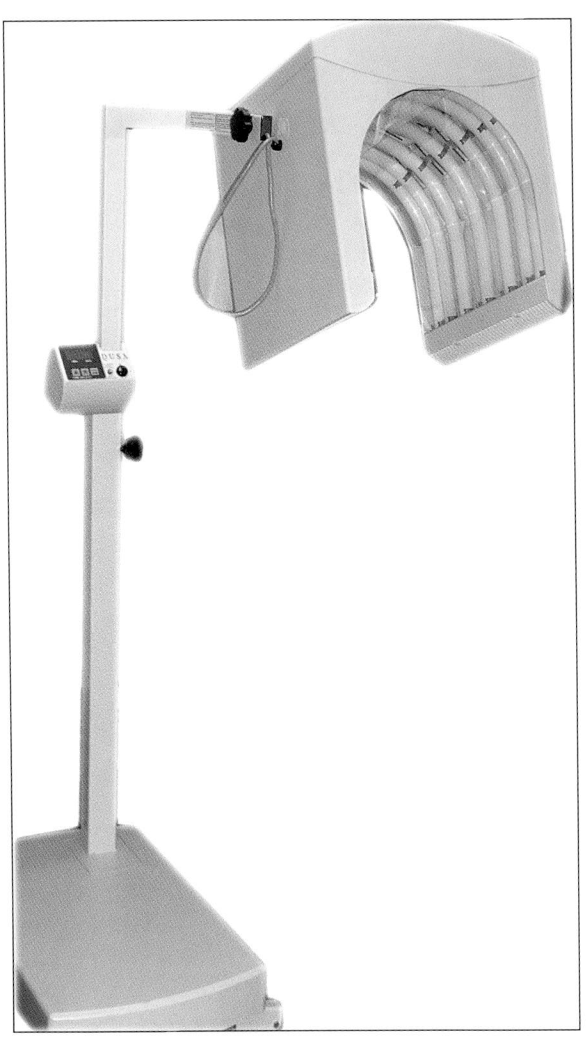

Fig. 6.7 BLU-U photodynamic illuminator

through damaged epidermis overlying tumors, as well as preferential uptake into proliferating, relatively iron-deficient tumor cells.

Laser-induced fluorescence of 5-amino-levulinic acid (ALA) induced PpIX formation demonstrates a signature fluorescence between 450 and 750 nm. When compared with normal tissue, BCC and SCC in situ demonstrates a higher intensity of PpIX fluorescence at 630 and 700 nm. A wide range of coherent and noncoherent light sources may be used (see Box 6.7). Most sources seek the 'red' 630 nm absorption peak of PpIX in order to maximize tissue penetration. The ALA-PDT treatment approved by the US Food and Drug Administration (for actinic keratoses) uses the Levulan Kerastick™ (Fig. 6.6) and the BLU-U lamp (Fig. 6.7) which emits 417 ± 5 nm. At present, no single light source is ideal for all possible indications for topical PDT.

Adverse effects of topical ALA-PDT include pain or discomfort, usually experienced as a burning, stinging, or prickling sensation in the treated area. This is felt to reflect nerve stimulation and/or tissue damage by reactive oxygen species. It lasts for hours, rarely a few days. Face and scalp lesions seem to be the most painful, as well as large and/or ulcerated lesions. Green light may be less painful than red, at least for facial actinic keratoses. Pain may be reduced by using topical and/or injected anesthetics, premedication with anxiolytics, fanning the patient, or spraying water on the patient. Erythema and edema are common after ALA-PDT treatment, and the development of crusts and erosions that heal in 2–6 weeks. Although histologic evidence of scar can be seen after PDT treatment, a clinically apparent scar is rarely seen. Post-inflammatory hyper- and hypopigmentation can be seen and resolve within the typical 6 months. Interestingly, permanent hair loss has been observed following ALA-PDT.

Light and laser treatment of actinic keratoses

Photodynamic therapy using ALA was shown to be effective in treating AKs in a pilot, dose-ranging study in 1997. Since then, PDT has rapidly become an established treatment modality for thin AKs. Recent literature indicates that approximately 50–90% of appropriately chosen patients with AKs experience a complete response, defined clinically as no residual visible or palpable lesions, within 4 weeks of treatment. In general, AKs of the head and neck area are more amenable to PDT than are AKs located on the distal extremities. These studies used 20% ALA in conjunction with either red or blue noncoherent light sources. Typically, most patients experience some degree of discomfort associated with treatment, usually described as itching or burning; this effect is more pronounced with longer application periods of the photosensitizer. The efficacy of PDT for treating AKs has also compared favorably with that of more conventional therapies such as topical 5-fluorouracil, demonstrating statistically comparable clearance rates. These comparisons included the use of short incubation PDT (1 hour) as well as both blue and red light sources.

Similar investigations, including prospective randomized trials, using methyl 5-ALA (160 mg/g) cream as the photosensitizer have proven the technique to be safe and effective in treating AKs. Methyl 5-ALA PDT, when used in conjunction with noncoherent red light, demonstrated a clear treatment advantage for AKs compared with placebo cream. In addition, the technique compared favorably to cryosurgery with liquid nitrogen, with both modalities exhibiting statistically equivalent response rates at a 3-month follow-up. Both modalities worked better for thinner lesions. In general, local adverse events were more commonly reported in those patients treated with methyl 5-ALA PDT than with liquid nitrogen, but PDT produced superior cosmetic results, with the vast majority of patients rating their cosmesis as good to excellent.

Disadvantages of PDT with noncoherent light include pain during the lengthy illumination period, which lasts approximately 16 minutes, as well as post-treatment erythema and crusting. A topical photosensitizer may also be used in conjunction with a coherent light source, such as a laser, in the treatment of AKs with PDT. Laser-mediated PDT may offer the advantages of the rapid treatment of large numbers of lesions with minimal discomfort, rapid recovery time, and improved cosmesis with diminished risk of hypopigmentation and scarring. Multiple lasers have been used in conjunction with PDT (see Box 6.7). Following the discovery that the absorption spectrum for PpIX peaks in the 585 nm range, recent investigations have focused on the use of the pulsed dye laser (PDL) for PDT. When used at non-purpuric parameters in conjunction with 20% 5-ALA, the long-pulsed PDL has shown great promise in the treatment of AKs, demonstrating at least equal efficacy when compared to noncoherent light sources. One group reported that the treatment was especially effective for AKs of the head with a 99.47% mean clearance at 10 days after one treatment. Ninety per cent of these patients remained clear at 8 months post-procedure. Treatment was also well-tolerated with excellent cosmesis noted.

Ablative laser therapy is another possible therapeutic option for AKs. Like dermabrasion, laser resurfacing allows for the removal of the epidermis and superficial dermis in a controlled manner, but with a relatively bloodless field. To our knowledge, no large multicenter clinical trials have examined the role of ablative laser therapy for the treatment of AKs. The Er : YAG laser (2940 nm) has been shown to be an effective treatment for AKs, with up to a 93% clinical and histologic improvement after one treatment, without significant adverse events reported. Follow-up duration of patients in some studies is limited, however. These findings are corroborated by reports of the successful prophylaxis against nonmelanoma skin cancer after carbon dioxide (CO_2) laser resurfacing. Compared to the Er : YAG laser, the carbon dioxide laser is associated with slower re-epithelialization and more prolonged erythema.

Laser and light treatment of actinic cheilitis

As with AKs, there are numerous well-established treatment options for actinic cheilitis (see Box 6.3), each with its own inherent risks. Carbon dioxide laser ablation of actinic cheilitis has been well-reported in the literature. According to some, carbon dioxide laser ablation seems to be as effective as vermillionectomy (surgical excision of the affected lip) with mucosal advancement, with clinical and histologic clearance rates similar at 4 years post-treatment. Laser ablation has been shown to be more effective than topical 5-fluorouracil or chemical peels with 50% trichloroacetic acid.

Laser and light treatment of basal cell carcinoma

While no published multicenter controlled clinical trials of carbon dioxide laser treatment for BCC exist, smaller studies have reported its success. Horlock et al performed CO_2 laser treatment prior to formal excision and histologic examination. Of 51 BCCs, two-thirds were completely ablated, although an extra two laser passes after visible tumor removal resulted in an 80% success rate. Superficial type BCCs responded best – all were completely ablated if lased to at least mid-dermis. Only 39% of nodular BCCs were completely ablated, although small nodular tumors less than 10 mm were completely ablated if lased to the lower dermis or subcutaneous tissue. Obviously, delayed healing is an issue once subcutaneous tissue is reached, diminishing the advantage of laser treatment in these cases.

The superpulsed CO_2 laser was used to treat BCC and combined with intraoperative histopathologic and cytopathologic exam. Before and after the laser treatment, scrape biopsies stained with the Papanicolaou method were used to check for residual tumor cells. One hundred and forty patients with superficial or small nodular BCCs (< 1.5 cm diameter) were treated. The laser parameters were duty cycle 2–3%, pulse duration 2–3 ms, frequency 10 Hz, 1–3 mm spots size. There was no clinical evidence of recurrence at 3 years in all 140 patients, and good aesthetic outcomes were achieved. Healing was rapid at 2–10 days. Interestingly, no anesthesia was used for either laser treatment or scrape biopsy.

Full-face CO_2 laser resurfacing can certainly be helpful in managing patients with numerous skin cancers, and arguably can be the best option for these patients. Patients with nevoid basal cell carcinoma syndrome may benefit from this option as other treatment options diminish.

A review of 12 studies totaling treatment of 826 superficial and 208 nodular BCCs showed a weighted average complete clearance rate after follow-up times of 3–36 months of 87% for superficial BCCs and 53% for nodular BCCs. Morpheaform and pigmented BCCs do not respond well to PDT.

Calzavara-Pinton treated 57 BCCs with 20% ALA-PDT emulsion under occlusion for 6–8 hours followed by exposure to a 630-nm dye laser. Treatments were continued every other day until tumor was no longer seen, erosion developed, or no lesion change with the last two treatments. One to eight treatments were required, and each light dose ranged from 60 to 80 J/cm^2. After a 24- to 36-month follow up, 86.9% (20 of 23) of superficial BCC and 50% (15 of 30) of nodular BCCs responded. Histopathologic evidence of fibrosis deeper in the dermis than the maximal pretreatment tumor thickness suggested that ALA-PDT failure may not be fully explained by lack of penetration.

Haller et al studied the effect of a double treatment regimen of superficial BCC using topical ALA-PDT, performed 7 days apart. The light source was 630 nm (120–134 J/cm^2, 50–100 mW/cm^2.) After an average of 27 weeks, this technique yielded a 96% clearance rate, and only 4% recurred (one out of 26 superficial BCCs). This same group had only a 50% clearance rate after a single treatment, suggesting the importance of double treatment.

Morton et al had an 85% clearance rate for large or multiple BCCs, and felt PDT to be superior to electrosurgery for large BCCs (>14 mm in diameter) and to excision in patients with multiple BCCs.

Rhodes et al performed a randomized prospective multicenter trial comparing methyl aminolevulinate (mALA) PDT using red light (570–670 nm) versus surgical excision with 5-mm margins in the treatment of nodular BCCs larger than 6 mm. Methyl ALA offers improved skin penetration and specificity for neoplastic cells over standard ALA. The PDT treatment included gentle debridement and application of mALA under occlusion for 3 hours prior to red light irradiation; a second treatment was given 1 week later and again at 3 months if needed. Three months after treatment, 91% of PDT lesions and 98% of surgically excised lesions showed complete clinical clearance. However, at 24 months, only 76% remained clear in the PDT group compared to 96% for the surgery group. Cosmetic outcomes were significantly better in the PDT group.

Current evidence supports the use of topical ALA-PDT as an effective therapy for superficial BCCs (< 2 mm thick), with superior healing, better cosmesis and at least equal efficacy compared with cryotherapy. It is especially effective for multiple and large superficial lesions. Unfortunately, ALA-PDT is less effective in the treatment of nodular BCCs, and not recommended for routine treatment. Debulking with a curette, repetitive treatments, and the use of penetration enhancers such as DMSO, or fractionated treatment may prove to increase clearance rates.

Light-based therapy may be considered in the treatment of SCC in situ (Bowen's disease), as these superficial cancers are routinely destructed without margin control and have a high cure rate. Due to varying thickness, hyperkeratosis and frequent follicular extension of SCC in situ, CO_2 laser ablation alone is not recommended. Residual tumor has been found in the majority of SCC in situ specimens subsequently excised after CO_2 treatment.

Topical 20% ALA-PDT therapy for SCC in situ has been extensively studied in 13 open and three randomized comparison studies. A single ALA-PDT treatment cleared 86%, and rose to 93% if treated once or twice more. The average recurrence rate was 12% at 3- to 36-month follow-up periods. Application time of the ALA was 3–6 hours for most studies. Red light seems to be preferred for the treatment of Bowen's disease, because it penetrates more deeply. Randomized studies have been conducted comparing topical ALA-PDT with cryotherapy and also with topical 5-fluorouracil. PDT was significantly better than cryotherapy in SCC in situ clearance after a single treatment (75 vs. 50%), and had no adverse events such as ulceration, infection, or scar. When compared with topical 5-fluorouracil, PDT was at least as effective at 8 months, with fewer adverse effects.

Erythroplasia of Queyrat (SCC in situ of the penis) can also respond to ALA-PDT treatment, but suffers from high recurrence rates. In three open studies of topical ALA-PDT in the treatment of SCC, clearance rates initially averaged 69% for superficial lesions, but recurrence rates averaged 24%, and were as high as 69% after 3–47 months. Because of the metastatic potential and high recurrence rates from the initial studies, PDT is not recommended for SCC.

Overview of Treatment Strategy

Treatment approach to actinic keratoses

Treatment of actinic keratoses has evolved over the years. Until approximately 10 years ago the vast majority of lesions were treated with LN2 or fluorouracil. The undesirable effects were accepted as part of the treatment course. The options now available give a broad range of choices for the patient and physician (Table 6.3). With patient education and a well thought out treatment plan, therapy can provide excellent, cost-effective removal of AKs with high patient and physician satisfaction.

Treatment approach to BCC and SCC

Any destructive mechanism can potentially be used in the treatment of BCC, and to a lesser degree SCC. Currently, curettage and desiccation and liquid nitrogen are the most utilized methods worldwide, as they are readily available and inexpensive. The main limiting factor to all destructive techniques is the lack of margin control and therefore higher potential for recurrence. The treatment of choice for most areas on the head is Mohs micrographic surgery as it has the highest cure rate while sparing the need for wide surgical margins. Relatively superficial lesions can be well treated by a variety of modalities, including light-based, with good results and excellent cosmesis. The ultimate choice should be made by the patient after education and guidance by the physician (Table 6.4).

Major determinants

Actinic keratoses and nonmelanoma skin cancer should be treated with light-based therapies in certain situations. Major issues in determining the proper treatment include: cost, cosmetic concern, time constraints, compliance, effectiveness, and concurrent medical problems. The cost of these new technologies may be prohibitive, especially if not covered by insurance. Topical creams and light-based therapy generally offer effective treatment with better cosmesis. Some patients may not be concerned by the hypopigmentation possible with liquid nitrogen or scarring with surgery. Light therapies avoid the difficulty in patient compliance that may be seen with the duration of therapy needed with topical treatment. Some types of light-based treatment may be more time-consuming for the physician than liquid nitrogen or surgery. In some instances, electrocautery is contraindicated (certain implanted electrical devices such as pacemakers), and surgery avoided.

AK approaches		
	Pro	**Con**
Liquid nitrogen	Quick and convenient Small numbers easily treated Insurance coverage	Zone treatment difficult Unsightly hypopigmentation
Topical diclofenac	Minimal reaction Excellent cosmesis Zone treatment possible Insurance coverage	Slow (3-month course)
Topical imiquimod	Excellent cosmesis Zone treatment possible Insurance coverage	Slow (1- to 4-month course) Moderate skin reaction
Topical fluorouracil	Excellent cosmesis Zone treatment possible Insurance coverage	Moderate length (2–4 weeks) Moderate–severe skin reaction
PDT	Excellent cosmesis Zone treatment possible Variable insurance coverage	Quick (same day treatment) Moderate skin reaction Photosensitivity
Laser vaporization/ resurfacing	Excellent cosmesis Zone treatment possible May improve photoaging	Wound healing for 1–2 weeks No insurance coverage

Table 6.3 AK approaches

BCC and SCC approaches		
	Pro	**Con**
Liquid nitrogen	Quick and convenient Best used with thermocouple Insurance coverage	Unsightly hypopigmentation No pathologic conformation
Electrodessication and curettage	Quick and convenient Insurance coverage	No pathologic confirmation Unsightly scar
Excisional surgery	Short procedure time Insurance coverage	Unsightly scar Non-tissue sparing Surgical complications
Mohs surgery	Best cure rate (98%) Outpatient day surgery Insurance coverage Tissue sparing	Unsightly scar Surgical complications
Topical imiquimod	Excellent cosmesis Insurance coverage	Slow (2–4 month course) Best for superficial lesions Moderate skin reaction
Topical fluorouracil	Excellent cosmesis Insurance coverage	Moderate length (2-4 weeks) Only for superficial lesions Moderate–severe skin reaction

Table 6.4 BCC and SCC approaches

Continued

BCC and SCC approaches—cont'd		
	Pro	**Con**
PDT	Excellent cosmesis Variable insurance coverage	Quick (same day treatment) Best for superficial lesions Moderate skin reaction Photosensitivity
Laser vaporization/ resurfacing	Good cosmesis	Wound healing for 1–2 weeks Insurance coverage minimal

Table 6.4, cont'd BCC and SCC approaches

Patient interviews

Once the diagnosis has been made, a frank discussion of the options available should be discussed. The patient should be made aware of the advantages and disadvantages of each modality. Patients concerned with appearance must be appropriately informed of the possible cosmetic outcome, effectiveness, downtime and cost. Some potential questions:

- Would a scar or discoloration bother you?
- Are you interested in options not covered by insurance?
- Can you take time off to recuperate?

Treatment Techniques

Photodynamic therapy

Patients

Photodynamic therapy can be used in nearly every patient. It may be especially beneficial in patients with a large number of actinic keratoses. Contraindications include photosensitivity, allergy to ALA, and porphyria. ALA is pregnancy category C and should be administered with caution in nursing mothers.

Equipment

Many types of light and laser sources within the visible light portion of the electromagnetic spectrum may be used to provide the photons needed (Box 6.7, see p. 79). The light sources may vary in exposure time depending on the intensity of the light provided. For example, the BLU-U Blue light photodynamic illuminator has a pre-set recommended exposure time of 16 minutes 40 seconds. Other lamps may have varying exposure times depending on lamp intensity and wavelength produced. Lasers and Intense Pulsed Light produce very high intensity of light in small areas within milliseconds. For nearly any light or laser treatment, appropriate eyewear is needed (Fig. 6.8).

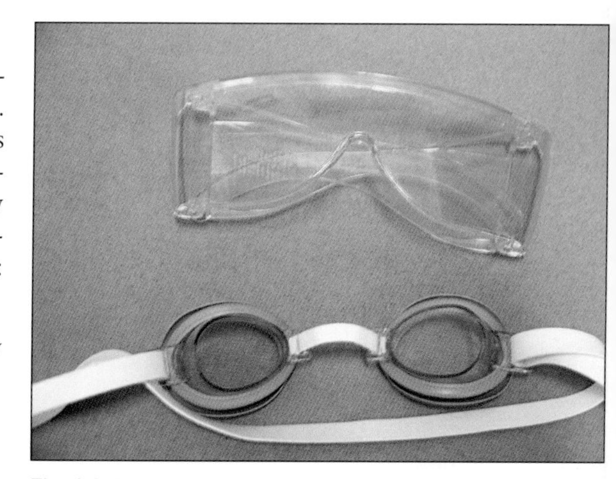

Fig. 6.8 BLU-U eye protection

Treatment algorithm

1. **Skin preparation.** None absolutely necessary. Some prefer cleansing with acetone or performing a microdermabrasion to enhance absorption of ALA. Curettage has been reported to debulk thicker lesions.
2. **Application of ALA.** Currently mainly used in the form of a Levulan Kerastick™. The Kerastick contains two glass chambers, one filled with ALA crystal, the other with a mixture of alcohol and polyethylene glycol (Fig. 6.9). When crushed, the ALA dissolves and is dispensed through the

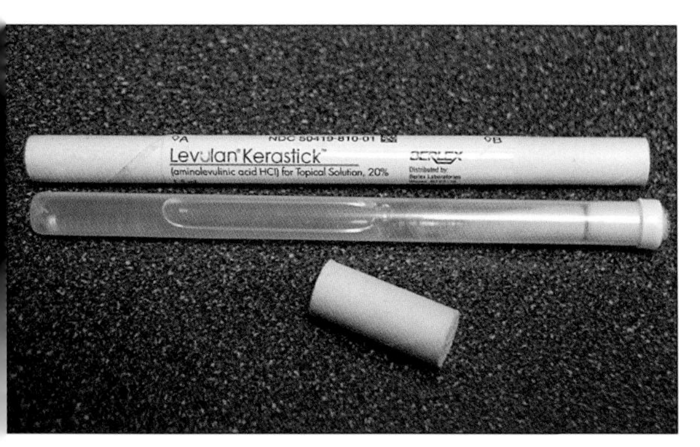

Fig. 6.9 Levulan® Kerastick™ removed from cardboard protective sleeve. Note the separate inner chambers separating the crystallized ALA from alcohol-based solution

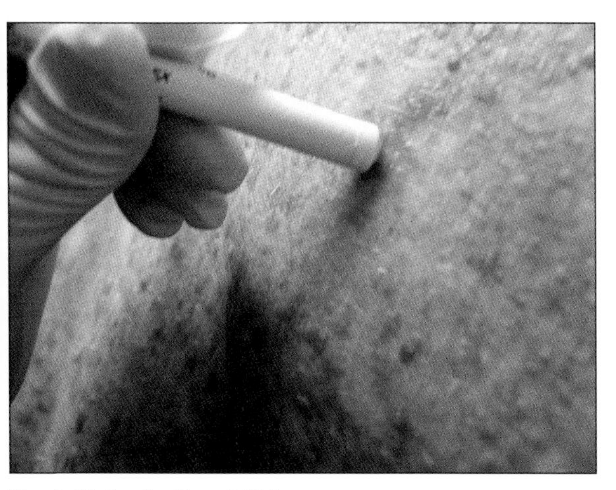

Fig. 6.10 Application of ALA

applicator tip. The ALA is then painted on the desired target, either for spot treatment or zone treatment (Fig. 6.10).

3. **Waiting period.** Originally 14–18 hours, many studies demonstrate comparable efficacy with a more tolerable treatment with shorter contact (30 minutes to 3 hours). Prior to treatment the area should not be exposed to sunlight or bright indoor lights.
4. **Immediately prior to treatment.** The area should be exposed and the patient properly positioned. Cleanse the skin surface to remove any residual ALA.
5. **Application of light.** A variety of light sources as described above may be used. Parameters needed depend on the light source. Proper positioning is important for patient comfort and treatment efficacy. When using the BLU-U™, the skin should be between 2 and 4 inches from the light source (Fig. 6.11). The BLU-U™ exposure time is 16 minutes 40 seconds (Fig. 6.12). Patients and technicians should wear protective eyewear.

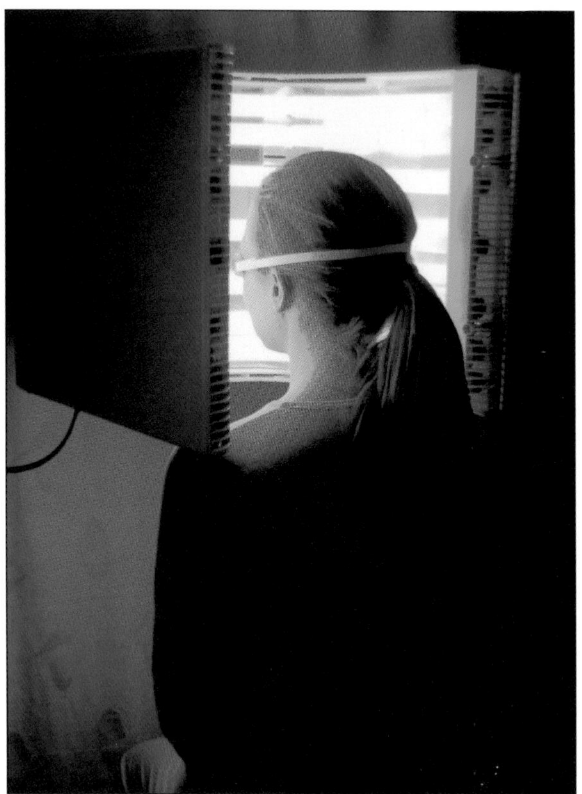

Fig. 6.11 BLU-U light exposure for photodynamic therapy

6. **Aftercare.** The skin is extremely photosensitive for at least 40 hours. The patient should be instructed to use a sunblock with broad-spectrum physical block (titanium, zinc) and photoprotective hats, hoods or suitable clothing. In addition, avoidance of the sun (including light from windows) and any bright lights (especially in the blue spectrum) is crucial to preventing a severe phototoxic reaction.

Troubleshooting

Absolute photoprotection for 40 hours after treatment is crucial. Patients should be given specific instructions before and after the treatment. Key strategies:

- sunblock with broad spectrum physical block (titanium, zinc)

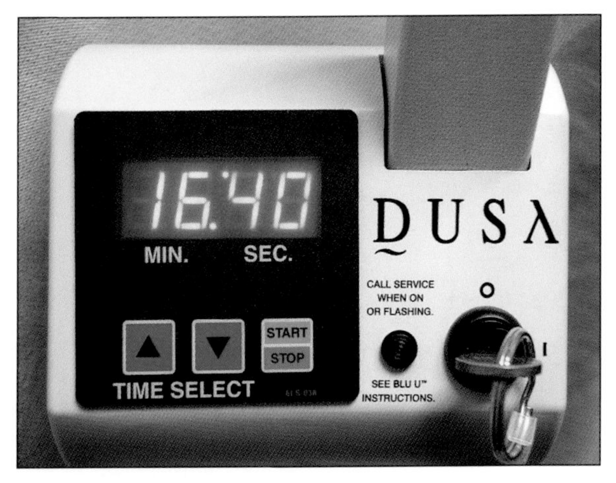

Fig. 6.12 Pre-set BLU-U timer

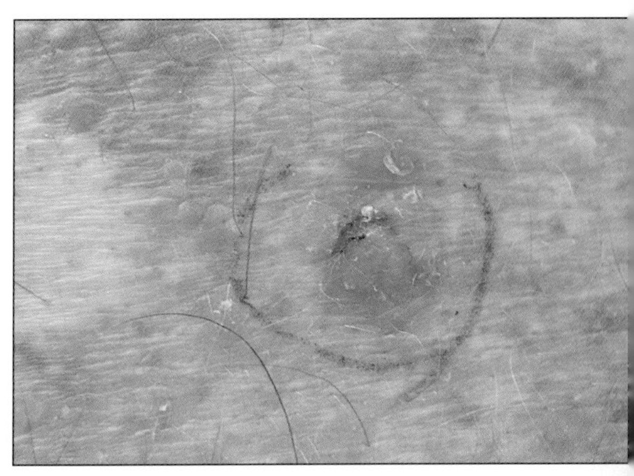

Fig. 6.13 BCC pre-ablative laser treatment with surrounding ink outline

- photoprotective broad brimmed hats, hoods or suitable clothing.
- avoidance of all sun exposure (including light from windows)
- avoidance of any bright lights (especially in the blue spectrum).

Side effects, complications, and alternative approaches

Prolonged incubation time of ALA on the skin (14–18 hours) prior to PDT results is a relatively painful treatment. Short-contact methods (30 minutes to 3 hours) have gained popularity due to convenience and much increased tolerability.

Photodynamic therapy is a moderate controlled phototoxic reaction in the skin. If excessive light exposure should occur, a severe phototoxic reaction may ensue, resulting in excessive burning, stinging, and swelling. Some physicians advocate the use of a short burst of oral steroids in an effort to prevent an excessive skin reaction.

Laser ablation

Patients

Ablative laser treatment is best for patients who have multiple actinic keratoses, actinic cheilitis, superficial BCC, or SCC in situ (Bowen's disease), especially if multiple lesions exist in an area. For best cosmetic results, it may be helpful to treat entire cosmetic units. Large areas may require prophylactic antibiotics and/or antivirals. The protocol for full face laser resurfacing will be covered elsewhere in this book.

Equipment

Ablative lasers that have been reported effective for nonmelanoma skin cancer include CO_2 laser and the Er:YAG laser. Because there is vaporization of skin, a smoke evacuator is helpful to suck in the plume and smoke. Protective eyewear and eyeshields are mandatory.

Treatment algorithm

1. **Setup.** Proper positioning of both patient and physician during the procedure is important for comfort and accessibility. All persons in the room should have protective eyewear during the entire procedure. Any flammable material should be kept away from the treatment site or covered with wet drapes.
2. **Skin preparation.** If a very small or thin tumor is being treated, anesthesia may not be required; however, most patients require at least topical anesthesia (LMX™ 4% or 5% or EMLA™) applied generously 30–90 minutes pre-procedure. Alternatively, individual tumors can be injected with local anesthetic such as 1% lidocaine with epinephrine. It may be helpful to outline the target lesion prior to anesthesia as local infiltration may obscure lesion visibility (Fig. 6.13).
3. **Treatment.** Settings vary with equipment, but using a CO_2 laser such as the Nova Pulse®, one can ablate the tumors and approximately 2 mm of surrounding skin with 7 W of power. Alternatively, a superpulsed CO_2 laser can be used with the following parameters: duty cycle 2–3%, pulse duration 2–3 ms, frequency 10 Hz, 1–3 mm spot size.

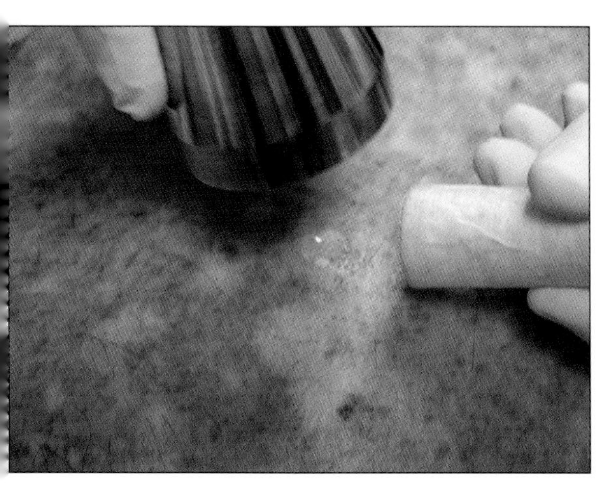

Fig. 6.14 During erbium laser treatment of BCC

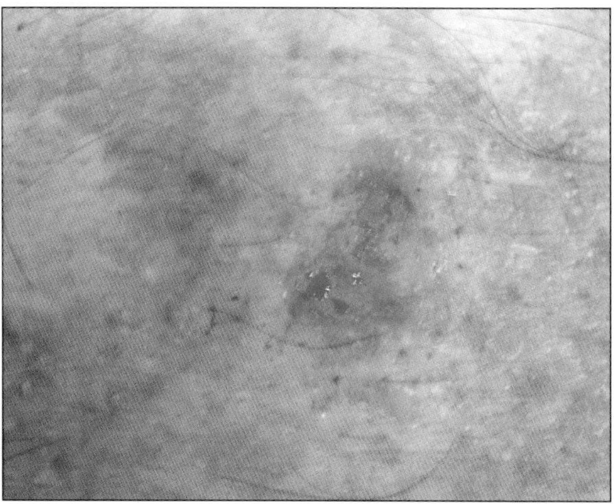

Fig. 6.15 Partially treated BCC demonstrating white dermis and pink residual tumor

Figure 6.14 demonstrates lesional ablation with a high-powered erbium laser set at 80 mμ of ablation per pulse. Note the close proximity of the smoke evacuator. After wiping away the char and blood with a damp gauze, residual tumor can often be visualized as a pinkish or reddish residue within a whitish dermis (Fig. 6.15). The latest generation CO_2 and erbium lasers developed for facial rejuvenation allow for more char free vaporization. Subsequent passes are performed until the pinkish residual tumor is no longer seen. This tumor-free dermis looks like a 'yellowish surface with big beams of fibers, similar to water-logged cotton threads,' meaning the deep dermis is reached (Fig. 6.16). For increased efficacy but at risk of increased scarring, two subsequent passes can be made after the disappearance of the tumor.

4. **Aftercare.** Postoperatively, a thin layer of Aquaphor™ or other ointment is applied to the treatment area and a pressure bandage is placed. Alternatively, several specialized dressings are available. Starting the next morning, the area should be gently cleansed with mild soap and water followed by frequent reapplication of Aquaphor. Healing time is generally 1 to 6 weeks. Sunscreen should be used to prevent post-inflammatory hyperpigmentation.

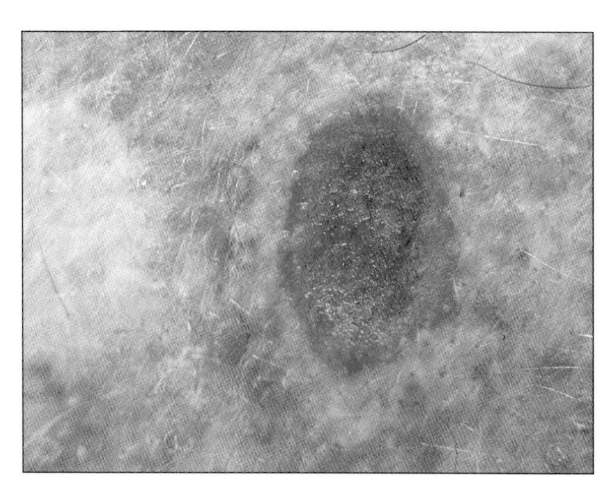

Fig. 6.16 Tumor-free deep dermis with a yellowish surface and large fibers after erbium laser treatment

Troubleshooting

If the areas to be treated are extensive, oral antibiotics or oral antivirals may be preferable. An assistant may be helpful to blot frequently so that blood in the field does not obscure the ability to differentiate tumor from normal dermis. If it is too difficult to distinguish the two, curetting the area either preoperatively or intraoperatively may aid in feeling the difference. If ablation reaches subcutaneous fat, then the distinction between tumor and normal dermis cannot be seen. Converting to excision in this case may be considered.

Side effects, complications, and alternative approaches

Side effects and complications are similar for ablative laser treatment of nonmelanoma skin cancer and actinic keratoses, and other destructive methods. These include pain, wound infection, risk of scarring, post-inflammatory hyperpigmentation, permanent hypopigmentation, prolonged healing, and potential for recurrence. Generally, ablative laser techniques have had less scarring than other traditional destructive modalities such as electrodessication and curettage or liquid nitrogen. Alternative approaches to laser ablation of nonmelanoma skin cancer can be found in Boxes 6.4 and 6.5 and Table 6.4.

Advanced Topics: Treatment Tips for Experienced Practitioners

For the best care of patients with multiple precancerous and cancerous lesions, often combination therapy can be useful. Therapeutic regimens can be tailored to body location. Cosmetically sensitive areas such as the face, neck, shoulders, upper chest and distal extremities can be treated with regimens less likely to scar or hypopigment. Relatively hidden areas may be treated with other modalities that may be quicker or more cost-effective. For example, in a cosmetically sensitive patient with financial limitations, laser-activated PDT might be used for multiple actinic keratoses on the face, while LN2 might be used on other AKs located on parts of the trunk.

Sequential therapy is often useful when patients present with large numbers of AKs. The majority can be removed with zone treatment via laser, PDT, and/or topical cream. When few remain they can be easily removed with selected application of liquid nitrogen or other spot treatment.

Further Reading

Alexiades-Armenakas MR, Geronemus RG 2003 Laser-mediated photodynamic therapy of actinic keratoses. Archives of Dermatology 139:1313–1320

Calpolim P, Brazzini B, Urso C 2002 Superpulsed CO2 laser treatment of basal cell carcinoma with intraoperatory histopathologic and cytologic examination. Dermatological Surgery 28(10):909–912

Calzavara-Pinton PG 1995 Repetitive photodynamic therapy with topical delta-aminolaevulinic acid as an appropriate approach to the treatment of superficial nonmelanoma skin tumours. Journal of Photochemistry in Photobiology 29:53–57

Cockerell CJ 2000 Histopathology of incipient intraepidermal squamous cell carcinoma ("actinic keratosis"). Journal of the American Academy of Dermatology 42:11–17

Fritsch C, Stege H, Saalmann G, Goerz G, Ruzicka T, Krutmann J 1997 Green light is effective and less painful that red light in photodynamic therapy of facial keratoses. Photodermatological Photoimmunological Photomedicine 13(5–6):181–185

Glogau RG 2000 The risk of progression to invasive disease. Journal of the American Academy of Dermatology 42:23–24

Gupta AK, Cooper EA, Feldman SR, Fleischer AB Jr 2002 A survey of office visits for actinic keratosis as reported by NAMCS, 1990–1999, National Ambulatory Medical Care Survey. Cutis 70:8–13

Haller JC, Cairnduff F, Slack G, et al 2000 Routine double treatments of superficial basal cell carcinomas using aminolaevulinic acid-based photodynamic therapy. British Journal of Dermatology 143(6):1270–1275

Horlock N, Grobbelaar AO, Gault DT 2000 Can the carbon dioxide laser completely ablate basal cell carcinomas? A histological study. British Journal of Plastic Surgery 53:286–293

Humphreys TR, Malhotra R, Scharf MJ, Marcus SM, Starkus L, Calegari K 1998 Treatment of superficial basal cell carcinoma and squamous cell carcinoma in situ with a high-energy pulsed carbon dioxide laser. Archives of Dermatology 134:1247–1252

Marmur E, Schmults CD, Goldberg DJ 2004 A review of laser and photodynamic therapy for the treatment of nonmelanoma skin cancer. Dermatological Surgery 30(2 pt 2):264–271

Morton CA, Brown SB, Collins S, et al 2002 Guidelines for topical photodynamic therapy: report of a workshop of the British Photodermatology Group. British Journal of Dermatology 146:552–567

Morton CA, Whitehurst C, Moseley H 1996 Comparison of photodynamic therapy with cryotherapy in the treatment of Bowen's disease. British Journal of Dermatology 135(5):766–771

Pariser DM, Lowe NJ, Stewart DM, Jarratt MT, Lucky AW, Pariser RJ, Yamauchi PS 2003 Photodynamic therapy with topical methyl aminolevulinate for actinic keratosis: results of a prospective randomized multicenter trial. Journal of the American Academy of Dermatology 48:227–232

Rhodes LE, de Rie M, Enstrom Y, et al 2004 Photodynamic therapy using topical methyl aminolevulinate versus surgery for nodular basal cell carcinoma: results of a multicenter randomized prospective trial. Archives of Dermatology 140(1):17–23

Salim A, Leman JA, McColl JH, Chapman R, Morton CA 2003 Comparison of photodynamic therapy with topical 5-fluorouracil in Bowen's disease. British Journal of Dermatology 148(3):539–543

Varma S, Holt PJ, Anstey AV 2000 Erythroplasia of Queyrat treated by topical aminolaevulinic acid photodynamic therapy: a cautionary tale. British Journal of Dermatology 142(4):825–826

7 Acne

E. Victor Ross Jr, Nathan Uebelhoer

Introduction

The combination of antibiotic resistance, the adverse effects of topical and systemic anti-acne medications, and the desire for 'high-tech' approaches, have all lead to new enthusiasm for light based acne treatments. Light based treatment of acne can be optimized by examining its pathophysiology. The sebaceous follicle is the site of lesion development. The most superficial portion of the follicle, the acroinfundibulum, shows similar anatomy and keratinization to the adjacent epidermis. Deposition of epidermal melanin, as seen in open comedones (blackheads), and the addition of ceramides to sebum, occur here. Melanin is also found in the acroinfundibulum but not below it. Deeper into the infundibulum at approximately 200 µm is the infrainfundibulum. This is the site of initial comedogenesis resulting from increased proliferation and accumulation of sloughed follicular keratinocytes mixed with sebum. As Plewig and Kligman note, it is the peculiar qualities of the infundibulum that provide insight into structural changes related to the development of acne. In the infrainfundibulum, the various *Propionibacterium* species act on triglycerides and release their cytokines. Changes in infundibular keratinization and inflammation follow their release. Most of the reddish-orange fluorescence seen on the face under 365 nm light is due to the coproporphyrin III produced by *P. acnes*. Further inferiorly, the infrainfundibulum splits into numerous sebaceous ducts which provide communication between the lobules of sebaceous glands and the infundibulum. Finally, the hair shaft itself extends through the sebaceous follicle and is characterized by an intermediate morphology between a vellus hair and a terminal hair shaft. This miniature melanized hair shaft may be subject to photothermal effects. 'Hyperfunctioning' sebaceous glands are one of the main contributors to acne. In an acne subject, sebaceous glands and the entire sebaceous follicle are much larger than in nonacne subjects. Their miniaturization results in a marked decrease in acne lesion counts and severity. Any long term acne cure most likely requires the participation of the sebaceous gland.

This chapter will teach you to treat acne with light based technologies. Most acne occurs on the face, however acne occurs on the back, chest, and neck as well. Our focus will be on the treatment of facial acne, as the anatomic regions are smaller and this is where one observes the greatest practical opportunities. The diagnosis of acne is straightforward and typically requires no special tests.

Patient selection

Which patient group benefits most from light treatment is unclear. Because prescriptive medical therapy is typically effective, the role of light will almost invariably be a complementary one. That is, as a monotherapy, with the exception of currently impractical therapies with deeply penetrating red light and long applications of photosensitizers or prodrugs, most light treatments only produce temporary benefits and incomplete acne remission. That being said, the ideal patient is one who might achieve 40–50% improvement with nonoral medical therapy. For example, if the patient is reluctant to use oral treatment, light might achieve a nearly complete remission in concert with appropriate topical therapy. Another group of 'light-appropriate' patients are those who enjoy 'active' acne treatments compartmentalized into a clinical appointment. In this way, patients feel that they are participating in therapy and may be more likely to be compliant with their home medical therapy.

Expected benefits

If one critically examines the literature and their own experiences, the likelihood of complete acne remission with any light based technology is small. With most light-based acne therapies, remission is incomplete and relapses are common. The scope of likely outcomes ranges from nearly imperceptible improvement to 70–80% clearing up to 3 months after treatment (see below). The few examples of complete and long term remissions with light based technologies occur in the singular regimen where photosensitizers work in combination with deeply penetrating red light. However, this regimen type is associated with significant side effects, such as desquamation, hyperpigmentation, crusting, and pain.

Objective data regarding efficacy, as well as the comfort and convenience of the various treatments, are described below. Overall, those procedures that involve low level photochemistry are painless and convenient in the sense that treatment times are short, and there is no downtime.

Overall the safety profile with the various strategies is overall good. However, there have been instances of prolonged erythema and hyperpigmentation with mid-infrared lasers. With photochemical approaches involving aminolevulinic acid, a not infrequent side effect is phototoxicity from inadvertent solar exposure on the day of or day after the procedure. In some cases, the exposure can result in long term hyperpigmentation. The cost of procedures varies widely, most practitioners charging between $200 and $500 per treatment depending on the type of treatment applied.

Due to the lack of long term research in light based acne treatment, it is difficult to predictably assess which treatments are best for which patients. Overall, small papules and pustules seem to respond best to light. Comedones and cysts respond poorly.

Equipment

There are now over 20 'machines' available for light based acne therapy. Also, most devices previously used for telangiectasias and pigment dyschromias have recently gained 'clearance' for acne from the FDA.

Using low level photochemistry requires either a continuous output blue light source or longer wavelength visible light source, as described below. These systems typically involve panfacial treatment with multiple banks of lights.

With pulsed light systems, low fluences can be used without or with a photosensitizer. With low fluence approaches such as low fluence pulsed dye laser or low fluence intense pulsed light (IPL) or potassium titanyl phosphate (KTP) lasers, the light doses are reduced to those that are only mildly uncomfortable or even painless. Treatment is carried out pulse by pulse until the area is completely covered. This will typically require anywhere from 5 to 15 minutes per treatment.

Using higher fluences with visible light technologies (without photosensitizers), the doses are in the typical range used for facial rejuvenation, i.e. treatments applied to telangiectasias and/or dyschromias. In this scenario, the practitioner delivers the pulses in a contiguous fashion so that the entire area of concern is covered. Pain will be proportional to fluence and the relative tolerance of the patient. In these cases, treatment times are roughly the same as their low fluence counterparts.

Using a photochemical approach with a photosensitizer or prodrug, such as aminolevulinic acid, there are various schemes. In the most common approach, the practitioner applies a solution of aminolevulinic acid approximately 1–3 hours prior to irradiation. During this time, the patient is required to stay away from any natural light. Either an acetone scrub and/or some type of microdermabrasion device enhance the penetration of the prodrug. A Wood's light is helpful to determine how much fluorescence is present pretreatment and is predictive of the amount of photosensitizer present in the skin.

With pulsed light, pain typically is similar to that observed without the application of aminolevulinic acid (ALA). However, the initial response with ALA is typically more robust as far as erythema and edema are concerned. With continuous light sources (with 10–15 minutes of panfacial exposures), such as the BLU-U light, pain is proportional to the time of application of the aminolevulinic acid, as well as the light dose. Patients typically appreciate the use of an air cooler (Zimmer, Germany) to make the treatment more tolerable.

Typical adverse effects are limited to those observed with like devices when applied for other indications; for example, overtreatment with pulsed light systems can result in blistering, dyspigmentation, and even scarring. The biggest concern for most practitioners is inadvertent phototoxicity with ALA. Most side effects have occurred in the postoperative period. Often the patient inadvertently exposes himself to a few minutes of sunlight. This can include sunlight through a skylight in the house or a car window. The patients must be coated with opaque sunblock on the way home.

General Approach and Basis for Treatment

Based on anatomy, one can photochemically and/or thermally alter 'trigger' points in acne's pathogenesis. Potential targets are the infundibulum, sebaceous gland, *P. acnes*, and any agents that might modulate the inflammatory response. Figure 7.1 shows a typical sebaceous follicle in an acne prone patient. The figure also shows how electromagnetic wave (EM) based treatment might attack one or more anatomic targets within the lesion. The physician should realize, as in the case of medical treatment, that therapy should be directed towards the prevention of new lesions. Even with a severe acne outbreak, lesional involvement comprises less than 1% of the surface area of the face. It follows that targeting active lesions should not be the emphasis of therapy.

Anatomically based approaches

When planning treatment approaches, one should consider the optical properties of the skin. Light is either absorbed or scattered in tissue. The wavelength specific depth of penetration (so called 'optical penetration depth', defined by the depth at which light is attenuated to 37% of its incident intensity), is experimentally determined and/or predicted by models. Light does not stop abruptly at the level of the 'penetration depth' but rather exponentially decays as it propagates through skin. As an example, consider a sebaceous gland 1 mm below the surface. At this depth, we would predict red light to be attenuated to about 20% of the surface fluence, whereas the blue light intensity would have decayed to almost zero. Even though blue light is 40 times as potent in porphyrin excitation, so little is available

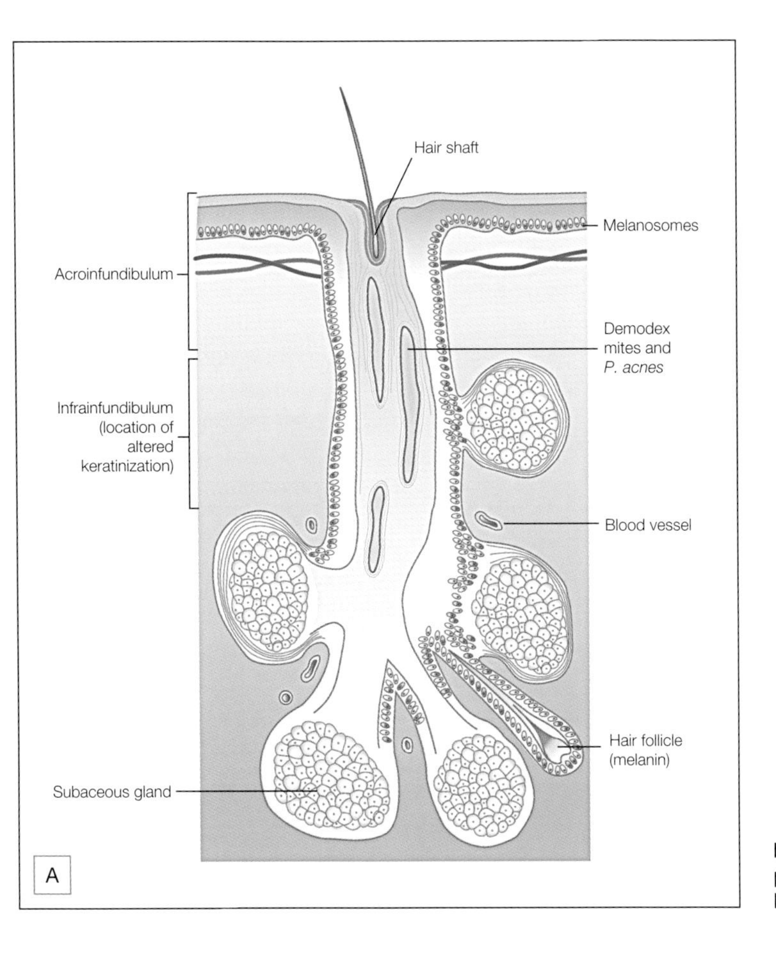

Fig. 7.1 (**A–C**) Sebaceous follicle in acne patient showing anatomic strategies in light based acne treatment *Continued*

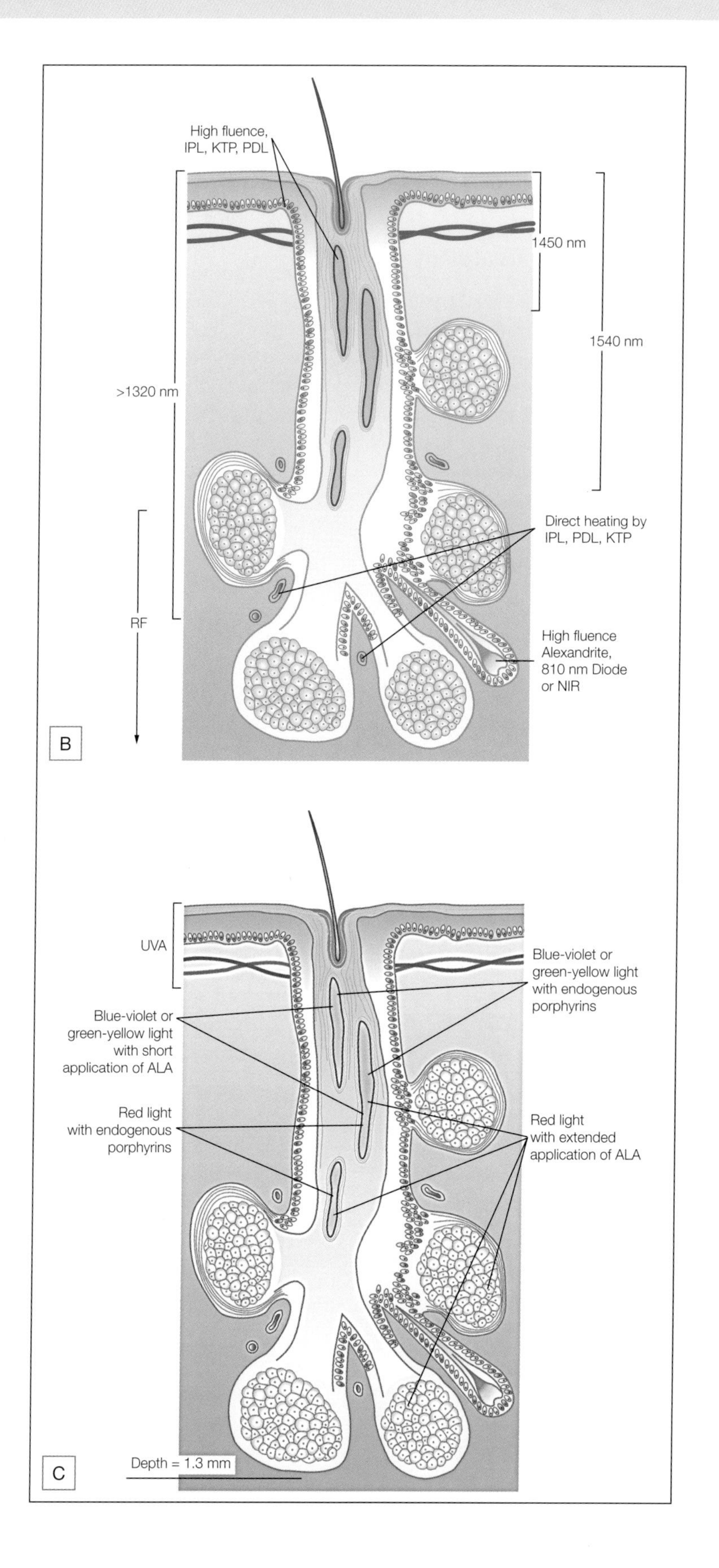
High fluence,
IPL, KTP, PDL
1450 nm
1540 nm
>1320 nm
Direct heating by
IPL, PDL, KTP
RF
High fluence
Alexandrite,
810 nm Diode
or NIR
B
UVA
Blue-violet or
green-yellow light
with endogenous
porphyrins
Blue-violet or
green-yellow light
with short
application of ALA
Red light
with endogenous
porphyrins
Red light
with extended
application of ALA
Depth = 1.3 mm
C

at the sebaceous gland that red light would be predicted to show a more robust photodynamic (PDT) effect.

UVA light

We start anatomically with UVA light (assuming UVB has little real antiacne activity nor will it be well tolerated due to the risk of burning). UVA light will penetrate to about 60 μm. Because of attenuation, UVA exposure alone likely only affects the upper infundibulum and epidermis. Exposure may lead to increased epidermal cell turnover and a mild desquamative effect. Also, superficially located *P. acnes* will be susceptible to both PDT and non-PDT bactericidal effects of UVA.

Violet and blue light

Violet and blue light will penetrate deeper (90–150 μm vs. 60 μm) than UVA light but its intensity rapidly decays in tissue (both due to melanin absorption and scatter). It follows that even with ALA application and preferential accumulation of ALA and Protoporphyrin IX (PpIX) production in the sebaceous gland (see below), it is unlikely that significant amounts of light will reach the gland itself. On the other hand, light will activate PpIX in the epidermis and acroinfundibulum, resulting in damage to these areas and some *P. acnes* killing. Subsequently, one might predict decreased inflammation, increased epidermal turnover, and possibly improved sebum outflow.

Green, yellow, and red light

Green, yellow and red light penetrate deeply enough (280, 450, and 550 μm, respectively) to have a primary effect on *P. acnes* in the infundibulum. With increasing power densities (beyond about 200 mW/cm^2), there is also direct heating of the epidermis, blood vessels, and possibly even the miniature pigmented hair shaft associated with sebaceous follicles. One would expect some light to reach the sebaceous gland, where, after ALA application, PpIX is formed.

Near-infrared (NIR) light

The 1064 nm laser has a unique place in the absorption spectrum of major skin chromophores. There are small but significant levels of melanin and HgB absorption. With pulse stacking and higher fluences, water will also be heated such that tissue damage will extend several millimeters into the dermis. One would expect only modest heating of the sebaceous gland. Severe damage to the gland in this setting (without selective heating) would cause considerable pain or possibly full thickness dermal necrosis and scarring.

Mid-infrared (MIR) lasers

These lasers can be tailored to heat different subsurface slabs of skin, depending on the cooling type, wavelength, pulse duration, and fluence. Water is the chromophore. For example, the 1450 nm laser equipped with cryogen spray cooling (DCD) heats from about 200 to 500 μm. The 1320 nm laser tends to heat a somewhat larger and deeper volume due to a lower absorption coefficient. In correlating the anatomy of acne with the depth of MIR effects, we have observed microscopic damage of superficially located (200–600 μm) sebaceous glands with the 1450 nm laser. However, in human skin this was only observed with high fluences and double passes. Most likely we are only mildly (and certainly not irreparably) heating the sebaceous gland with practical settings with these devices. According to the sebum absorption curve (Fig. 7.2) there is no selectivity for sebum over water in this range (1320–1540 nm). It follows that sebaceous glands are damaged only if and because they are embedded within the volume of tissue water heated. If one were to design a light source for selective sebaceous gland heating, it would emit around 1.2 or 1.7 μm. However, even for these wavelengths, the ratio between water and sebum is still small. On the other hand, because the sebaceous gland should cool more slowly than the surrounding skin, one might be able to optimize parameters for selective destruction of the gland.

Mechanisms of electromagnetic wave based treatment

We now examine EM based therapies from a mechanistic viewpoint. Four broad approaches are addressed, as below:

1. Pure photochemical:
   a. UV
   b. visible light—low power density.
2. Combined approaches. Possible synergy between photothermal and photochemical mechanisms.

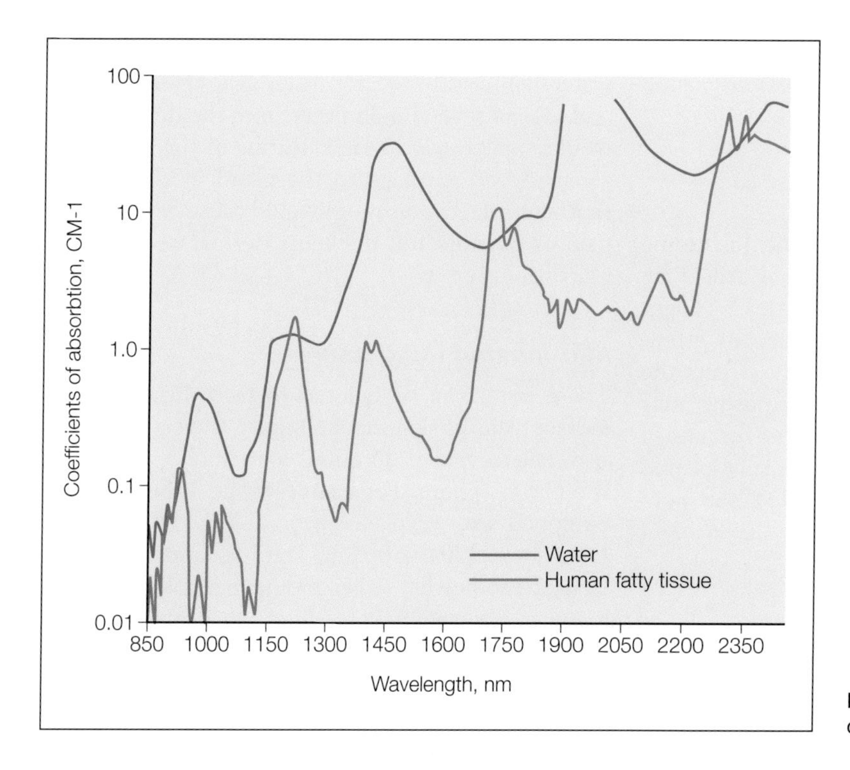

Fig. 7.2 Sebum and water absorption curves

3. Photosensitizer assisted photochemical and/or photothermal approaches:
   a. ALA with light
   b. indocyanine green (ICG) dye with light.
4. Pure photothermal approaches:
   a. hair removal laser (>670 nm)
   b. MIR.

Photochemical tissue interactions (without an exogenous photosensitizer)

Photochemical treatment of acne using endogenous porphyrins is founded on the principle of *P. acnes* photoinactivation. *P. acnes* produces coproporphyrins and protoporphyrins. The intercellular porphyrin stores will, under long wavelength UVA and certain visible light wavelengths, cause cell killing through membrane damage. This PDT effect has been demonstrated in vitro. However, the efficiency of bacterial killing with endogenous porphyrins is low, and consecutive in vitro illuminations are necessary to reduce viability by four or five orders of magnitude. When supplied with ALA (a prodrug that creates PpIX), *P. acnes* produces more porphyrins than it produces naturally, and the bacteria are inactivated by several orders of magnitude more than without ALA. The sebaceous gland proper is sterile. It follows that any significant photochemical damage to the gland itself requires an exogenous porphyrin (or a prodrug such as ALA). Any blue, red, or green color light source alone might result in *P. acnes* killing but should not cause significant sebaceous gland damage.

Johnsson found that the extruded contents of the sebaceous follicle yielded a spectrum with an excitation peak ranging from 381 to 405 nm. Penetration arguments not withstanding, this finding supports violet-blue light as an excellent color scheme for killing *P acnes*. Less absorptive 'Q bands' are other logical pumping wavelengths. They are 504, 538, 576, and 630 nm (Fig. 7.3).

UVB and UVA light have been shown to have no long term efficacy in acne (at least not better than what might be expected from topical remedies and even placebo effects). UVA is the least beneficial. However, UV light may have some anti-inflammatory effect in acne, and 70% of patients believe sunlight to be beneficial in acne (probably due to acute effects of drying the skin). Even though the action spectrum favors shorter wavelengths for *P. acnes* killing (i.e. UV vs blue light), visible light penetrates better and, unlike UVA, is not carcinogenic. Also, long term exposure to UVA light enlarges the sebaceous glands.

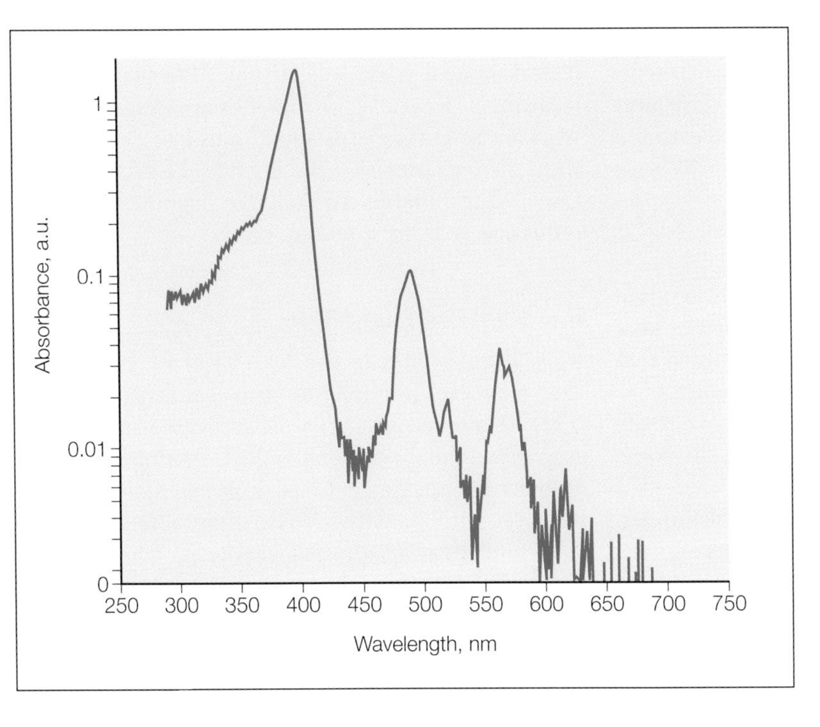

Fig. 7.3 A typical porphyrin absorption spectrum

Recently the focus in acne therapy has been on blue-violet light continuous wave (CW) sources. These devices emit light in the mW/cm^2 range, use exposure times of 10–20 min, and are painless. The working theory is that endogenous porphyrins (produced as byproducts of *P. acnes* metabolism) are excited and singlet oxygen is formed. Overall, the results have been variable and the endurance of endogenous porphyrin based treatment (with power densities of <100 mW/cm^2) has not been well defined. In one study, 34 patients were treated with a blue light device. Patients were divided into two groups (based on high vs low dose) and treated with a high energy high pressure blue light (400–420 nm). They found that after 10 of 20 treatments (10 minutes a day at ~55 mW/cm^2, 4×/week for 5 weeks) there was 'very good' acne improvement. The total light dose in the larger group was 650 J/cm^2. Interestingly, improvement did not increase between 10 and 20 treatments. Also, the lower dose group showed greater improvement. In this study, subjects were not followed past the last treatment. In another study, 107 patients were randomized into four treatment groups: blue light, blue-red light, cool white light, and benzoyl peroxide. Treatment sessions lasted 15 minutes and the cumulative doses over 12 weeks of daily treatments were 320 J/cm^2 for the blue light and 202 J/cm^2 for the red light. White light was used as a control. Overall, the blue–red light combination was superior, showing 75% reduction in inflammatory lesions after 12 weeks. The blue light and benzoyl peroxide produced similar improvement of about 60% after 12 weeks. Low output white light (a room light 'control') was associated with a 25% decrease in counts.

In another study patients were treated three times a week for a total of 20 sessions. Treatments required about 20 minutes. Three types of light were used: (i) 'full spectrum', a mix of UVA, violet, and green light; (ii) 'violet light', a mix of UVA and violet light with a small contribution of green light; (iii) 'green light', a mix of mostly green light with a small contribution of violet light. The investigators observed a final reduction of acne severity of 14%, 30%, and 22% at the end of 20 sessions with full spectrum, violet, and green light respectively. Overall, the violet light group did best, but the differences were not significant. As in most studies, the light effects were primarily on inflammatory lesions, with little effect on comedones and papules. Kawada et al treated 30 patients using a blue light source (metal halide source, Clear light, Lumenis), which has a peak emission between 407 and 420 nm. The irradiance was 90 mW/cm^2, with two treatments per week for up to 5 weeks. There was an overall 55% reduction in the number of lesions (all types). Seventy seven per cent of the patients either 'improved' or 'markedly improved', with 20% either worsening or remaining unchanged. One month after the final treatment most of the improvement was sustained.

Pulsed light sources and PDT

Short pulses are at odds with one condition that optimizes PDT, that is, long application times that allow for oxygen availability. It has been shown that lower irradiances demonstrate a more robust PDT effect. Although pulsed light sources have been shown to be equivalent to CW sources in some experiments, the PDT effect was only equivalent if the light doses and average irradiances were similar. Most pulsed light sources in dermatology are below the theoretical PDT saturation threshold ($4 \times 10^8 W/m^2$). All of this suggests that an optimal pulsed light therapy for acne (at least, with PDT as a mechanism) might require multiple passes with blue, green, yellow, or red light. The interval between passes should be designed such that the average irradiance is similar to that of CW devices with similar emission spectra.

Photochemical and photothermal

The visible light devices cited above work exclusively through photochemical mechanisms. That is, singlet O_2 production by long exposures results in *P. acnes* killing. The irradiances are insufficient to achieve significant temperature elevations in or around the acne lesion or normal skin. The following studies involve irradiances and fluences where there is at least a slight temperature elevation as well as a possible PDT mediated antibacterial effect.

Pulsed dye laser (PDL)

Seaton et al examined the effects of low fluence PDL treatment (585 nm, 1.5 or 3 J/cm^2, 1 pass, one treatment session) with a follow up of 12 weeks. They found that acne severity improved markedly vs controls (53% lesion count decreases in treatment areas vs only 9% in controls). There was no difference between the high and low fluence groups. They postulated that the laser might directly kill bacteria and also alter the immunologic response to the bacteria. It was also suggested that the laser might somehow alter the comedonal environment or alter follicular wall maturation. Although low fluence PDL will also transiently heat microvessels, it is unknown what role, if any, this plays in acne treatment. Recently Orringer et al presented their work on acne laser treatment, and like Seaton et al, they also examined low fluence PDL. However, they were unable to achieve significant lesion reduction in their split face study.

Intense pulsed light (IPL)

Most devices emit in the 500–1200 nm range, with the greatest portion of the spectrum in the 530–700 nm range. IPLs have been used in two scenarios, the first using higher settings normally applied for rosacea and photorejuvenation. These settings, with or without ALA, are able to achieve sufficient heating of telangiectasia and pigment dyschromias to diminish their appearance. Published studies of IPL with 'high' fluences (without ALA) have shown a reduction in redness and acneform papules. In our own experience with traditional IPL treatments, we have observed a reduction in redness associated with acne/rosacea, and patients have remarked that they observe fewer lesions in the postoperative period. In this first 'high setting' scenario, two potential mechanisms might be operative. One is temperature elevation in the hyperemic acne lesions as well as the dermo-epidermal junction. Because of 'pumping' of endogenous porphyrins in the Q bands (see above), a second mechanism might be photoactivation and singlet O_2 creation.

In another scenario, lesser settings are used with multiple pulsing. In this second application type, lower settings presumably will change the ratio in favor of photochemical over photothermal mechanisms. There are newer pulsed light sources that use low energies and a spectrum that allows for considerable violet-blue and/or green-yellow-red light. These handpieces are able to pump most if not all of the absorption bands for PpIX. For example, we have used an IPL emitting mostly green-yellow light (Lux G, 525–1200 nm, Palomar Medilux, Palomar, Burlington, MA, USA) or mostly violet-blue light violet (Lux V, 400–700 nm and 870–1200 nm) in weekly treatments (up to four) without ALA. In this split face study comprising four weekly treatments, patients were randomized into the 'green-yellow' light or 'violet' light groups. Both groups showed about 85% inflammatory lesion reduction during treatment (Fig. 7.4). The control sides improved by about 30%. However, within 8 weeks after the final treatment, the acne counts began to return to baseline level. There was a slight warm sensation during our IPL treatments, indicating at least a mild thermal effect. However, no obvious thermal side effects were observed (i.e. microcrusting). Dierickx used the same system with both violet and green light handpieces and found significant clearing of lesions (after up to five treatments over 5–15 weeks). Follow up to 3–6 months resulted in only a partial return of lesion counts in most patients.

Another flash lamp device (Clear touch™, Radiancy Inc., Orangeburg, NY, USA) uses the green-yellow part of the spectrum for *P. acnes* killing and a 'heat' pulse to 'reduce inflammation'. A recent study of 50 patients showed 50% reduction in inflamed lesions at the end of the study. Full faces were treated and compared to controls in a crossover design. There were two treatments per week over 4 weeks.

Demodex can be selectively coagulated via IPL, most likely through primary heating of the melanized chitinous exoskeleton. It follows that primary heating of the mites might contribute to the success of IPL treatments.

KTP laser

Selectively heating pigment and blood, as well as possibly exerting a primary PDT effect, the KTP laser has been used to treat acne and rosacea. In a study of 11 patients with acne vulgaris, subjects were treated in a split face trial. Four treatments were delivered over 2 weeks. Using fluences of 7–9 J/cm^2, a 4 mm spot, and contact cooling (6–10 passes, cumulative fluence of 20–50 J/cm^2), acne clearance was 36% on the treated side 1 month after the last treatment vs a 2% increase on the control (cooling only) side. Presumably, heating of the vasculature as well as potential photochemical effects are active with this approach. Lee reported treatment of 25 patients with a KTP laser alone. Using multiple passes with a fluence per pass of 6–12 J/cm^2 and contact cooling, she observed clearing of 60–70% after six treatments. However, she reported that patients treated with laser alone showed more post-treatment flares, decreased clearance, and faster relapses than in other arms of her trial where lasers were used in tandem with topical and oral medications.

Exogenous photosensitizer assisted PDT

ALA PDT

The preferential accumulation of ALA and production of PpIX in sebaceous glands has been shown in various studies. However, the selectivity and accumulation in the glands will depend on the vehicle and application time. Most likely at least 3–4 hours will be required for significant accumulation in the gland itself. When light is delivered to ALA treated skin, PpIX is excited to a triplet

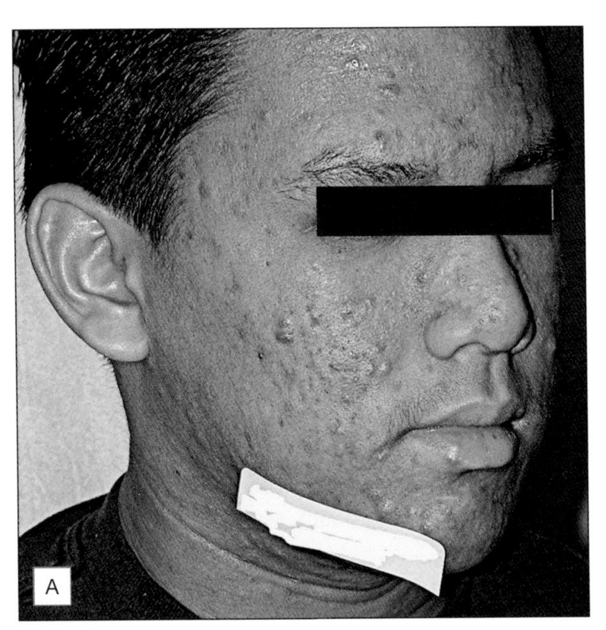

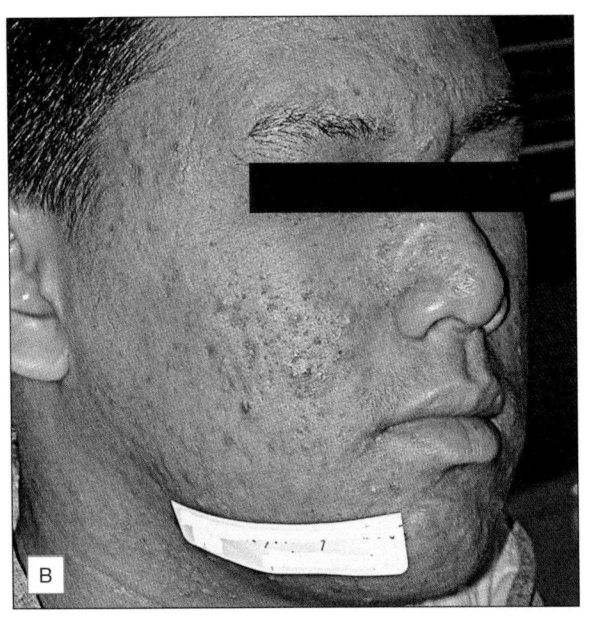

Fig. 7.4 (**A**) Pretreatment. (**B**) 2 weeks after two treatments with Lux V handpiece (9 J/cm^2, 100 ms, double pulse, 1 pass)

state, indirectly creating singlet O_2. ALA has been used with CW light sources for a broad array of skin maladies, including acne. More recently, ALA is being promoted as a 'booster' for IPL and PDL. The working theory is that the combination of ALA and photorejuvenation settings with PDL and IPL can achieve acne clearance while simultaneously reducing brown and red dyschromias. Three treatment sessions are typically advised at 4 week intervals. ALA is applied for 1–2 hours after which light is applied. While there is evidence that this approach reduces acne lesions, and while it is possible that ALA plays a role, the likelihood that the pulsed light source results in large amounts of immediate singlet O_2 formation is small. It is more likely that that IPL-PDL reduces redness through well established photothermal mechanisms or that there might be some synergy between PDT and photothermal action.

PDT effects can be observed with these MS (millisecond) domain IPL and PDL pulses. However, only moments of sun exposure will create more singlet O_2 than the 5–30 J/cm^2 of pulsed green or yellow light. This will be truer if the IPL or PDL exposure occurs too early after ALA application (before there is time for sufficient PpIX production). No study thus far has shown selective sebaceous gland damage after short contact (0–2 hour) ALA pulsed light PDT.

Itoh used an excimer pulsed dye laser (635 nm) and showed long term remission in facial acne after 20% ALA application (for 4 hours). Using the laser at 5 J/cm^2, he showed complete remission in acne 8 months after one treatment. In another study of 13 patients, Itoh found good improvement in acne after ALA treatment with a halogen source (600–700 nm).

Goldman and Boyce treated 22 patients in a study with the BLU-U light (10 mW/cm^2 at 417 nm). They treated one group of patients for 6 min without ALA (two treatments, 1 week apart, with follow up after 2 more weeks). In the second group, they applied ALA for 15 min and then treated with the light (two treatments, 2 weeks apart, with evaluation after 2 more weeks). Overall, they found a 25% reduction in acne severity in the first group and 32% in group 2. There was no pain. Some patients did report a sunburn reaction from inadvertent outdoor exposure.

There have been other novel approaches with ALA assisted treatment of acne. In a recent clinical roundtable discussion, a list of options was proposed for acne and rosacea treatment. Among them were PDL and ALA, IPL and ALA, and BLU-U and ALA. Most of these approaches combine short contact (30–60 min) with ALA (Levulan, DUSA) followed by light exposures with one of the aforementioned devices. In most cases, physicians will use similar settings as they would without ALA. Some will reduce the setting by 10–20% to allow for the more robust reaction observed after ALA. Some typical parameters are outlined below: (i) PDL: 595 nm, 7 J/cm^2, 6–10 ms, 10 mm spot, 30/20 DCD; (ii) PDL: 595 nm, 3 J/cm^2, 10 mm, 10 ms, 30/30 DCD; (iii) PDL: 40 ms, 12 mm, 595 nm, 6 J/cm^2, 3 passes (18 J/cm^2 total fluence); (iv) IPL (Quantum, Lumenis): 2.4 – 2.4 ms (double pulse), 10 ms delay, 550 nm filter, total fluence 24–27 J/cm^2. Most of these treatments are performed monthly for 3 months. One concern by all of the panelists was the need for sun protection after treatment. Many physicians are advocating 48 hours of sun avoidance/protection after the procedure.

It is clear that the use of ALA will expand in acne treatment. In the future we may see various application times, vehicles, and light sources. Presently a challenge is to achieve preferential accumulation of ALA in the sebaceous gland versus the epidermis. With short contact times (<2 hours), most of the PpIX formation will be in the infundibulum and upper epidermis. On the other hand, with longer times and frequent wiping of the surface, one might achieve preferential penetration into the sebaceous follicle without epidermal compromise.

ALA assisted light treatment may work in several ways. In addition to direct photokilling of *P. acnes*, there may be PDT mediated injury to the gland (inhibiting sebum production). Finally follicular obstruction might be altered by changing keratinocyte shedding and hyperkeratosis (likely the mechanism with short application times). Long term acne improvement does appear to be correlated with decreased sebum production. However, ALA mediated sebum inhibition requires more aggressive treatment than ALA mediated killing of *P. acnes*.

ICG dye and sebaceous gland damage

Two studies have reported the use of indocyanine green (ICG) dye to damage sebaceous glands. In this scenario, the ICG is applied topically. Then an 805 nm diode laser was used in a low or high power mode to cause photodynamic or photothermal damage to the sebaceous gland. Likewise, Lloyd showed preferential accumulation of ICG suspension after 24 hours application. Then, applying an 810 nm light at 40 J/cm² and 50 ms, she showed selective damage of the sebaceous gland and long term improvement in back acne (up to 10 months after the final treatment).

'Pure' photothermal tissue interactions

Manuskiatti et al reported focal damage to the sebaceous gland after ruby laser treatment on the thigh and back. They speculated that the loss of hair might improve sebum outflow and therefore acne. Perhaps damage to the sebaceous gland via the hair shaft is one mechanism.

Mid-infrared lasers

Three wavelengths (1320, 1450, and 1540 nm) have all been applied to active acne in some form of clinical trials. Ross et al examined the use of the 1450 nm laser in the treatment of back acne and observed marked decreases in the number of inflammatory lesions 12 weeks after once weekly treatments for 1 month. However, the number of lesions in the treated zones was small, and the durability of the results beyond 12 weeks was unclear. In a later human split face study, they found a 47% reduction in acne lesions on the treated side and 18% on the control side (6 weeks after the final treatment) (Fig. 7.5). A more recent full face study showed 75% reduction in acne counts 6 weeks after the final treatment. A review of MIR selective dermal heating can be found in a recent article by Painthankar et al. A biopsy is presented in Figure 7.6 and a representative patient in Figure 7.5. One should note that most *P. acnes* and enlarged sebaceous glands will lie below the level of maximal heating with 1450 nm (maximum heating in combination with DCD is about 300–400 μm below the surface). It follows that the 1450 nm laser might work through direct heating of the infundibulum. We

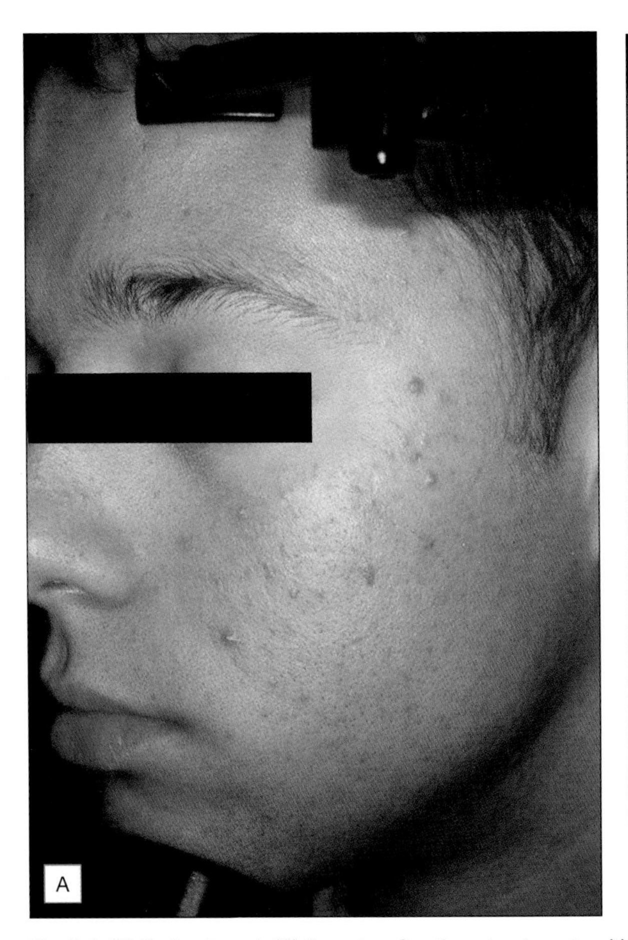

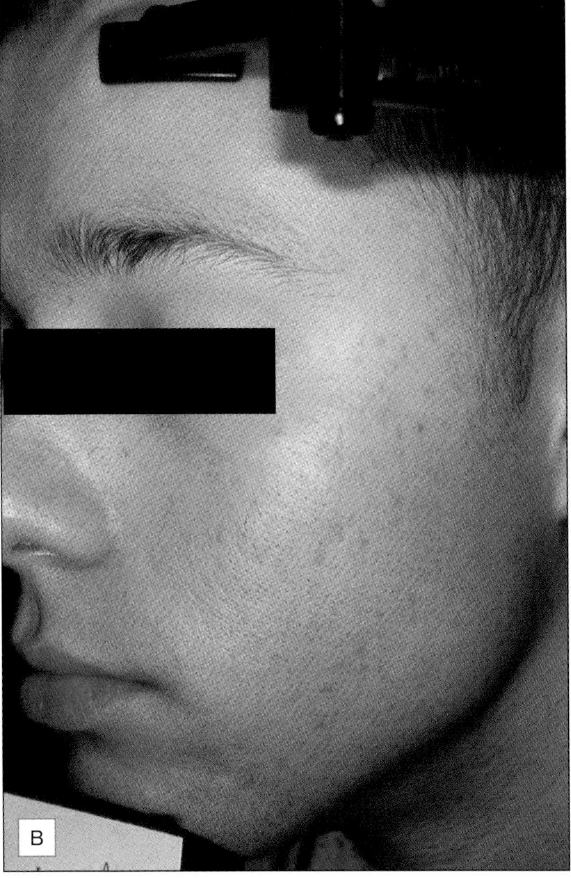

Fig. 7.5 (**A**) Pretreatment. (**B**) 6 weeks after three treatments with 1450 nm laser (14 J/cm², 1 pass, 6 mm spot, 45 ms DCD)

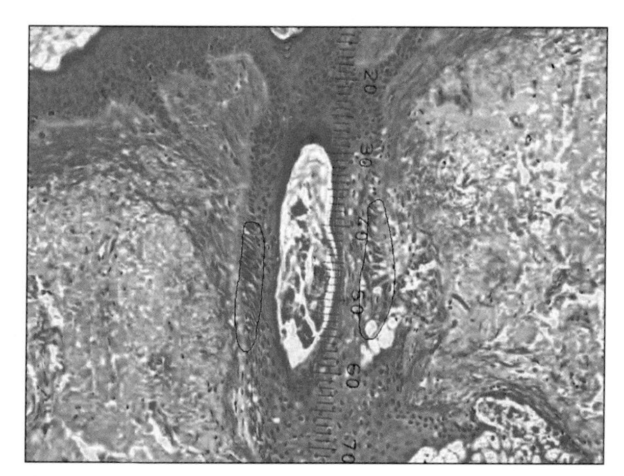

Fig. 7.6 Microscopic view of sebaceous follicle just after treatment with 1450 nm laser (2 passes, 16 J/cm^2, 6 mm spot, 50 ms DCD). Encircled areas show thermal damage to infundibulum

speculate that this might improve sebum outflow and 'reset' the keratinization pattern in the follicle.

Friedman reported an 80% mean reduction in inflammatory lesions after three monthly treatments with the 1450 nm laser. The 19 patients were allowed to continue whatever medications they were on prior to accessioning into the study. Patients were not followed after the end of treatments.

Boineau et al used the 1540 nm laser (four treatments at 4 week intervals) in 25 patients. Twelve weeks after the final treatment, they observed a 78% reduction in acne lesions. Patients reported that their skin was less oily.

A radiofrequency device

A radiofrequency device (Thermage, Hayward, CA, USA) has recently been reported to be effective in the treatment of acne vulgaris. Twenty-two patients were treated and most showed a good response (>75% reduction in lesions in over 90% of patients). However, some subjects used other therapies at the time of treatment, and no controls were performed. Although selective fat heating has been shown with this device, selective sebaceous gland heating has not been demonstrated microscopically.

Conclusions

Despite great enthusiasm for new physical modalities in acne, one should remember that many results are often temporary and not 100% effective. As a home light therapy system, available low power red and blue light sources might prove practical for teenagers and others who are willing to self-treat for about 15 minutes a day. However, visible light sources alone can probably only achieve mild acne improvement. On the other hand, the patient might be able to use the light in combination with a topical agent such as benzoyl peroxide and negate the need for an oral antibiotic.

What approaches are most likely to yield long term success in EM based acne therapy? We know that sebum output returns to normal after isotretinoin and *P. acnes* comes back. However, the infrainfundibulum keratinization process is still normalized, pointing to this as a possibly more important feature in any long term acne solution. However, as Plewig and Kligman point out, sebum 'fuels' the acne fire, and successful long term EM based strategies have included damage to the gland. Acne does not occur when sebum output is low (but does not always occur when it is high). We will see in the near future more sebum-selective light sources and other improved ways to achieve selective accumulation of photosensitizer in the gland.

One could argue that all acne can be improved without the use of electromagnetic waves. The cost of these therapies, particularly for office based approaches, might always limit their use as a first line approach. However, as Cunliffe recently suggested, despite the 'smorgasbord' of therapies, light based technologies may fill a current void within the treatment spectrum in a potentially 'medication-sparing' role.

Further Reading

Alexiades-Armenakas M, Alster T, Dover JS, et al 2003 Levulan clinical roundtable. Aesthetic Buyer's Guide May/June:22–27

Boineau D, Angel S, Auffret N, Dahan S, Mordon S 2004 Treatment of active acne with an erbium glass (1.54 micron) laser. Lasers in Surgery and Medicine 16(suppl):55 (abstract)

Bowes L, Manstein D, Anderson R 2003 Effects of 532 nm KTP laser on acne and sebacous glands. Lasers in Medical Science 18(suppl 1):S6–7

Cunliffe WJ, Goulden V 2000 Phototherapy and acne vulgaris. British Journal of Dermatology 142:855–856

Divaris DX, Kennedy JC, Pottier RH 1990 Phototoxic damage to sebaceous glands and hair follicles of mice after systemic administration of 5-aminolevulinic acid correlates with localized protoporphyrin IX fluorescence. American Journal of Pathology 136:891–897

Elman M, Lebzelter J 2004 Light therapy in the treatment of acne vulgaris. Dermatologic Surgery 30(2 Pt 1):139–146

Elman M, Slatkine M, Harth Y 2003 The effective treatment of acne vulgaris by a high-intensity, narrow band 405–420 nm light source. Journal of Cosmetic and Laser Therapy 5:111–117

Friedman PM, Jih MH, Kimyai-Asadi A, Goldberg LH 2004 Treatment of inflammatory facial acne vulgaris with the 1450-nm diode laser: a pilot study. Dermatologic Surgery 30(2 Pt 1):147–151
Goldman MP, Boyce SM 2003 A single-center study of aminolevulinic acid and 417 nm photodynamic therapy in the treatment of moderate to severe acne vulgaris. Journal of Drugs in Dermatology 2:393–396
Gregory A, Thornfeldt C, Leibowitz K, Lane M 2004 A study on the use of a novel light and heat energy system to treat acne vulgaris. Cosmetic Dermatology 17:287–300
Hongcharu W, Taylor CR, Chang Y, et al 2000 Topical ALA-photodynamic therapy for the treatment of acne vulgaris. Journal of Investigative Dermatology 115:183–192
Itoh Y, Ninomiya Y, Tajima S, Ishibashi A 2000 Photodynamic therapy for acne vulgaris with topical 5-aminolevulinic acid. Archives of Dermatology 136:1093–1095
Kawada A, Aragane Y, Kameyama H, Sangen Y, Tezuka T 2002 Acne phototherapy with a high-intensity, enhanced, narrow-band, blue light source: an open study and in vitro investigation. Journal of Dermatological Science 30:129–135
Lloyd JR, Mirkov M 2002 Selective photothermolysis of the sebaceous glands for acne treatment. Lasers in Surgery and Medicine 31:115–120
Mark KA, Sparacio RM, Voigt A, Marenus K, Sarnoff DS 2003 Objective and quantitative improvement of rosacea-associated erythema after intense pulsed light treatment. Dermatologic Surgery 29:600–604
Mills OH, Kligman AM 1978 Ultraviolet phototherapy and photochemotherapy of acne vulgaris. Archives of Dermatology 114:221–223
Mutzhas MF, Holzle E, Hofmann C, Plewig G 1981 A new apparatus with high radiation energy between 320–460 nm: physical description and dermatological applications. Journal of Investigative Dermatology 76:42–47
Paithankar DY, Ross EV, Saleh BA, Blair MA, Graham BS 2002 Acne treatment with a 1450 nm wavelength laser and cryogen spray cooling. Lasers in Surgery and Medicine 31:106–114
Papageorgiou P, Katsambas A, Chu A 2000 Phototherapy with blue (415 nm) and red (660 nm) light in the treatment of acne vulgaris. British Journal of Dermatology 142:973–978
Ross E, Blair M, Saleh B, Graham B, Paithankar D 2002 Laser treatment of acne through selective dermal heating. Lasers in Surgery and Medicine 14(suppl):23 (abstract)
Ruiz-Esparza J, Gomez JB 2003 Nonablative radiofrequency for active acne vulgaris: the use of deep dermal heat in the treatment of moderate to severe active acne vulgaris (thermotherapy): a report of 22 patients. Dermatologic Surgery 29:333–339; discussion 339
Seaton ED, Charakida A, Mouser PE, Grace I, et al 2003 Pulsed-dye laser treatment for inflammatory acne vulgaris: randomised controlled trial. Lancet 362:1347–1352 [see comment]
Sigurdsson V, Knulst AC, van Weelden H 1997 Phototherapy of acne vulgaris with visible light. Dermatology 194:256–260
Tuchin VV, Genina EA, Bashkatov AN, et al 2003 A pilot study of ICG laser therapy of acne vulgaris: photodynamic and photothermolysis treatment. Lasers in Surgery and Medicine 33:296–310
Uebelhoer N, Paithankar DY, Ross E 2003 Laser treatment of facial acne with a 1450 nm diode laser. Lasers in Surgery and Medicine 15(suppl):29 (abstract)

8 Psoriasis

Ming H. Jih, Paul M. Friedman

Introduction

Psoriasis

Psoriasis is a chronic skin disorder characterized by dermal inflammation and keratinocyte hyperproliferation that affects an estimated 1–3% of the population. Recent studies have established that psoriasis is fundamentally an inflammatory condition in which activated T lymphocytes initiate and maintain an inflammatory milieu. Understanding the immunologic disturbances that cause psoriasis has contributed to the development of specific targeted therapies.

Clinical variants of psoriasis include plaque, guttate, pustular, inverse, palmoplantar, and erythrodermic. The plaque type is most common and is characterized by sharply demarcated, erythematous plaques with silvery scale. The classic locations are elbows, knee, scalp, and lower back, but lesions can occur in any anatomic location and are usually symmetrically distributed (Fig. 8.1).

The diagnosis of psoriasis is usually made clinically and ancillary tests are rarely necessary (Box 8.1). The clinical differentials are also listed in Box 8.1. However, the chronic nature, characteristic distribution, and the typical scaly plaques distinguish psoriasis from other papulosquamous disorders. A family history of psoriasis and characteristic nail changes can also aid the diagnosis (Fig. 8.2). Where diagnosis is uncertain, a biopsy may be performed (Box 8.2, Fig. 8.3). Psoriatic arthritis, affecting 5–30% of patients with psoriasis, is progressive and mutilating. Thus, patients with symptoms of arthritis should undergo radiologic, serologic, and rheumatologic evaluation (Box 8.2).

Light source and laser treatment for psoriasis

Although the use of lasers to treat psoriasis is relatively novel, light based energy was one of the earliest treatment modalities. Sunlight was known to improve psoriasis even in ancient times, and climatotherapy still thrives today as an effective treatment. Phototherapy using ultraviolet (UV) light was initially introduced in 1925 and has become standard therapy for psoriasis.

The psoriasis action spectrum is defined as the range of UV wavelengths (295–365 nm) therapeutic for psoriasis. Photochemotherapy with psoralens and ultraviolet A (320–400 nm) (PUVA) and broad band ultraviolet B (BB-UVB) (290–320 nm) were introduced in the 1970s (Fig. 8.4). More recently, narrow band ultraviolet B (NB-UVB) with peak emissions between 311 and 313 nm has been shown to be highly effective with fewer adverse effects than PUVA. All conventional phototherapy systems are limited by the need to initiate treatments at low doses with incremental increases due to concurrent UV exposure of normal skin.

The initial use of lasers to treat psoriasis was driven by the search for more effective and potentially safer treatment alternatives. Various lasers and light sources have been used for the treatment of psoriasis (Box 8.3, Fig. 8.5). The first use of a laser to treat psoriasis was reported in 1986 and treatments focused on ablation of psoriatic plaques using the carbon dioxide (CO_2) or erbium yttrium–aluminum–garnet (Er : YAG) laser. The rationale for use of ablative lasers was based on the 'reverse Koebner phenomenon' observed after removal of both the epidermis and papillary dermis which resulted in clearing and prolonged remissions

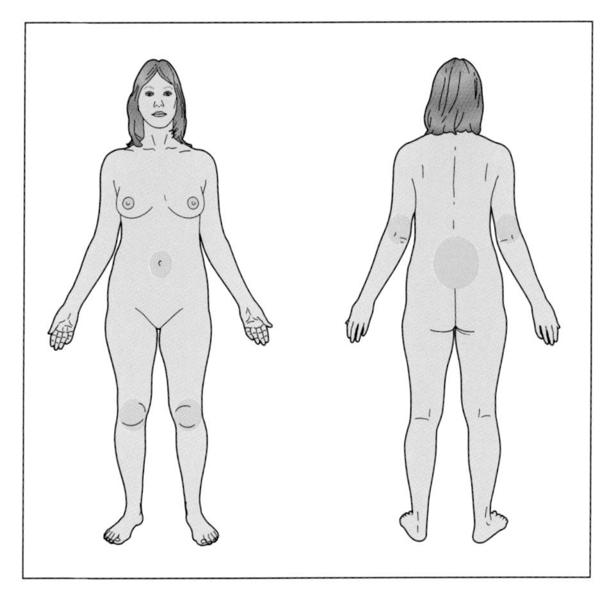

Fig. 8.1 Typical symmetric distribution of plaque type psoriasis includes the elbows, knees, scalp, buttocks, umbilicus, and hands and feet

Clinical findings and clinical differential for classic plaque type psoriasis

Clinical findings for classic plaque type psoriasis

- Erythematous well demarcated plaques
- Silvery 'micaceous' adherent scale
- Nail findings: pits, oil spots, onycholysis, hyperkeratosis
- Typical symmetric anatomic distribution
- Family history of psoriasis

Clinical differentials for plaque type psoriasis

- Atopic dermatitis
- Seborrheic dermatitis
- Tinea
- Mycosis fungoides
- Pityriasis rubra pilaris
- Subacute cutaneous lupus erythematosus
- Pityriasis rosea
- Secondary syphilis

Box 8.1 Clinical findings and clinical differential for classic plaque type psoriasis

Ancillary diagnostic procedures

Procedures	Findings
Skin biopsy: a punch biopsy should be obtained for the most accurate diagnosis of inflammatory skin disorders	Acanthosis, elongation of the rete ridges, reduced or absent granular layer, parakeratosis, polymorphonuclear cells in the scale crust and epidermis forming micropustules, and dermal edema with dilated blood vessels in the dermal papillae (Fig. 8.3)
Radiological testing for joint disease in cases of suspected psoriatic arthritis	'Fluffy' periosteal bone formation, digital tip erosions, pencil-in-cup deformity, acroosteolysis, bony ankylosis
Serologic testing for joint disease in cases of suspected psoriatic arthritis	Elevated erythrocyte sedimentation rate, elevated C-reactive protein, negative rheumatoid factor

Box 8.2 Ancillary diagnostic procedures

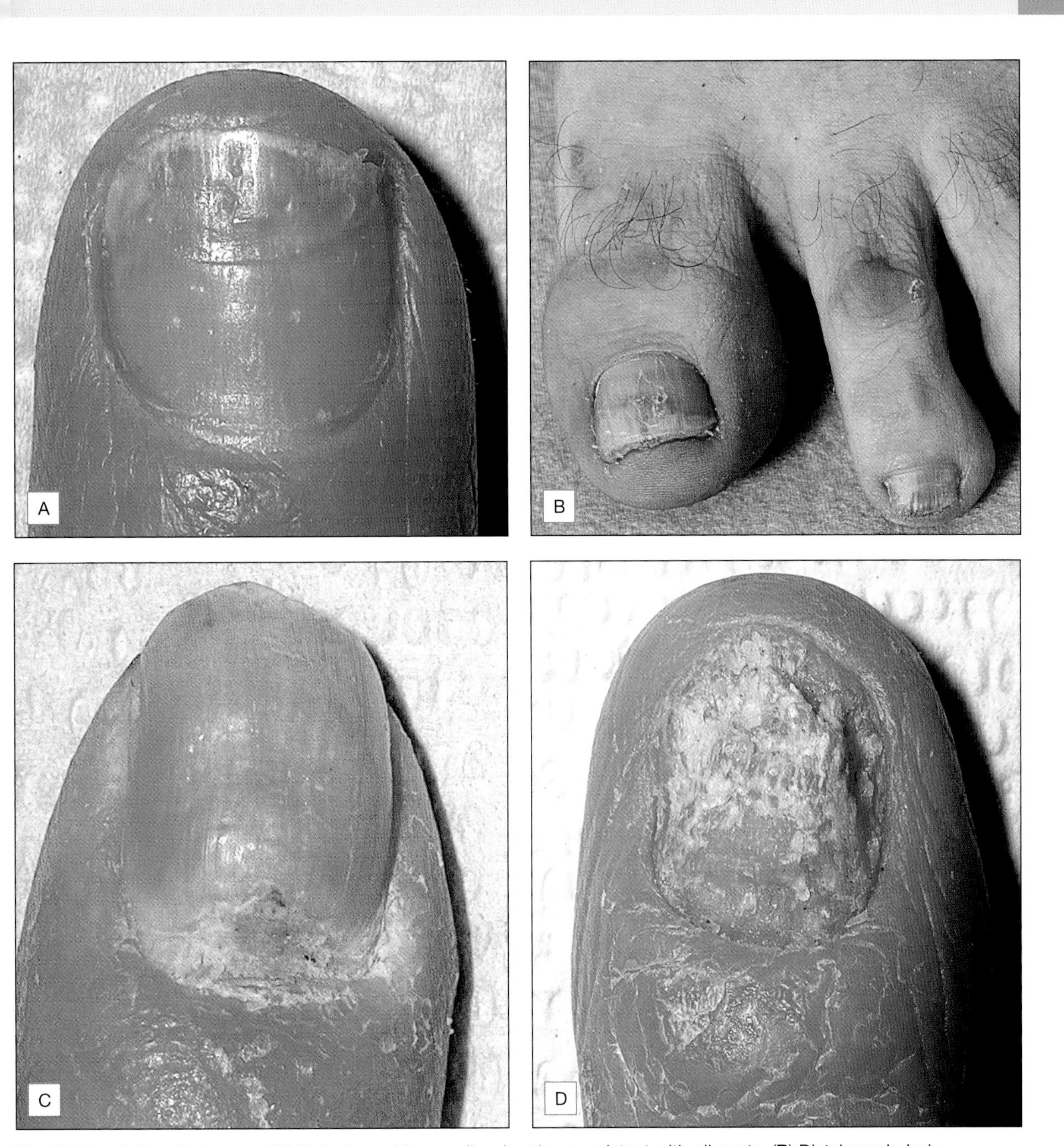

Fig. 8.2 Psoriatic nail changes. (**A**) Nail pits and brown discoloration consistent with oil spots. (**B**) Distal onycholysis, thickening and yellowing of nail. (**C**) Proximal hyperkeratosis. (**D**) Distal hyperkeratosis with partial loss of the nail. (Photographs courtesy of Bruce Strober, MD)

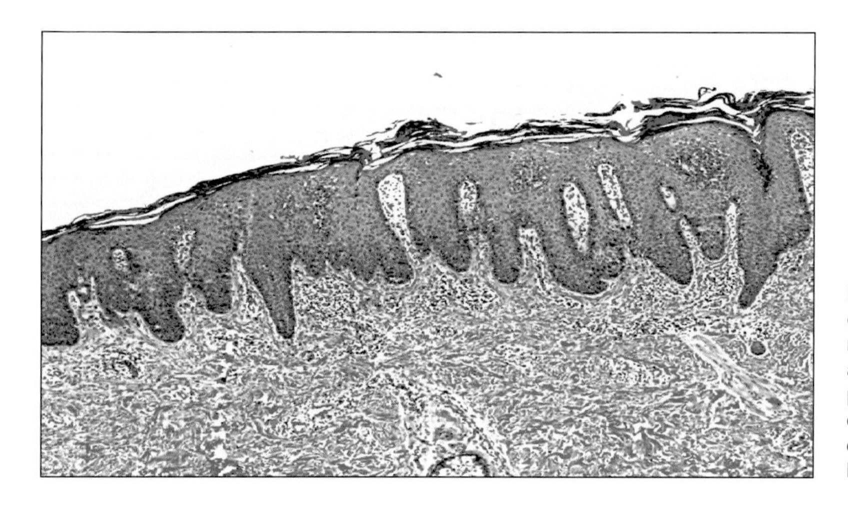

Fig. 8.3 Histology: parakeratosis, epidermal acanthosis with elongated rete ridges and loss of granular layer, and dilated, tortuous superficial papillary vessels consistent with chronic plaque psoriasis. (Photograph courtesy of Fitzgeraldo A. Sanchez Negron, MD and Hideko Kamino, MD)

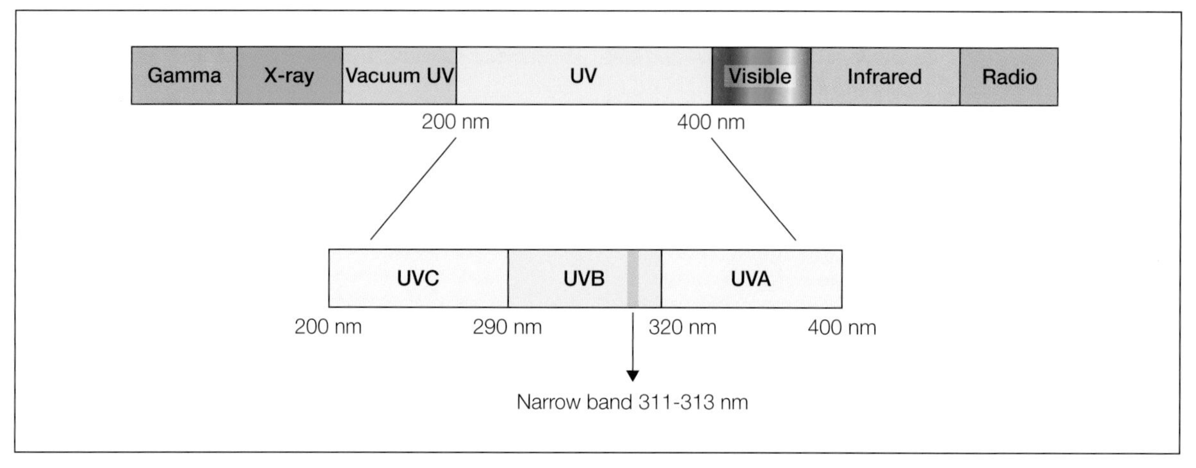

Fig. 8.4 Electromagnetic spectrum

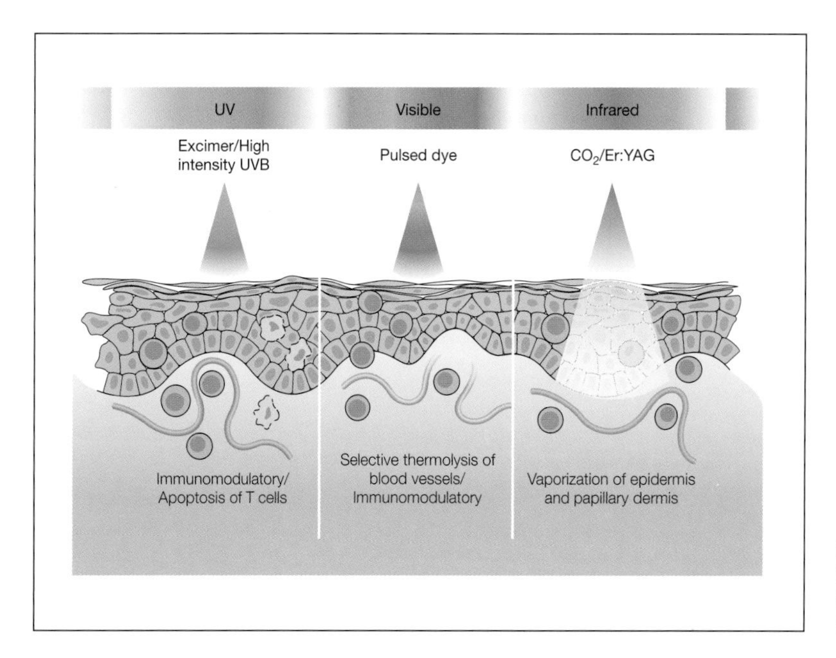

Fig. 8.5 Electromagnetic spectrum: mechanisms of lasers and light sources utilized for the treatment of psoriasis

Laser and light source and proposed mechanisms of action

CO_2/Er:YAG lasers
- Ablation of diseased epidermis and papillary dermis with depletion of epidermal/dermal inflammatory cells and mediators

Pulsed dye laser
- Selective ablation of papillary dermal vasculature
- Reduction of dermal inflammatory cells/mediators

Photodynamic therapy
- Sublethal damage to keratinocytes and/or inflammatory cells
- Damage to papillary dermal vasculature

Excimer laser/high intensity UVB light source
- Apoptosis of inflammatory T cells
- Depletion and/or suppression of Langerhans cells
- DNA damage with inhibition of keratinocyte proliferation

Box 8.3 Laser and light source and proposed mechanisms of action

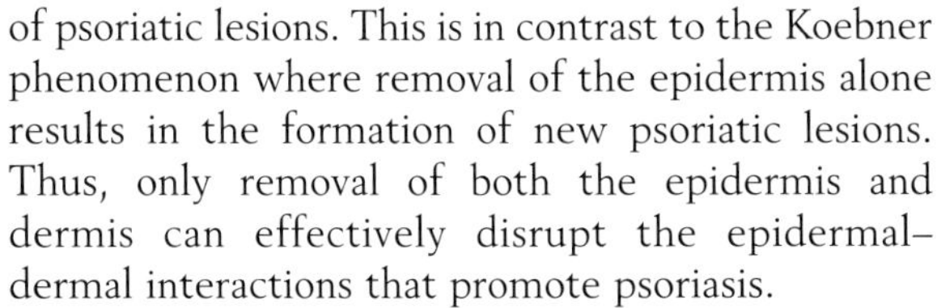

of psoriatic lesions. This is in contrast to the Koebner phenomenon where removal of the epidermis alone results in the formation of new psoriatic lesions. Thus, only removal of both the epidermis and dermis can effectively disrupt the epidermal–dermal interactions that promote psoriasis.

An alternative strategy targeted the hypervascularity of psoriatic lesions via selective vascular photothermolysis using the pulsed dye laser (PDL). Dilated, elongated, tortuous capillary loops, and increased capillary volume, are typically seen in psoriasis. These microvascular changes are postulated to contribute to the pathogenesis of psoriasis through promotion of inflammation and proliferation.

Photodynamic therapy (PDT) utilizing light and a photosensitizer has also been utilized for psoriasis. During the photodynamic reaction, a photosensitizer is excited by light, resulting in the generation of intracellular reactive oxygen species that selectively damage cells accumulating the photosensitizing agent. The most commonly used photosensitizer in dermatologic procedures is 5-aminolevulinic acid (5-ALA).

Recently, laser treatment of psoriasis has come full circle to focus again on wavelengths in the UVB range which are clinically proven to treat psoriasis by inducing apoptosis of disease mediating inflammatory T cells. The new high intensity UVB laser and light systems combine the proven clinical efficacy of UVB phototherapy with the advantages of focused, high dosage, lesion specific treatment minimizing the adverse effects of UV radiation. Uniform localized delivery of higher fluences also results in faster clearances with fewer treatments compared to conventional phototherapy.

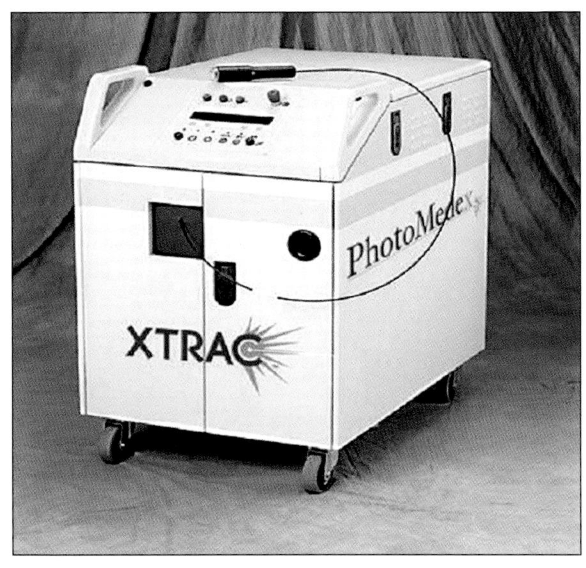

Fig. 8.6 The XTRAC excimer laser. (Reproduced with permission from PhotoMedex Inc, Radnor, PA, USA)

The excimer laser (Fig. 8.6) was the first clinically utilized system to provide localized high intensity UVB. The word excimer is based on two terms, 'excited' and 'dimmer'. When an inert gas such as xenon (Xe) and a reactive halide such as chloride (Cl) are bound in excited states, the diatomic molecules have short life spans and rapidly dissociate. This allows the molecules to act as a 'dimmer' with release of the excitation energy as highly coherent 308 nm UV light.

More recently, light sources utilizing a filtered mercury vapor arc lamp have been developed to provide high intensity incoherent UVB light (Fig. 8.7). The unit's peak irradiance of 311–315 nm overlaps with the therapeutic NB-UVB range.

Patient selection

Although lasers offer a novel treatment for psoriasis, the choice of therapy for each individual patient should be ultimately based on the type of lesion, their locations, and the body surface area involved. Although we will not address the myriad of topical,

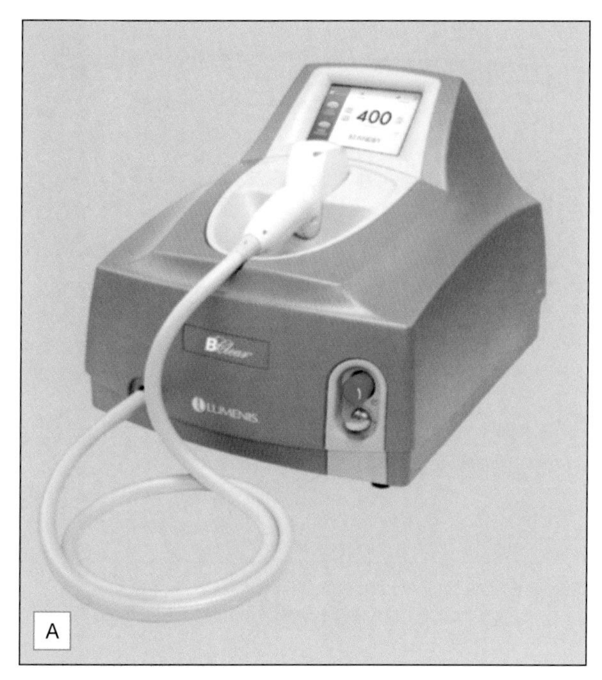

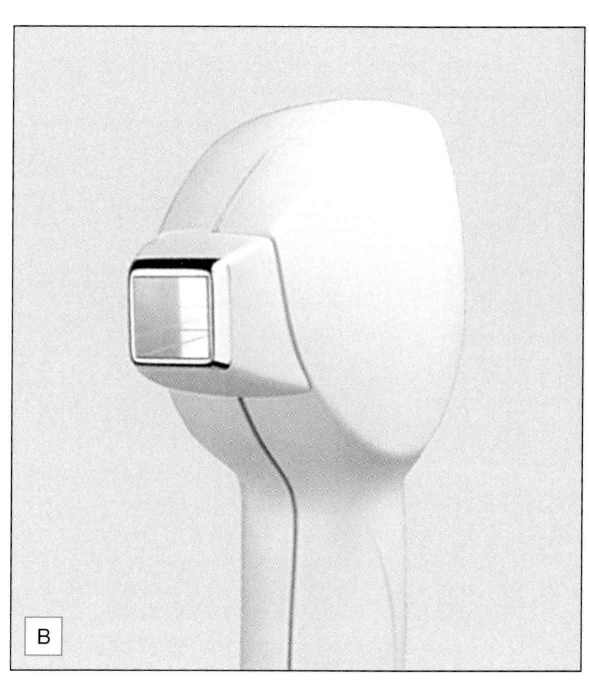

Fig. 8.7 The B*Clear* high intensity UVB photosystem. (Reproduced with permission from Lumenis Inc., Santa Clara, CA, USA)

Topical and intralesional agents in the treatment of psoriasis	
Treatment	**Disadvantage**
Emollients	Time consuming, messy, minimal clinical efficacy
Topical corticosteroids	Time consuming, messy, transient response, skin atrophy, striae, telangiectasia, HPA (hypothalamic–pituitary axis) suppression
Intralesional corticosteroids	Time consuming, transient response, skin atrophy, striae, telangiectasia, HPA suppression, painful, hypopigmentation at injection sites
Tar	Time consuming, messy, malodorous, transient response
Anthralin	Time consuming, messy, transient response, skin irritation
Topical retinoids	Time consuming, messy, transient response, skin irritation
Topical calcipotriene	Time consuming, messy, transient response, skin irritation
Keratolytics	Time consuming, messy, transient response, skin irritation

Table 8.1 Topical and intralesional agents in the treatment of psoriasis

systemic or biologic treatments currently used for psoriasis, a brief overview of available treatments is provided in Tables 8.1–8.4.

The ideal patient for laser treatment is one with chronic, stable, limited, well demarcated plaque or inverse type psoriasis. Patients who are recalcitrant to topical treatments, those seeking an alternative to frequent application of topical agents, or those who desire treatment offering longer term remissions should also be considered. Supplemental laser treatment can be used for select resistant plaques in patients receiving other systemic medications.

In terms of limitations, plaque type psoriasis involving large surface areas warrants systemic

Systemic agents in the treatment of psoriasis	
Treatment	**Disadvantages**
Methotrexate	Hepatotoxicity, myelosuppression, reactivation of phototoxic reactions Routine liver biopsies Laboratory monitoring
Acitretin	Teratogenicity, hepatotoxicity, hyperlipidemia Laboratory monitoring
Hydroxyurea	Myelosuppression Laboratory monitoring
Cyclosporin	Renal toxicity, hypertension Laboratory monitoring
Mycophenolate mofetil	Gastrointestinal side effects, leukopenia Laboratory monitoring
6-Thioguanine	Myelosuppression Laboratory monitoring

Table 8.2 Systemic agents in the treatment of psoriasis

Biologic agents in the treatment of psoriasis	
Treatment	**Disadvantage**
Infliximab	Intravenous infusions Immunosuppressive Laboratory monitoring, screening for tuberculosis
Etanercept	Subcutaneous injection Possibly immunosuppressive
Efalizumab	Subcutaneous injection Possibly immunosuppresive, thrombocytopenia Laboratory monitoring for platelet counts
Alefacept	Intravenous or intramuscular administration Immunosuppresive (lowered CD4 count) Laboratory monitoring for lymphocyte counts

Table 8.3 Biologic agents in the treatment of psoriasis

Phototherapy treatment of psoriasis	
Treatment	**Disadvantage**
PUVA	UV irradiation to uninvolved normal skin Nausea, photosensitivity Mandatory eye protection for 24 hours after each dose of psoralens Need to undress, need to cover face and genitalia Claustrophobia from enclosed light box Photoaging of normal skin Long term carcinogenicity (increased risk of squamous cell carcinomas, malignant melanomas, and Merkel cell carcinomas)
BB-UVB/ NB-UVB	UV irradiation to uninvolved normal skin Need to undress, need to cover face and genitalia Claustrophobia from enclosed light box Photoaging of normal skin Potential long term carcinogenicity

Table 8.4 Phototherapy treatment of psoriasis

Expected clinical outcomes		
Laser/light source	**Range of clinical outcomes**	**Maximum reported duration of remission**
CO_2/Er : YAG laser	Variable improvements to complete clearing	Up to 3.5 years reported
Pulsed dye laser	Gradual improvement to complete clearing depending on fluence, frequency, and number of treatment sessions	Up to 3 years reported
PDT	Gradual improvement to complete clearing depending on fluence, frequency, and number of treatment sessions	No long-term follow up data available
Excimer laser	Gradual improvement to complete clearing depending on fluence, frequency, and number of treatment sessions	Up to 2 years reported
High intensity UVB system	Gradual improvement to complete clearing depending on fluence, frequency, and number of treatment sessions	Up to 6 months reported

Table 8.5 Expected clinical outcomes

medications and/or conventional phototherapy. Similarly, patients with unstable disease who continually develop new lesions should be avoided, as UV irradiation of individual psoriatic plaques will not limit development of new lesions.

Expected benefits

A summary of expected benefits and objective data regarding the efficacy of treatment for each system is summarized in Tables 8.5 and 8.6. The potential complications from laser and light source treatments are summarized in Table 8.7.

CO_2 and Er : YAG laser

The CO_2 and Er : YAG lasers emit at wavelengths of 10 600 nm and 2940 nm, respectively. Both are strongly absorbed by water with resultant vaporization of tissue. In psoriasis, the best clinical outcomes with the CO_2 and Er : YAG lasers occur when ablation extends to the level of the papillary dermis, inducing the 'reverse Koebner' phenomenon.

Previous studies with the CO_2 laser have shown remissions of up to 3.5 years. Preprocedure anesthesia is necessary and multiple passes (2 to 22 reported) are necessary to achieve the clinical end point of papillary dermal ablation (Fig. 8.8, see p. 112).

Laser and light source: cost and expected reimbursement		
Laser/light source	**Cost of device**	**Reimbursement (cost/benefit ratio)**
CO_2 laser	Variable: $70 000 and up	Variable
Er : YAG laser	Variable: $70 000 and up	Variable
Pulsed dye laser	Approximately $85 000	Variable
PDT	Cost of 5-ALA + cost of laser or light source	Variable
Excimer laser (XTRAC, PhotoMedex, Radnor, PA, USA)	Laser is loaned by the company at $45–85 per treatment charge	Approximate reimbursement of laser treatment for inflammatory skin disease: $325–410 per treatment CPT 96920 (<500 cm^2) CPT 96921 (250–500 cm^2) CPT 96922 (>500 cm^2)
High intensity UVB system (BClear, Lumenis, Santa Clara, CA, USA)	Approximately $60 000	Approximate reimbursement for phototherapy: $45 per treatment CPT 96910

Table 8.6 Laser and light source: cost and expected reimbursement

Laser and light source and possible complications	
Laser/light source	**Possible complications**
CO_2/Er : YAG laser	Pigmentary alteration Persistent erythema Wound infection Atrophic or hypertrophic scarring
Pulsed dye laser	Blistering/erosion Pigmentary alteration Atrophic or hypertrophic scarring
PDT	Blistering/erosion Hyperpigmentation Atrophic or hypertrophic scarring
Excimer laser	Blistering/erosion Hyperpigmentation
High intensity UVB system	Blistering/erosion Hyperpigmentation

Table 8.7 Laser and light source and possible complications

Wound healing occurs over 2–6 weeks depending on the anatomic area treated and depth of tissue ablated. Biopsies of healed lesions reveal reversal of acanthosis and restoration of the granular layer (Fig. 8.8). Mild hypopigmentation is the most common complication seen, with only two occurrences of scarring on the lower extremities reported.

Pulsed dye laser

The rationale for using the pulsed dye laser for treating psoriasis is based on selective thermolysis of blood vessels. In addition, treatment with the pulsed dye laser has been shown to significantly reduce inflammatory T lymphocytes (Fig. 8.9), as well as levels of intracellular adhesion molecule 1 (ICAM-1) which are critical for attachment and migration of lymphocytes from blood vessels. Disruption of the interaction between the vasculature and inflammatory cells appears to be one of the key mechanisms of action of the pulsed dye laser.

Clearance is achieved in most cases after several (three to five) treatment sessions (Fig. 8.10). The degree of improvement is contingent on the fluence used, with fluences under 5–7 J/cm^2 minimally effective. Treatment is quick and preoperative anesthesia is usually not required. Most published reports of the pulsed dye laser for the treatment of psoriasis have utilized the 585 nm pulsed dye laser. A recent report indicates that similar effects can be achieved with the 595 nm long-pulsed dye laser when used at purpuragenic settings.

Photodynamic therapy

The use of PDT to treat psoriasis was first reported in 1937 with systemically administered hematoporphyrin and ultraviolet radiation. Porphyrin precur-

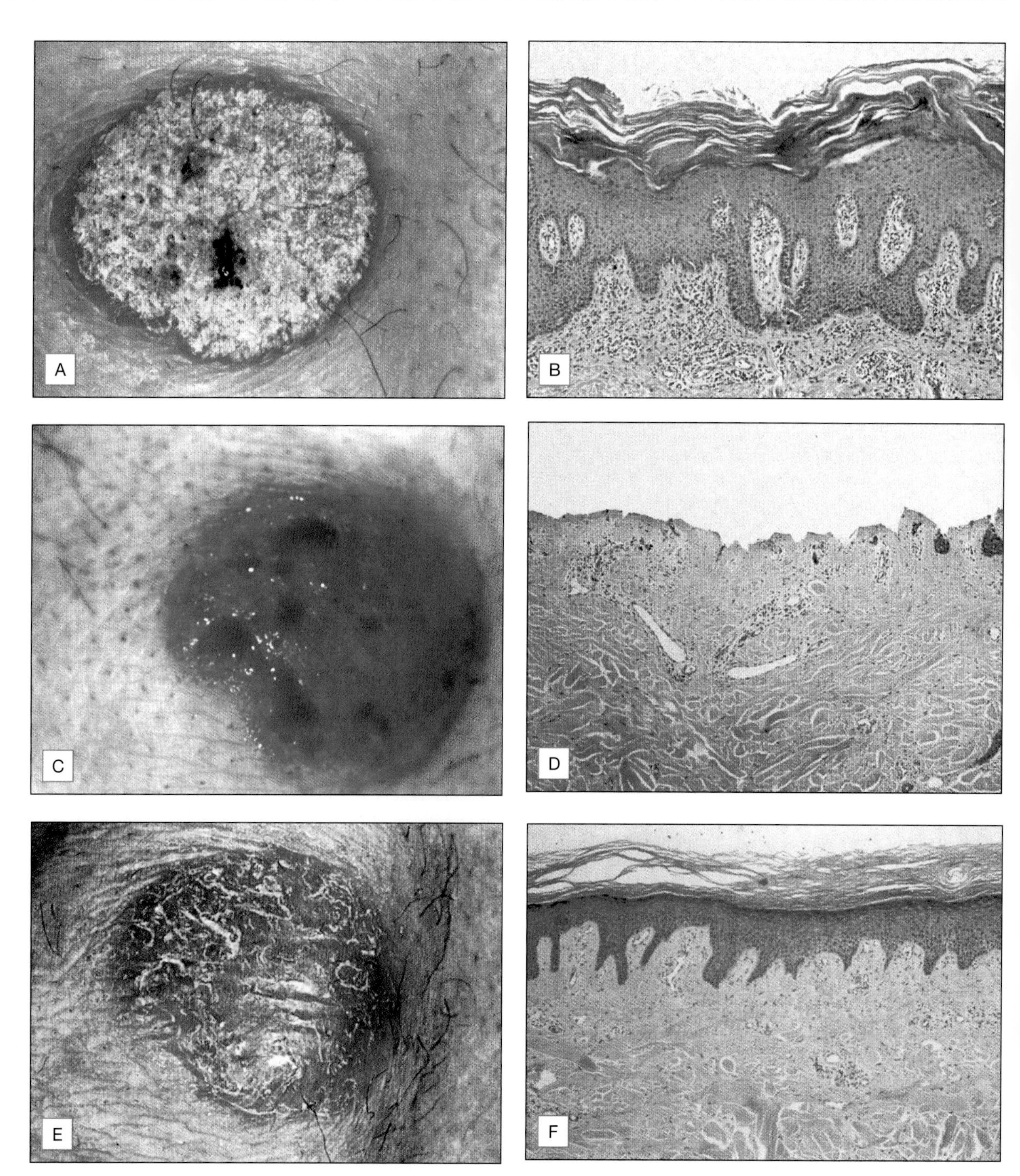

Fig. 8.8 (**A,B**) Psoriatic plaque on knee and corresponding histology prior to therapy. (**C,D**) Clinical finding and histology immediately after Er : YAG laser therapy. (**E,F**) 4 weeks after treatment. (Reproduced with permission from Boehncke WH, Ochsendorf F, Wolter M 1999 Ablative techniques in psoriasis vulgaris resistant to conventional therapies. Dermatologic Surgery 25:618–621)

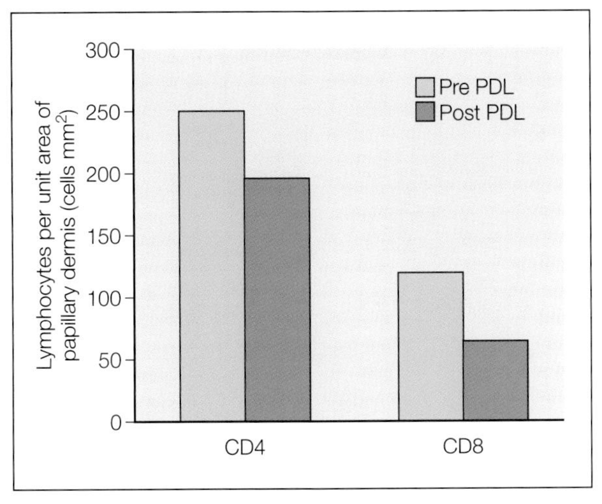

Fig. 8.9 CD4 and CD8 T lymphocytes in the superficial dermis, before and after pulsed dye laser (PDL) treatment. (Modifed from Hern S, Allen MH, Sousa AR, et al 2001 Immunohistochemical evaluation of psoriatic plaques following selective photothermolysis of the superficial capillaries. British Journal of Dermatology 145:45–53)

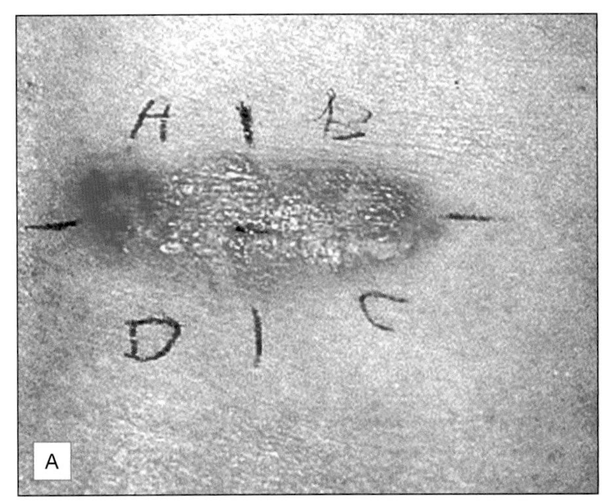

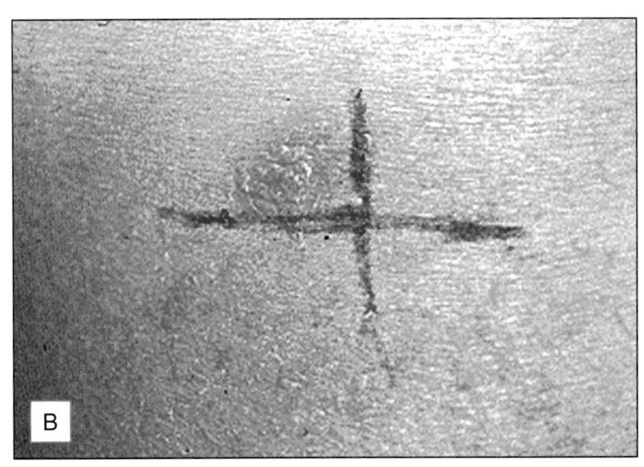

Fig. 8.10 Psoriatic lesions: (**A**) Baseline. (**B**) 6 months after 3 treatments with the pulsed dye laser: Left upper quadrant (A) - control; Right upper quadrant (B) - 585 nm pulsed dye laser at 7 J/cm; Right lower quadrant (C) - 595 nm pulsed dye laser at 10 J/cm, without dynamic cooling device; Left lower quadrant (D) - 595 nm pulsed dye laser at 10 J/cm with dynamic cooling device 30 ms with 10 ms delay. Note persistence of psoriasis lesions in control area on left upper quadrant. (Courtesy of JM Mazer, MD)

sors or derivatives, with peak absorption in the 400–650 nm range, are used as the photosensitizers. Most recently, 5-ALA, a porphyrin precursor converted intracellularly to protoporphyrin IX, has been used clinically. It has the advantage of a short half-life, reducing the risk of prolonged systemic photosensitivity.

5-ALA has been shown to selectively localize to psoriatic plaques and to induce apoptosis of lesional T lymphocytes. Topical ALA is applied 4–5 hours prior to photoactivation with lasers or light sources in the 400–700 nm range. A series of treatments is usually necessary with variable clinical response. To date, long term follow up has not been reported.

Excimer laser and high intensity localized UVB systems

The excimer laser produces 308 nm monochromatic ultraviolet light. The light is delivered unattenuated through a fiberoptic delivery system. A high intensity localized UVB photosystem is also available which produces incoherent light with peak irradiance between 311 and 315 nm.

The use of the excimer laser and high intensity UVB photosystem for psoriasis is based on the effects of UVB radiation on keratinocyte proliferation and its ability to induce apoptosis of inflammatory T lymphocytes (Fig. 8.11). The prolonged remittive effect of UV light is due primarily to depletion of inflammatory T cells. Recent studies have demonstrated greater T cell apoptosis with the excimer laser versus conventional NB-UVB which correlates with the improved clinical efficacy of the excimer laser.

Two basic treatment paradigms can be utilized. Either high fluences are administered during few treatment sessions, or low to medium fluences are administered over multiple sessions with incremental dosage increases similar to conventional photo-

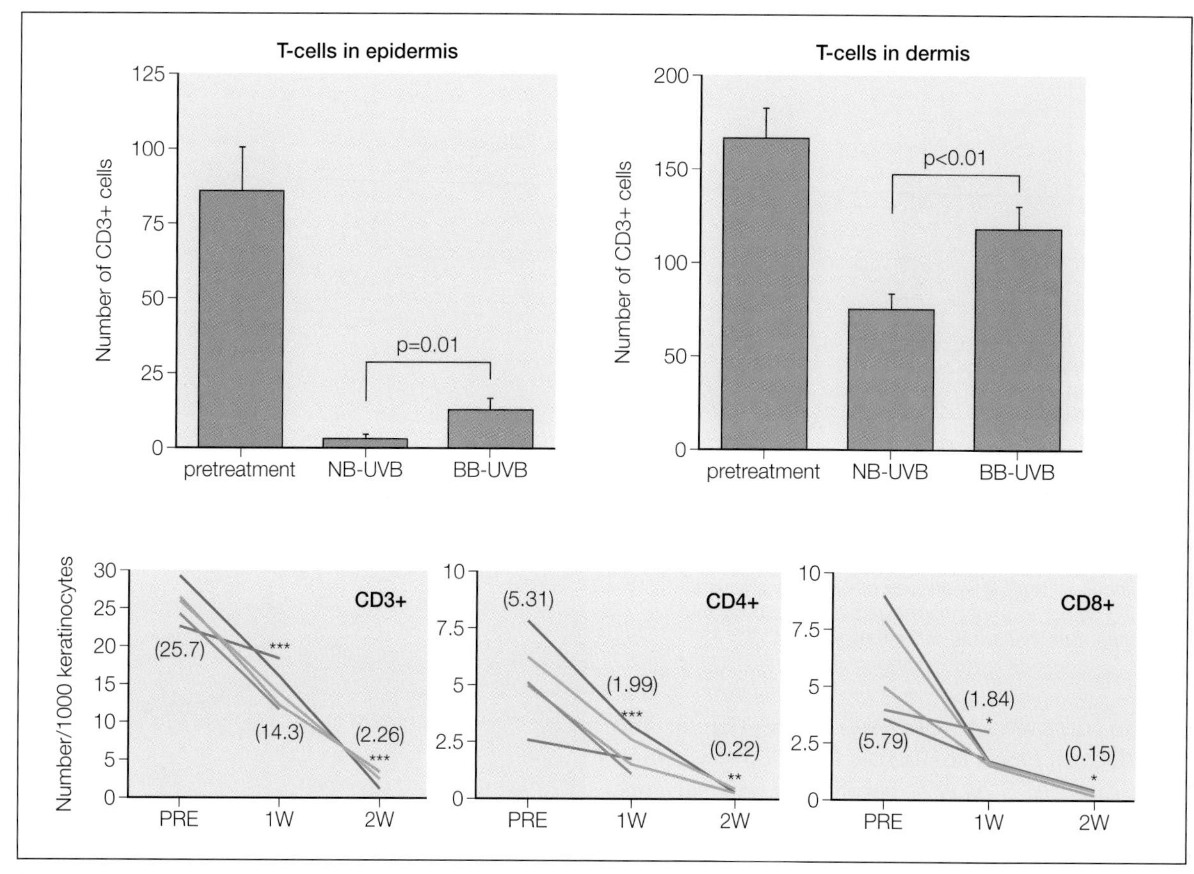

Fig. 8.11 Quantitative analysis of T cell infiltration in psoriatic skin before treatment and after treatment with NB-UVB and BB-UVB. (Reproduced with permission from Ozawa M, Ferenczi K, Kikuchi T, et al 1999 312-nanometer ultraviolet B light (narrow-band UVB) induces apoptosis of T cells within psoriatic lesions. Journal of Experimental Medicine 189:711–718)

therapy (Figs 8.12–8.14). Higher fluences may produce faster and longer remissions, but are associated with greater risk of phototoxic reactions. The clinical performance of the excimer and high intensity localized UVB systems are similar with regard to the rate and extent of clearance. The ability of these systems to focally deliver UVB radiation has been utilized to treat inverse (Fig. 8.15, see p. 117) and scalp psoriasis (Fig. 8.16, see p. 117), which are typically not amenable to conventional phototherapy.

In comparison to NB-UVB which can achieve 78.5% improvement over 20 sessions with a mean cumulative dose of 15.1 J/cm^2, the excimer laser achieved similar improvements over only 10 sessions with a mean cumulative dose of 8.75 J/cm^2. Remissions of up to 2 years have been reported. Fluence appears to be the single most important factor for clinical clearance. A recent review showed faster clinical clearing with the excimer laser than with topical medications, conventional phototherapy, and even systemic agents (Table 8.8, see p. 18).

Overview of Treatment Strategy

A thorough patient evaluation should be performed prior to treatment with lasers or light sources (Box 8.4, see p. 18). A history of current medical conditions, medications, allergies, and past surgeries including problems with bleeding or wound healing should be obtained. In the case of ablative laser treatment, any recent history of retinoid use or a history of herpes simplex at or near the treatment area should be elicited. With the high intensity UVB systems, use of medications that are photosensitizing or that decrease the thickness of psoriatic plaques should be noted. In addition, any history of photosensitizing conditions would preclude treatment with ultraviolet radiation.

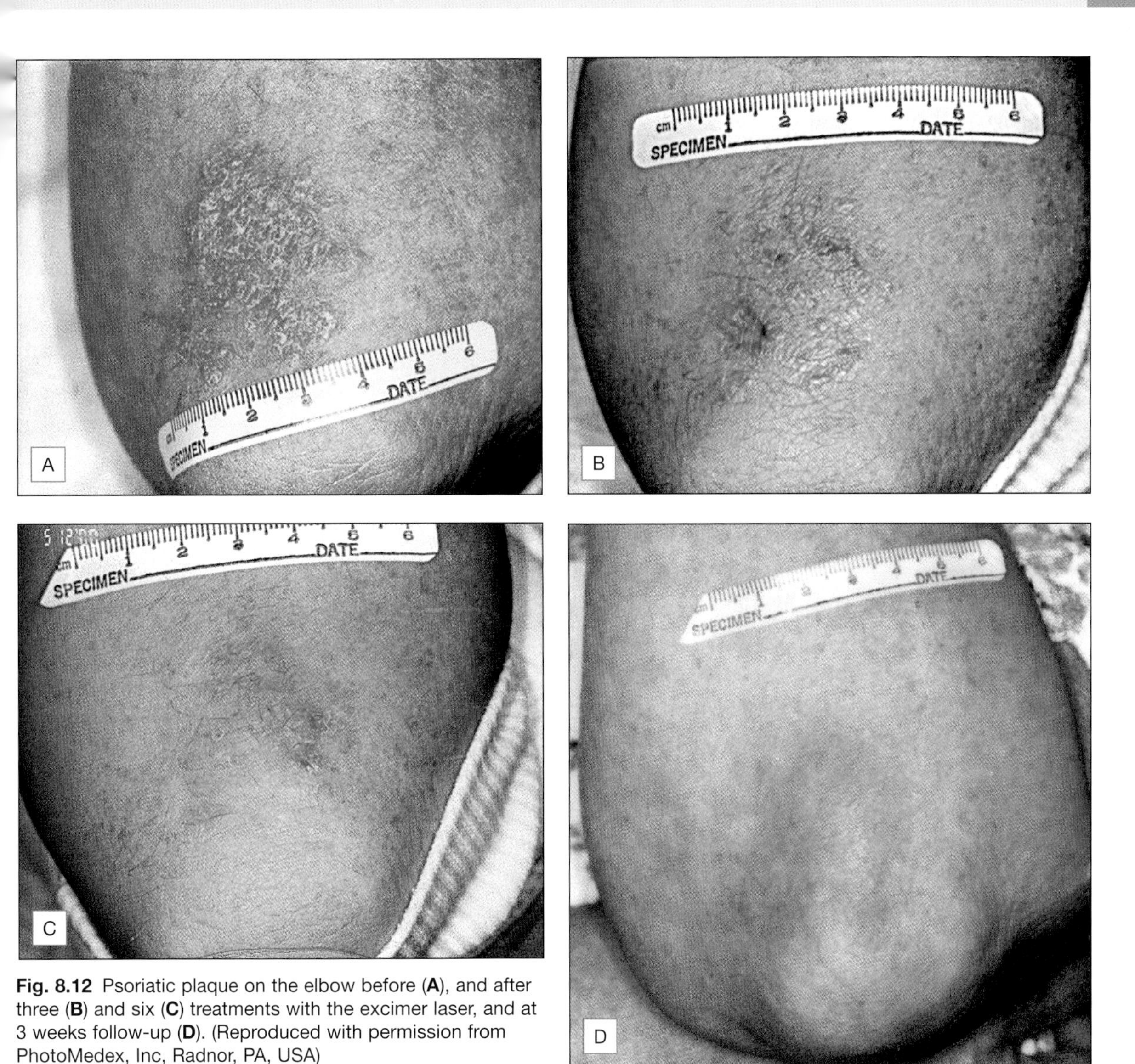

Fig. 8.12 Psoriatic plaque on the elbow before (**A**), and after three (**B**) and six (**C**) treatments with the excimer laser, and at 3 weeks follow-up (**D**). (Reproduced with permission from PhotoMedex, Inc, Radnor, PA, USA)

In reality, the availability of and costs associated with procuring and/or using the equipment may be the major determining factor for the use of laser and high intensity light sources for the treatment of psoriasis. For ablative and pulsed dye lasers, their primary use for other indications likely determines whether a practice procures the equipment. With the excimer laser and high intensity UVB systems, the cost of the laser or light source is less, but because these systems can be used only for the treatment of psoriasis and vitiligo, it is important to assess the volume of patients that would utilize these systems prior to making the investment.

Treatment Techniques

Patients

The proper selection of patients is the critical first step (Box 8.5, Fig. 8.17, see pp. 118 and 119). Patients with stable plaque or inverse psoriasis with limited body surface area involvement can be considered for treatment. Also in patients with widespread skin disease but with few recalcitrant plaques, laser treatment can be used as a supplement to conventional treatments. The patient should be counseled to have realistic expectations in terms of possible outcomes and the number of treatment sessions,

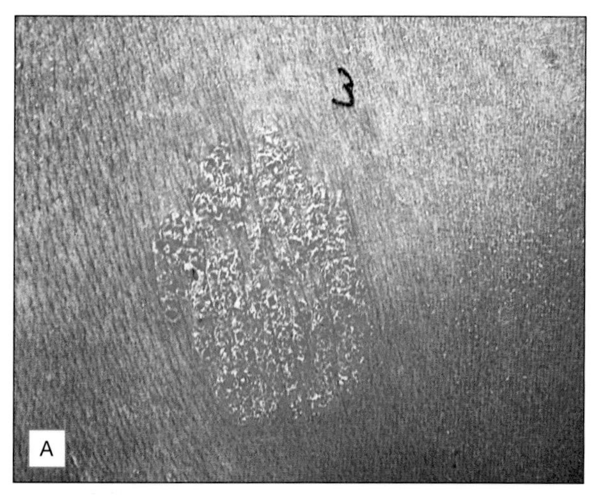

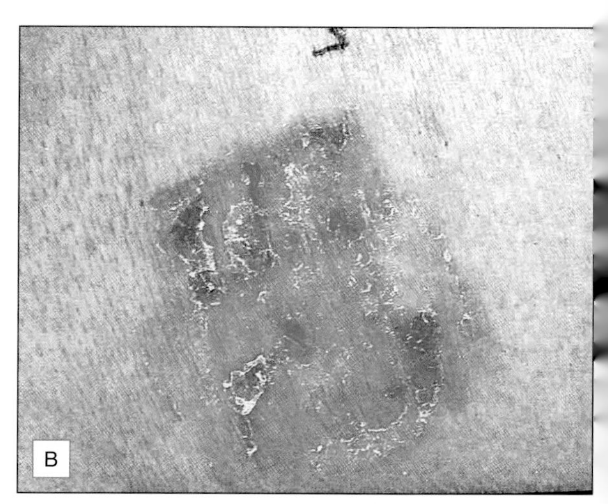

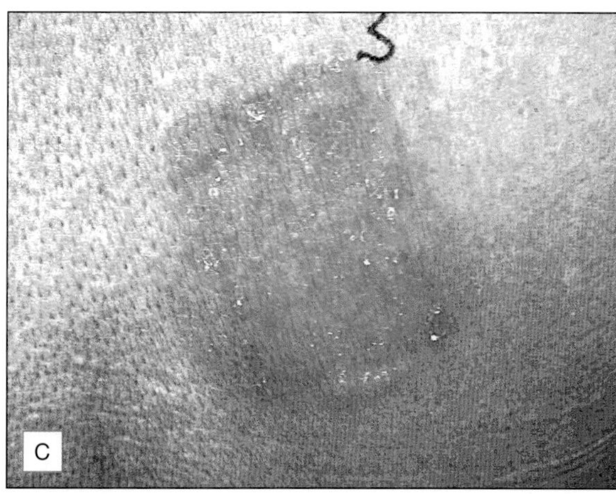

Fig. 8.13 Psoriatic plaque at baseline (**A**) and after two (**B**) and six (**C**) treatments with the B*Clear* high intensity UVB photosystem at 3× MED. (Photographs courtesy of and with permission from Christine Dierickx, MD and Lumenis Inc.)

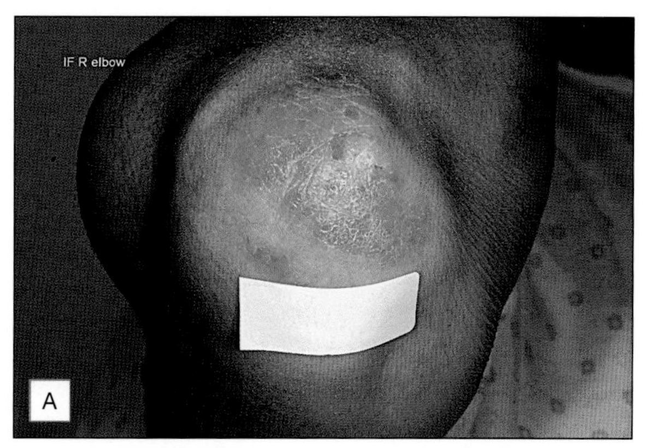

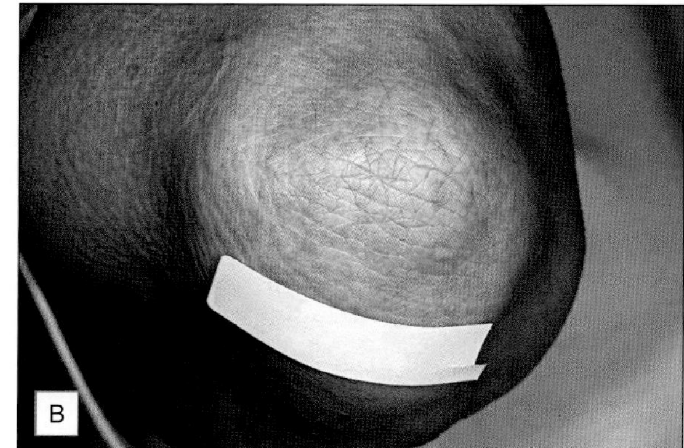

Fig. 8.14 Psoriatic plaque on the elbow at baseline (**A**) and after three treatments (**B**) with the B*Clear* high intensity UVB photosystem with a total cumulative dose of 12 MED (Photographs courtesy of and with permission from Emil A. Tanghetti, MD and Lumenis Inc.)

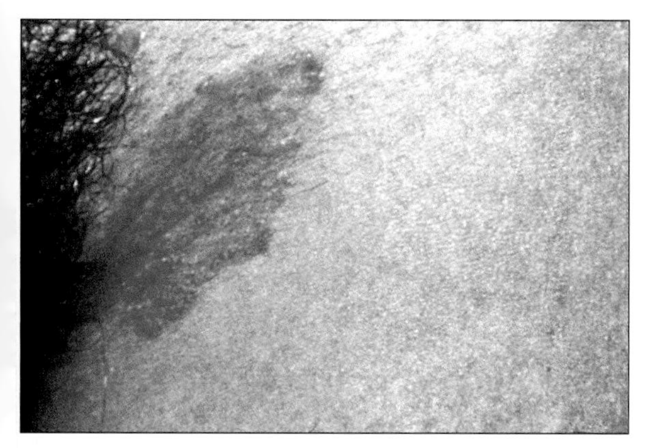

Fig. 8.15 Inguinal area with erythematous, elevated, inverse psoriatic plaque at baseline. (Reproduced with permission from Mafong E, Friedman PM, et al 2002 Treatment of inverse psoriasis with the 308 nm excimer laser. Dermatologic Surgery 28:530–532)

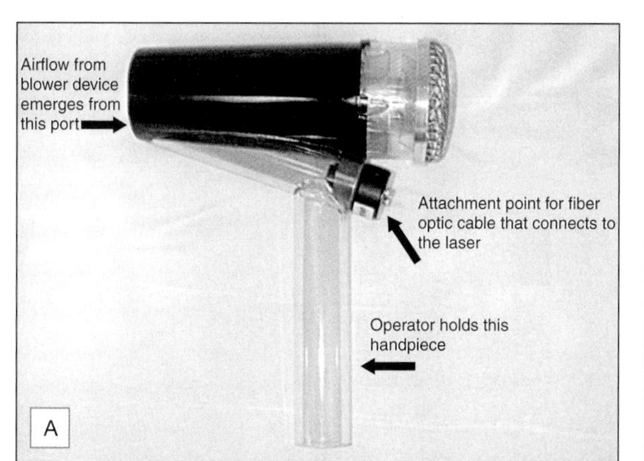

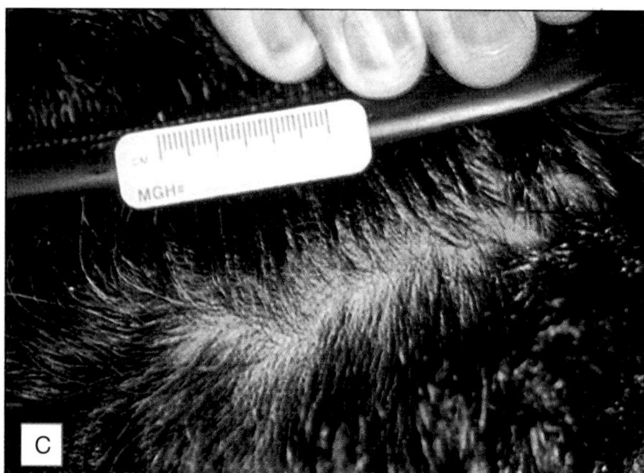

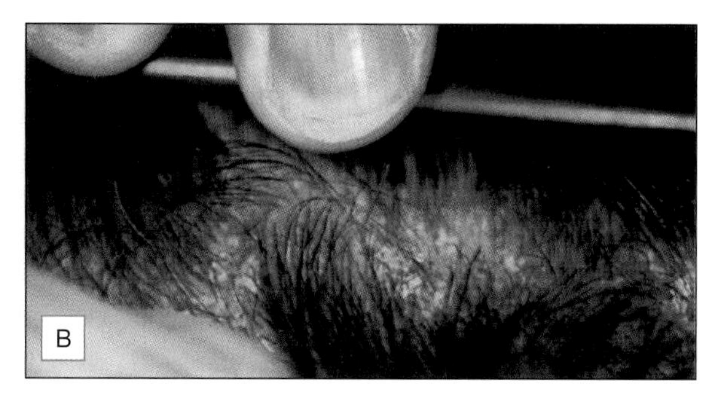

Fig. 8.16 (**A**) Air blower device adaptor on the excimer laser hand piece allowing for treatment of scalp psoriasis. (**B**) Scalp psoriasis before treatment. (**C**) Scalp after 23 treatments with the excimer laser. (Reproduced with permission from Taylor CR, Racette AL 2004 A 308-nm excimer laser for the treatment of scalp psoriasis. Lasers in Surgery and Medicine 34:136–140)

Comparison of UVB laser to various treatments for psoriasis		
Treatment	**Percent achieving 75% improvement**	**Number of days to 75% improvement**
UVB laser	72	36
Calcipotriene 0.005%	70	56
Tazarotene 0.1%	58	84
Fluocinonide 0.05%	68	84
Acitretin 50–75 mg	25	56
PUVA	80	98
Ciclosporin 2.5–3 mg/kg/day	50	84–252
Etanercept 25 mg	26	56
Infliximab 5 mg/kg	82	28

Table 8.8 Comparison of UVB laser to various treatments for psoriasis. (Adapted from Rodewald EJ, Housman TS, Mellen BG, et al 2002 Follow-up survey of 308-nm laser treatment of psoriasis. Lasers in Surgery and Medicine 31:202–206)

Patient interview checklist

- How long have you had psoriasis?
- What treatments are you currently using for your psoriasis?
- What past treatments have you used for psoriasis?
- Have you had a biopsy to confirm the diagnosis?
- Is there any family history of psoriasis?
- What are your current medications (any photosensitizing medications, any use of isotretinoin in the past 6 months)?
- Are you able to come for regular treatment sessions two or three times per week? (for excimer laser and high intensity UVB systems)
- Do you have any joint pain or swelling?
- Is there any previous personal or family history of skin cancers?
- Do you have any photosensitizing conditions (lupus erythematosus, porphyria, etc.)?
- If treating ablatively – do you have any history of locoregional herpes?

Box 8.4 Patient interview checklist

Patient characteristics

Ideal patient

- Has stable plaque or inverse psoriasis
- Understands treatment protocol and associated risks
- Has realistic expectations
- Willing to comply with postoperative care and follow up

Problematic patient

- Has widespread or unstable plaque psoriasis, guttate, pustular or erythrodermic psoriasis
- Unable to understand treatment protocol or associated risks
- Has unrealistic expectations that lasers can 'cure' psoriasis
- Needs to travel long distances and unable to appear for follow up or frequent treatments

Box 8.5 Patient characteristics

and should be aware of prolonged healing times that can be associated with some of the laser procedures.

Equipment

CO_2 and Er : YAG laser treatment

CO_2 lasers can be divided into two general groups: pulsed or scanned. Both can be used to effectively vaporize psoriatic plaques. There are also many different Er : YAG lasers currently available and any of these can be effectively used. The ultimate decision of which laser to obtain will rely largely on what other procedures the lasers will be utilized for. Ancillary supplies necessary for the treatment with the CO_2 or Er : YAG lasers are listed in Box 8.6.

Pulsed dye laser treatment

The 585 nm and the longer pulsed 595 nm lasers are highly versatile, and used in the treatment of vascular lesions as well as nonvascular lesions such as warts, striae, and hypertrophic scars. Although previously published reports using the pulsed dye laser for psoriasis have utilized the 585 nm pulsed

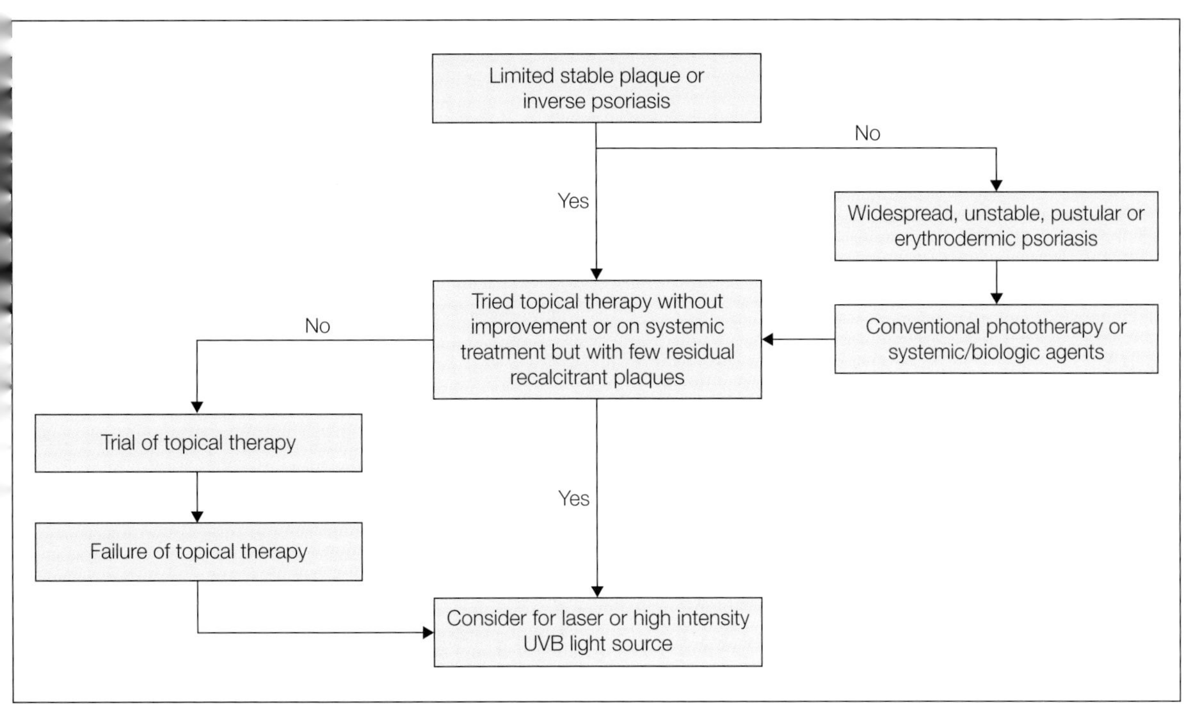

Fig. 8.17 General treatment approach guideline: flow chart

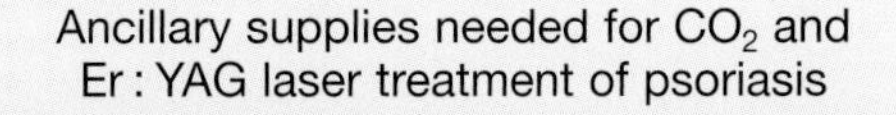

Ancillary supplies needed for CO_2 and Er : YAG laser treatment of psoriasis

- Safety goggles for operating personnel and protective eye shields for the patient
- Local anesthesia: injectable lidocaine (lignocaine), syringes, 30 gauge needle for injection
- Wet drapes to protect adjacent nontreated areas
- Procedure tray: saline or water soaked gauze, dry gauze, cotton tip applicators
- Hydrophilic petrolatum or antibiotic ointment
- Nonadherent dressing

Box 8.6 Ancillary supplies needed for CO_2 and Er : YAG laser treatment of psoriasis

Ancillary supplies needed for pulsed dye laser treatment of psoriasis

- Safety goggles for operating personnel and protective eye shields for the patient
- Topical anesthetic cream if treating at higher fluences or over larger areas
- Mineral oil to enhance laser penetration
- Hydrophilic petrolatum or antibiotic ointment
- Nonadherent dressing or hydrogel dressing

Box 8.7 Ancillary supplies needed for pulsed dye laser treatment of psoriasis

dye laser, similar clinical efficacy has been recently reported with the 595 nm laser. The pulsed dye laser is well tolerated and only occasionally requires the use of topical anesthesia. The use of a hydrogel dressing such as Vigilon (Bard, Seton Healthcare Group, Oldham, UK) is useful after treatment to minimize pain and purpura. Ancillary supplies necessary for treatment with the pulsed dye laser are listed in Box 8.7.

Photodynamic therapy

Many different lasers and incoherent light sources (400–700 nm) can be used for photodynamic therapy (Box 8.8). In fact, one of the most commonly used light sources to activate 5-ALA is an inexpensive modified slide projector. Topical treatment with 5-ALA is preferable and associated with less systemic side effects. 5-ALA can be prepared as 5–20% emulsions and is also commercially available

Common light sources used for PDT

- Argon laser
- Gold vapor laser
- Copper vapor laser
- Q-switched Nd : YAG laser
- Potassium-titanyl-phosphate (KTP) laser
- Pulsed dye laser
- Light emitting diode (LED)
- Red light
- Blue light
- Intense pulsed light devices
- White light from a modified slide projector

Box 8.8 Common light sources used for PDT

as a topical 20% solution (Levulan Kerastick, Dusa, Wilmington, MA, USA). Treatment may be associated with significant pain, and it may be prudent to use topical anesthesia prior to treatment. Ancillary supplies necessary for PDT are listed in Box 8.9.

Ancillary supplies necessary for topical PDT

- 5–20% ALA emulsion
- Local anesthesia: topical anesthetic cream or injectable lidocaine (lignocaine), syringes, 30 gauge needle for injection
- Appropriate eye protection for operating personnel and protective eye shields for the patient
- Procedure tray: water, gauze
- Hydrophilic petrolatum or antibiotic ointment
- Nonadherent dressing

Box 8.9 Ancillary supplies necessary for topical PDT

UVB lasers and light sources

The XTRAC excimer laser (PhotoMedex, Radnor, PA, USA) and the high intensity UVB light source currently marketed as the B*Clear* Targeted PhotoClearing System (Lumenis Inc, Santa Clara, CA, USA) are the most common localized UVB systems currently used. Treatments with both systems are well tolerated. Ancillary supplies required for treatment are listed in Box 8.10.

Ancillary supplies necessary for excimer laser or high intensity UVB light treatment of psoriasis

- Appropriate eye protection for operating personnel and protective eye shields for the patient
- Mineral oil to enhance penetration
- Procedure tray: gauze to wipe off mineral oil

Box 8.10 Ancillary supplies necessary for excimer laser or high intensity UVB light treatment of psoriasis

Treatment algorithm

The specific treatment parameters for each laser or light source will depend on many different factors, including anatomic area being treated, the patient's skin type, and individual response to treatment. General guidelines for treatments and potential avoidable pitfalls are outlined in Table 8.9 and Box 8.11.

Preprocedure planning

The patient should be informed on all aspects of the procedure as well as the risks and benefits of the procedure, and written consent should be obtained prior to treatment. Written postoperative instructions and potential costs involved should also be provided in writing. Photographs can be obtained at baseline and at appropriate intervals to monitor progress. In general, the use of keratolytics for 1–2 weeks prior to treatment can thin the plaques and improve laser penetration.

CO_2 and Er : YAG laser

Pretreatment

Antiviral prophylaxis should be provided to patients with a history of herpes outbreaks around the treatment area. Treatment should start 1 day prior to laser treatment and continued for 10 days. Oral antibiotics can be considered if larger areas are treated, and particularly if lower extremity lesions are treated. The areas to be treated should be anesthetized with lidocaine (lignocaine) injections prior to treatment.

Treatment technique

The actual number of laser passes will depend on the anatomic area and the thickness of the lesion. A first pass with minimal overlap should be performed, followed by gentle wiping with moist gauze until all coagulated debris is removed. For thick plaques, several initial passes may be necessary to remove the hyperkeratotic epidermis. Subsequent passes are made until the pink-gray color

Laser/light	Pretreatment	Anesthesia	Post-treatment
CO_2/Er : YAG	Keratolytics for thick plaques prior to treatment Consider antiviral prophylaxis if any history of locoregional herpes Consider antibiotic prophylaxis if treating larger areas, particularly on the lower extremity	Injection with lidocaine (lignocaine) and epinephrine (adrenaline)	Wound care with saline soaked gauze two times per day and dressing changes with hydrophilic petrolatum or antibiotic ointment Sun avoidance
Pulsed dye	Keratolytics for thick plaques prior to treatment Mineral oil to enhance laser penetration	None or topical numbing cream	Hydrogel dressing, hydrophilic petrolatum, or antibiotic ointment if any blistering or erosions develop Sun avoidance
PDT	Keratolytics for thick plaques prior to treatment Application of topical ALA 5–20% 4–5 hours prior to treatment	May consider topical numbing cream or injection with lidocaine (lignocaine) and epinephrine (adrenaline)	Hydrogel dressing, hydrophilic petrolatum or antibiotic ointment if any blistering or erosions develop Sun avoidance
Excimer/high intensity UVB systems	Keratolytics for thick plaques prior to treatment Obtain MED Mineral oil to enhance laser penetration	None	Hydrophilic petrolatum or antibiotic ointment if any blistering or erosions develop

Table 8.9 Laser and light source: pretreatment, anesthesia, and post-treatment care

Common pitfalls to avoid

- Inappropriate patient selection: unstable or widespread psoriasis
- Not obtaining a MED prior to start of treatment with the excimer laser or high intensity UVB light source
- Not pretreating thick plaques with keratolytics or using mineral oil for thick plaques
- Not adjusting the dosage of laser or light source delivered once plaques begin to thin or hyperpigment

Box 8.11 Common pitfalls to avoid

of the papillary dermis disappears and is replaced by a yellow color consistent with the reticular dermis. Ablation of both the epidermis and the papillary dermis is critical in order to obtain local remission.

Postoperative care

Wound care should be performed twice daily by cleansing the treated areas with saline soaked gauze. The areas should be covered with hydrophilic petrolatum or antibiotic ointment and a non-adherent dressing for the first 2–3 days after the procedure, and thereafter kept moist to promote healing. The treated skin will exhibit erythema and edema, and serous exudates will be present for several days. Healing should be closely monitored, particularly since nonfacial areas can take longer to heal.

Side effects and complications

Side effects of ablative CO_2 or Er : YAG laser treatments can be minimized with good preoperative preparation and fastidious postoperative care. Some erythema at the treated site is common during the healing process and can last 1–3 months. While there is residual erythema, sun avoidance will reduce the risk of postinflammatory hyperpigmentation. Hyperpigmenation can be improved with the use of bleaching creams, as well as strict sun avoidance. Permanent hypopigmentation can also occur less commonly with deeper ablation into the reticular dermis. Bacterial infections are minimized with the use of prophylactic antibiotics when appropriate. Pain, swelling, persistent erythema, failure to heal, and purulent drainage from the treated sites should prompt a search for an underlying infection. Yeast infections, particularly candidiais, can also occur as a complication. The risk of scarring is generally small but may be higher on the lower extremities.

Pulsed dye laser

Pretreatment

There is usually minimal treatment pain and anesthesia is not necessary. However, depending on the fluence, anatomic area to be treated, and patient preference, a topical numbing cream may be applied 30–60 minutes prior to treatment to decrease discomfort. Mineral oil may be applied to the lesion to enhance penetration of the laser prior to treatment.

Treatment technique

There should be minimal overlap between treatment pulses. For the 585 nm pulsed dye laser (450 μs pulse duration, 5 mm spot size), a starting fluence of 7–8 J/cm^2 is recommended. A higher starting fluence of 10 J/cm^2 with a short pulse duration of 1.5 ms is recommended for the 595 nm pulsed dye laser. The high fluence and short pulse duration are necessary to achieve purpura, which appears necessary for the successful treatment. Several treatments (three to five) at intervals between 2 and 3 weeks are typically necessary to obtain clinical improvement. Fluences may be kept unchanged or fluence can be incrementally increased by 0.5 J/cm^2 per treatment, as tolerated, until clinical clearing.

Postoperative care

The skin may appear purpuric and edematous, but the purpura will typically resolve in 7–14 days. A hydrogel dressing (Vigilon) is helpful in minimizing post-treatment pain and edema. At higher fluences, some patients can develop superficial erosion and crusting, requiring wound care with topical antibiotic ointment or hydrophilic petrolatum until the areas heal. To prevent hyperpigmentation, the treated area should be kept out of sunlight and protected with sunscreen.

Side effects and complications

Side effects of the PDL are uncommon, with transient hyperpigmentation being the most likely adverse event. The hyperpigmentation can be managed as discussed previously. Rarely, blistering can occur at treated sites if excessively high fluences are used or there is excessive overlapping of laser pulses. Scarring from PDL treatment is extremely rare but may occur on the lower extremities.

Topical ALA-PDT

Pretreatment

Topical 5-ALA should be applied and left on for 4–5 hours prior to treatment. Once 5-ALA is applied, the areas should be protected from excessive ambient light. For the treatment of actinic keratoses, 20% ALA solution (Levulan Kerastick™) has been shown to be effective with as little as a 3 hour application. However, this accelerated protocol has not yet been tested on psoriasis lesions. There is usually pain associated with treatment and anesthesia with topical or injectable lidocaine (lignocaine) prior to the treatment may be advisable particularly if large areas are treated.

Treatment technique

The appropriate light source or laser should be used to activate the porphyrins.

Postoperative care

The skin may appear erythematous, purpuric and edematous after treatment. Although hydrophilic petrolatum or antibiotic ointment can be applied postoperatively, a cool hydrogel dressing (Vigilon) can minimize pain. Topical antibiotic ointment or hydrophilic petrolatum can be applied if any blisters or erosions form. To avoid phototoxic reactions, the patient should avoid any sunlight or intense visible light for 24 hours. Sun avoidance and sunscreens will prevent hyperpigmentation.

Side effects and complications

Potential side effects of PDT vary with the photosensitizer and light source used. Cutaneous photosensitivity is common and patients should avoid exposure to any intense light for 24 hours after application of the photosensitizer to avoid a 'sunburn' reaction. Occasional blistering may occur and hyperpigmentation can occur at treated sites. Very rarely scarring can occur particularly on the lower extremities. A single case of allergic contact dermatitis has been reported with topical 5-ALA methylester but not 5-ALA.

Excimer laser or high intensity UVB light source

Pretreatment

The skin type of the patient should be determined and minimal erythema dose (MED) testing should be performed on non-sun-exposed areas of the skin such as the inner arm or buttock at least 1 day prior to treatment. Suggested fluences for MED test spots are shown in Table 8.10. Patients return 24 hours later and the minimal dosage resulting in obvious erythema is designated as the MED (Fig. 8.18).

Weekly or biweekly treatments are typically required (Fig. 8.19). Treatments are quick and take less than 2–3 minutes for a 10 cm^2 lesion. Most patients feel no sensation or only mild warmth at the treatment site. As such, anesthesia is not necessary.

Proposed MED range for test spots (mJ/cm^2) for high intensity UVB system			
MED test spot	**Skin types I–II**	**Skin types III–IV**	**Skin types V–VI**
1	100	150	200
2	130	190	250
3	160	230	300
4	190	270	350
5	220	310	400
6	260	350	450

Table 8.10 Proposed MED range for test spots (mJ/cm^2) for high intensity UVB system

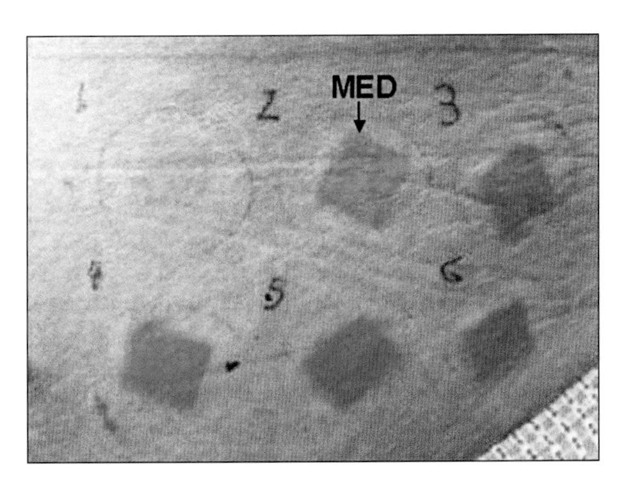

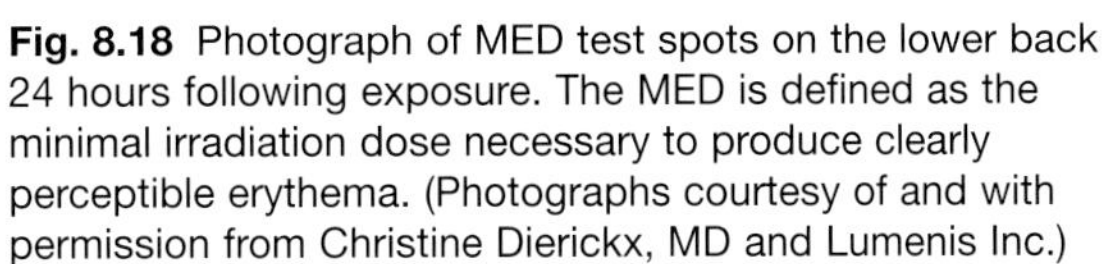

Fig. 8.18 Photograph of MED test spots on the lower back 24 hours following exposure. The MED is defined as the minimal irradiation dose necessary to produce clearly perceptible erythema. (Photographs courtesy of and with permission from Christine Dierickx, MD and Lumenis Inc.)

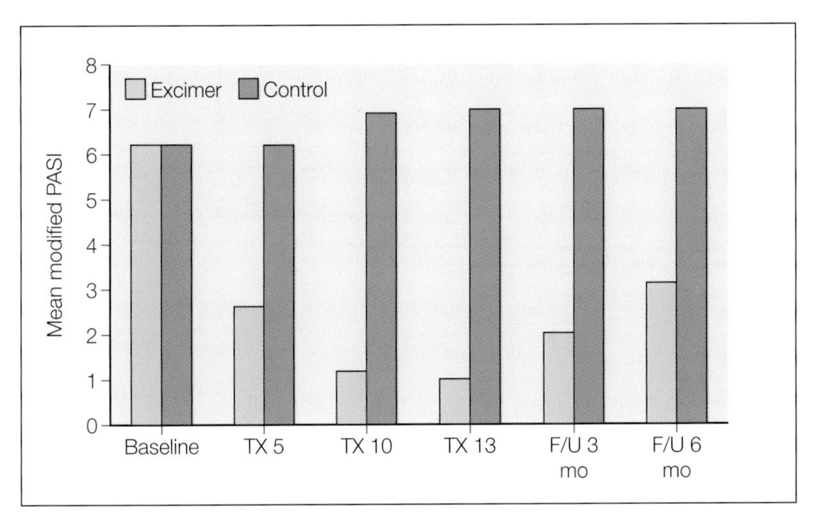

Fig. 8.19 Mean modified psoriasis area and severity index (PASI) scores after treatment with the excimer laser. (Modified from Taneja A, Trehan M, Taylor CR 2003 308-nm excimer laser for the treatment of psoriasis: induration-based dosimetry. Archives of Dermatology 139:759–764)

Combination treatment with topical and/or oral therapies is likely to yield improved clinical outcomes. Previous studies have shown more rapid improvement in clinical disease with the combined NB-UVB and topical calcipotriene, anthralins or retinoids compared to NB-UVB alone. A recent report has shown that topical calcipotriene in combination with high intensity UVB light source can also have synergistic effects.

Treatment technique

The two basic treatment paradigms employed are high dose versus low dose UVB. Most studies have shown that higher fluences can induce faster clearing and longer remissions. However, high fluences are also associated with significantly greater risk of phototoxic reactions and blistering which are associated with longer healing times and post-procedure pain. There may be some instances where a single treatment with high fluence UVB may be the treatment of choice. If there are only one or two isolated recalcitrant plaques, and the patient understands the risk of blistering versus the benefit of needing only a single or very few treatments, then high dose UVB treatment can be attempted. High dose UVB (8× to 16× MED) has been reported to induce blistering but can achieve clearing with long term remissions even following a single treatment.

Low or medium dose UVB treatment follows a protocol similar to that for conventional UVB phototherapy with weekly or biweekly treatments. Sessions can be maintained at the same initial dose until clinical improvement is achieved, or dosage can be incrementally increased. Appropriate withholding or adjustment of the UVB dose can be made in the event of clinical improvement, blistering, or pigmentation. In a similar way to conventional phototherapy, because the high intensity UVB light source is not a laser, treatment can be potentially delivered by trained nonphysician personnel. However, since clinical thinning of the plaque occurs very rapidly, close follow up by the physician is necessary to prevent inadvertent phototoxicity. A sample suggested treatment schedule is given in Fig. 8.20.

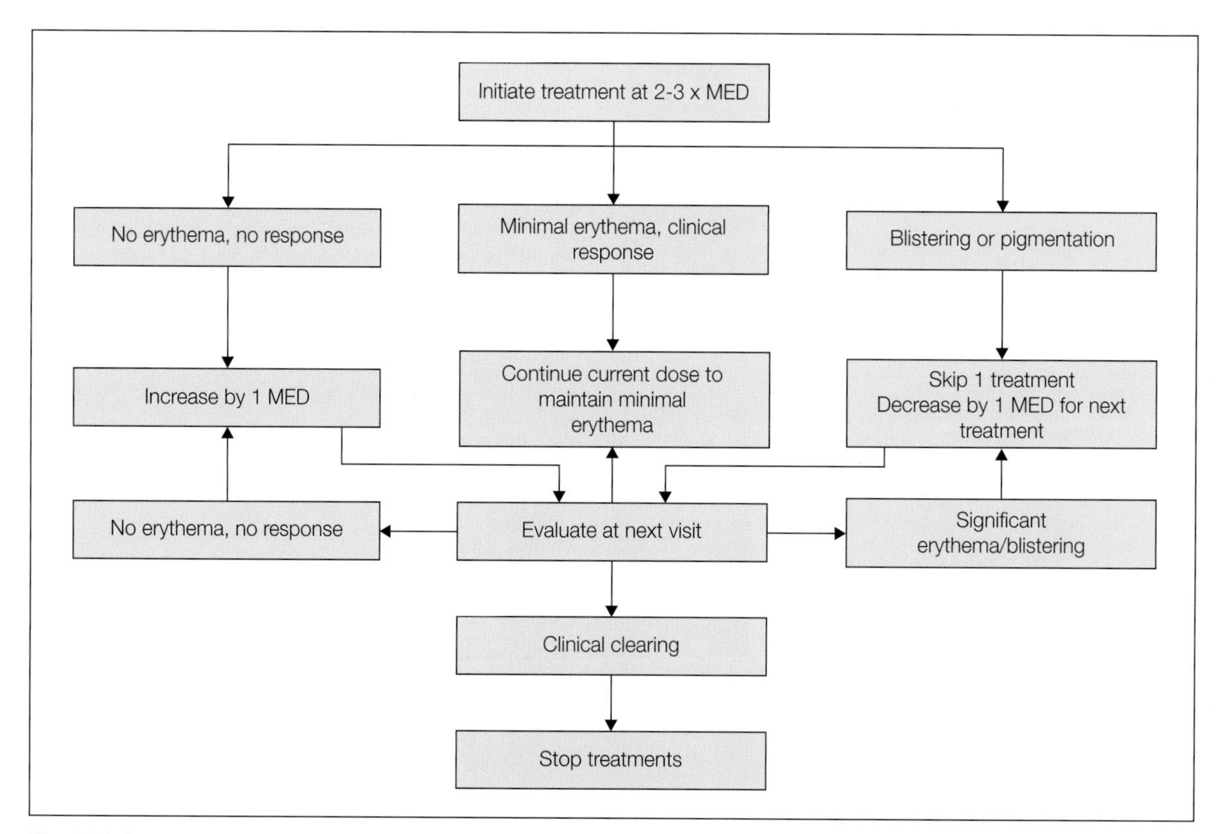

Fig. 8.20 Suggested sample treatment protocol for medium dose UVB for the excimer laser or high intensity UVB light source

Treatment should be delivered in nonoverlapping pulses over the target lesion and mineral oil can be applied to enhance UV penetration.

Postoperative care

After treatment, there is typically mild erythema. At higher fluences blistering can occur, mimicking a severe sunburn reaction. If any blistering or erosions occur, the area should be covered with antibiotic ointment or hydrophilic petrolatum until healed. There have been no reports of the Koebner phenomenon following such blistering, and a blistering reaction seen at higher fluences may actually contribute to improved clearance. Severe phototoxic reactions can occur if appropriate reductions in fluence are not made as treated plaques begin to thin.

Side effects and complications

Tanning is the most common side effect in patients with skin types amenable to tanning. Occasional blistering may occur at higher fluences and hyperpigmentation can occur at treated sites. No cases of scarring have been reported after treatment with the excimer laser or high intensity UVB photosystems.

Conclusions and Alternatives

There are many currently available options for laser or light source treatments of psoriasis, all of which are effective for limited and stable plaque or inverse psoriasis, particularly if the lesions are recalcitrant to conventional topical medications, and of such limited extent that systemic treatments are not necessary. Prolonged clearing and remission of disease rarely achieved with either topical or systemic treatments can occur following laser and light treatments. Indeed, although lasers and light sources may not be considered first line treatments for psoriasis, the high rate of clinical response and remissions achieved with these treatments may translate to overall shorter treatment times and lower treatment costs for persistent lesions that could otherwise require treatment for months or years with conventional therapies. Thus, for select psoriasis lesions, lasers and light sources may be highly effective and viable therapeutic options.

Further Reading

Asawanonda P, Anderson RR, Taylor CR 2000 Pendulaser carbon dioxide resurfacing laser versus electrodesiccation with curettage in the treatment of isolated, recalcitrant psoriatic plaques. Journal of the American Academy of Dermatology 42:660–666

Bissonnette R, Tremblay JF, Juezenas P, et al 2002 Systemic photodynamic therapy with aminolevulinic acid induces apoptosis in lesional T lymphocytes of psoriatic plaques. Journal of Investigative Dermatology 119:77–83

Boehncke W-H, Ochsendorf F, Manfred W, et al 1991 Ablative techniques in psoriasis vulgaris resistant to conventional therapies. Dermatologic Surgery 25:618–621

Bonis B, Kemeny L, Dobozy A, et al 1997 308 nm UVB excimer laser for psoriasis. Lancet 22:1522

Christophers E, Mrowietz U 2003 Psoriasis. In: Freedberg IM, Eisen AZ, Wolff K, eds. Fitzpatrick's dermatology in general medicine. McGraw-Hill, New York, pp 407–427

Dierickx C 2003 Optimalization of treatment of psoriasis with B Clear system. Lasers in Surgery and Medicine (suppl 15):37

Feldman SR, Mellen BG, Housman TS, et al 2002 Efficacy of the 308-nm excimer laser for the treatment of psoriasis: results of a multicenter study. Journal of the American Academy of Dermatology 46:900–906

Hern S, Allen MH, Sousa AR, et al 2001 Immunohistochemical evaluation of psoriatic plaques following selective photothermolysis of the superficial capillaries. British Journal of Dermatology 145:45–53

Honigsmann H, Schwartz T 2003 Ultraviolet light therapy. In: Bolognia JL, Jorizzo JL, Rapini RP, eds. Dermatology. Elsevier, London, pp 2109–2120

Mazer J-M, Fayard V 2004 Response of psoriasis plaques to pulsed dye lasers: predictive criteria. Lasers in Surgery and Medicine (suppl 16):68

Parrish JA, Jaenicke KF 1981 Action spectrum for phototherapy of psoriasis. Journal of Investigative Dermatology 76:359–362

Richards HL, Fortune DG, O'Sullivan TM, et al 1999 Patients with psoriasis and their compliance with medication. Journal of the American Academy of Dermatology 41:581–583

Rodewald EJ, Housman TS, Mellen BG, et al 2002 Follow-up survey of 308-nm laser treatment of psoriasis. Lasers in Surgery and Medicine 31:202–206

Tanghetti EA, Alvarado SL, Gillis PR 2002 Comparison of localized UVB phototherapy systems for high dose treatment of stable plaque psoriasis. The Lumenis Group of Companies, Santa Clara, CA, USA

Weinberg JM 2003 An overview of infliximab, etanercept, efalizumab, and alefacept as biologic therapy for psoriasis. Clinical Therapeutics 25:2487–2505

Yamauchi PS, Rizk D, Kormeili T, et al 2003 Current systemic therapies for psoriasis: where are we now? Journal of the American Academy of Dermatology 49:S66–77

Zanolli M 2003 Phototherapy treatment of psoriasis today. Journal of the American Academy of Dermatology 49:S78–86

Zelickson BD, Mehregan DA, Wendelshfer-Crabb G, et al 1996 Clinical and histologic evaluation of psoriatic plaques treated with a flashlamp pulsed dye laser. Journal of the American Academy of Dermatology 35:64–68

9 Cooling

E. Victor Ross Jr, Dilip Paithankar

Introduction

Surface cooling has expanded the breadth of laser-treatable conditions. Applications are less dependent on patient pigmentation so that darker patients can now enjoy the benefits of laser. In most pulsed laser applications in dermatology, selective heating is desirable and achieved by the proper choice of wavelength and pulse duration. With melanocytic and vascular lesions, efficacy and safety are optimized when absorption is at least tenfold that of surrounding normal skin. However, in darker skinned patients, this ratio decreases so that the window between under- and overtreatment is quite narrow.

Before the availability of surface cooling, fluence thresholds for efficacy and epidermal damage were often perilously close, even in mildly pigmented skin. It follows that the operator was sometimes walking a tightrope between lack of efficacy and epidermal injury. A classic example was the olive colored Hispanic patient with a port wine stain (PWS) treated with pulsed dye laser (PDL). The patient would be treated at 5 J/cm^2 with little to no improvement, then at the next visit the fluence would be increased to 6 J/cm^2 and one would observe focal crusts and pigmentary changes. With cryogen spray cooling, this patient can now be treated at fluences up to 8 and 9 J/cm^2 with little risk of epidermal damage.

Visible light technologies (especially green-yellow light sources such as intense pulsed light (IPL), potassium-titanyl-phosphate (KTP), and PDL) have become increasingly popular for skin rejuvenation. They are also the wavelength ranges where epidermal damage is most likely. The epidermis is an innocent bystander in cutaneous laser applications where the intended targets, such as hair follicles or blood vessels, are located in the dermis. Specifically, absorption of light by epidermal melanin causes epidermal heating. Melanin is distributed throughout the epidermis but is especially concentrated in the basal cell layer. Melanin absorption of visible light causes heating of melanosomes and through thermal diffusion, subsequent damage to the entire epidermis. This is especially true for green-yellow light, but the risk of selective DE (dermal–epidermal) junction derived epidermal injury extends to wavelengths as long as 1064 nm. Overall, shorter wavelengths pose a greater risk to the skin surface, because the ratio of epidermal to dermal heating is higher. The reasons for this phenomenon are twofold: (i) there is higher absorption of melanin by shorter wavelengths; (ii) there is a tendency for photon scatter to limit penetration of shorter wavelengths. This leads to an accumulation of energy near the DE junction.

Beyond visible light (green, yellow, and red) sources, surface cooling also has been employed in near-infrared (NIR) and mid-infrared (MIR) lasers. With NIR lasers surface cooling is important, but not only because of DE junction derived epidermal heating. In addition, deep beam penetration may cause catastrophic bulk heating. With MIR lasers (1.32, 1.45, and 1.54 μm), the chromophore is water. It follows that with even very low fluences, surface cooling is imperative. Without cooling, water's ubiquitous nature in the skin causes laser induced top to bottom injury. There is no discrete heating.

There are six types of practical cooling technologies that are subsets of three broader categories (contact, cold air, and cryogen spray). There are advantages and drawbacks of each approach. All of the techniques are susceptible to operator error and device failure.

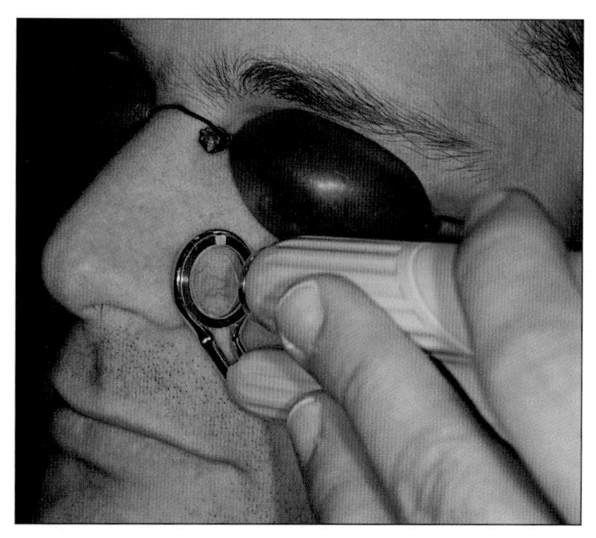

Fig. 9.1 Sapphire window chilled by circulating cold water at 4°C. In this case, water cools the metal ring which in turn chills the window

Cooling

There are three primary objectives of surface cooling. The first and intuitively simple goal is preservation of the epidermis. Unintentional heating of the basal cell layer can lead to vesiculation, crusting and, at times, scarring. The laser induced temperature rise of the epidermis is proportional to the fluence and the wavelength-specific absorption by melanin. The value of ΔT, $(T_f - T_i)$ is similar to the case without cooling. But with cooling, the initial temperature, T_i, is reduced, thus rendering a reduced temperature at the end of the laser pulse, T_f. Besides protection of the DE junction from pigment 'unfriendly' wavelengths, sometimes bulk cooling is required because the volume heated is large and there is a risk for large volume overheating and catastrophic scarring (i.e. with 1064 nm).

The second and related goal of surface cooling is to allow for delivery of higher fluences to the intended target (i.e. the hair bulb and/or bulge or a subsurface blood vessel). By cooling the epidermis, higher fluences and therefore higher temperature elevations are possible in the targeted structures in the dermis. Thus, surface cooling strategies improve efficacy as well as safety.

A third goal of surface cooling is analgesia, as almost all cooling strategies will provide some pain relief.

Another tissue-related issue is the timing of the cooling relative to the laser pulse. Cooling can be before the laser pulse (pre), during the pulse (parallel), or after the pulse (post). All three cooling periods are important. For example, postcooling may prevent retrograde heating (i.e. from the vessel back to the epidermis) from damaging the skin surface.

It should be noted that heating from the laser pulse is instantaneous, whereas cooling is slow. The rate-limiting step to rapid cooling, particularly in the case of contact cooling, is keeping the cooling medium 'cold'. Once in contact with the skin, the medium (e.g. a sapphire window (Fig. 9.1)) tends to warm. The ability of it to remain cool depends on many factors, among which is the thermal conductivity of the cooling substrate. For example, copper is a better conductor than sapphire, which is better than quartz or glass.

There are some scenarios where cooling is unlikely to prove beneficial:

- When the absorption of the wavelength is so strong by water (i.e. erbium Er : YAG and CO_2 lasers), the cooling and heating volumes tend to be collocated so that preservation of epidermal viability is unfeasible.
- When using Q-switched lasers in the range from 532 to 1064 nm, cooling achieves pain reduction but is unlikely to reduce the high peak temperatures generated by these ultrashort pulses in melanin and exogenous inks (tattoos).

Cooling Methods

Cooling can broadly be categorized temporally (pre, parallel, and post cooling), by technique (contact, cryogen spray, or cold air), and/or by level of integration with the laser (integrated versus non-integrated). An example of a nonintegrated chiller is the CoolRoller (Fig. 9.2), which is completely separate from the laser. Finally cooling can be active or passive. 'Active' implies that the cooling medium is 'actively' cooled (i.e. sapphire window chilled continuously by circulating water) versus 'passive' (e.g. placing an ice pack on the skin).

Contact cooling

Most skin cooling approaches include placement of a cooled medium in contact with the skin. The rate of heat extraction depends on the temperature difference and the 'thermal contact' between the skin and cooling medium. The simplest cooling

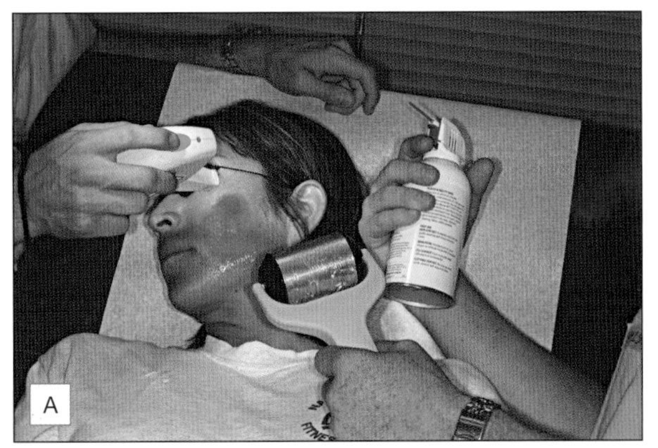

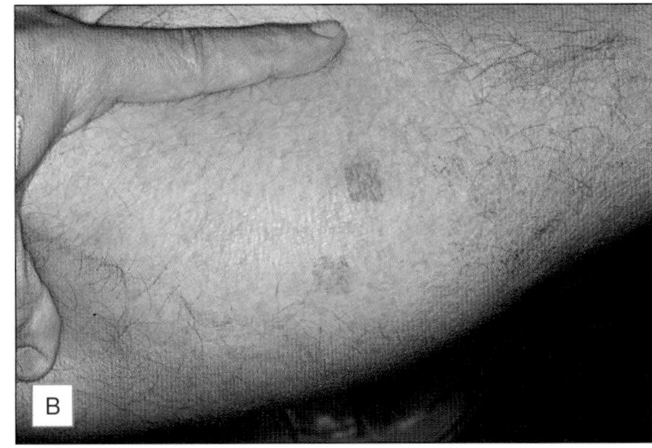

Fig. 9.2 (**A**) The CoolRoller used with an IPL. This is rolled over the skin back and forth like a rolling pin. It should be repeated after every few pulses. (**B**) Two days after treatment with green IPL handpiece. Heavy crust is observed at site without roller precooling. Lighter crust is observed at site precooled by 5 seconds of back and forth rolling

method is pre-icing of the skin. A more typical modern active integrated cooling system is a chilled sapphire window cooled to 4°C. The scheme includes a precooling period of about 250 ms (as one slides the window across the skin). The precooling time depends on the size of the beam relative to the window and the repetition rate. There is also parallel cooling in this configuration. With shorter pulses this is not too important, but with pulses longer than 100 ms, parallel cooling becomes relevant. Finally, there is usually some postcooling as the handpiece is moved across the skin. Sapphire is a good thermal conductor but requires an efficient external cooling medium (such as chilled water between two sapphire plates). Otherwise, the sapphire warms with sustained contact with irradiated skin.

Copper is an excellent conductor and is about tenfold more conductive than sapphire. Because copper is such a good conductor, despite the lack of parallel cooling, the skin surface remains cool during and after the pulse (Fig. 9.3). The lack of parallel cooling (and postcooling) can become a drawback if one inadvertently stacks pulses or if one is treating a large vessel that requires several seconds to cool.

Precooling with an aluminum roller, ice, or cold gels is a form of nonintegrated, passive cooling. A recently introduced chiller is the CoolRoller. This aluminum 'rolling pin' (see Fig. 9.2) possesses a high thermal conductivity. With about 10 back and forth rolls over 10 seconds, the DE junction temperature can be reduced by about 10–15°C. Moreover, some bulk cooling and analgesia are achieved.

Convective air cooling

Cold air is commonly used in skin chilling. The Zimmer (Cyro 5, Zimmer MedizinSysteme, Ulm, Germany) directs –10°C air at the skin at a rapid rate (1000 L/min).

Cryogen spray cooling (DCD)

The DCD^{TM} (dynamic cooling device) is best able to achieve rapid temperature reduction at the skin surface (Fig. 9.4). The heat transfer rate is about twice that of contact cooling. The cooling agent, tetrafluoroethane, boils at –26°C but is associated with temperatures as low as –44°C at the skin surface. With a single continuous spurt as long as 80–100 ms, the DCD does not induce cryoinjury. However, with sequential spurts unopposed cooling has been shown to cause erosions and hyperpigmentation. There is more heat flux with sequential sprays.

It has been suggested that the cyrospray impedes the laser beam. However, with single spurts and the typical delay between spray and laser pulse, laser emission is not affected by the spray. Another issue is the frost that forms after the spray. Experiments have proven that this frost forms as a result of condensation of ambient water vapor on the cooled surface of human skin. This phenomenon occurs approximately 100 ms after the end of a 30 ms spray. The incident laser light dose delivered for therapy is not affected by optical scattering due to frost because the delay is regularly chosen to be

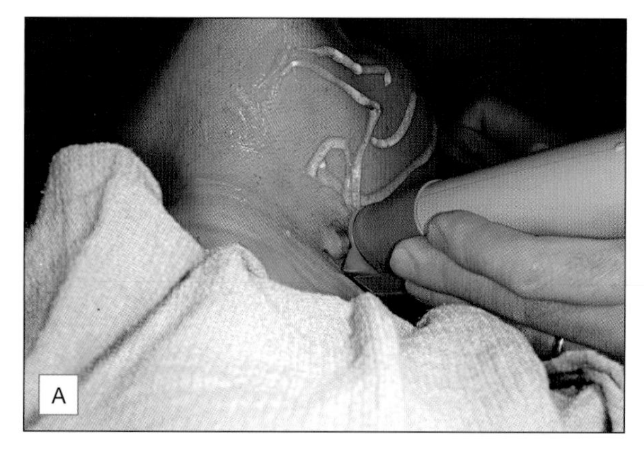

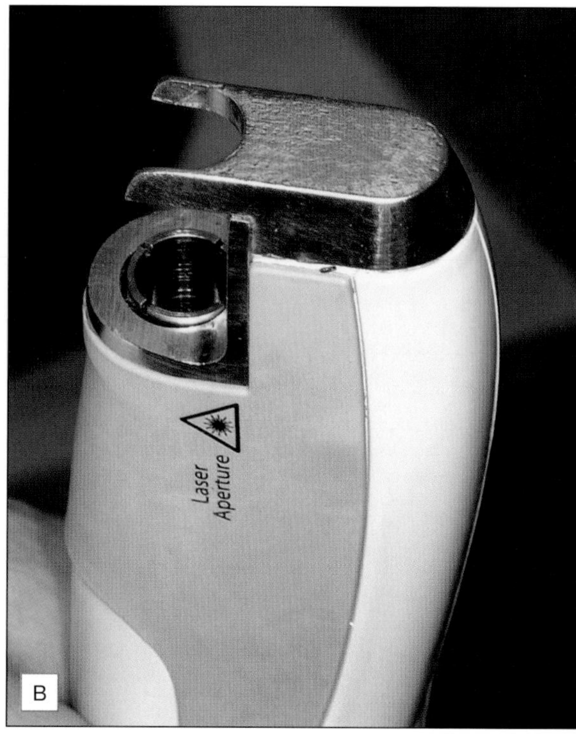

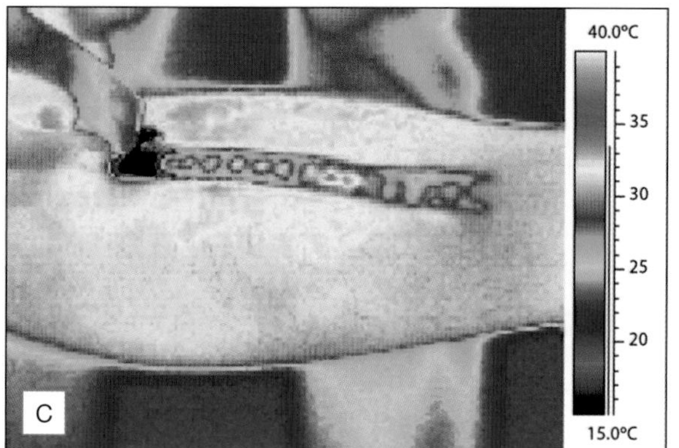

Fig. 9.3 (**A,B**) Copper plate in action with Nd : YAG laser in laser hair removal. This is an example of precooling only (however, the plate can be used after treatment to postcool by sliding the handpiece back and forth without laser pulsing). (**C**) Thermal camera image showing 'cool' trail after copper plate

much shorter than 100 ms. However, during clinical work, the laser handpiece typically is moved from a given site to an immediately adjacent spot. With a 1.5 Hz repetition rate and longer spray duration, frost may occur at the beginning of the next pulse. Therefore it is important to maneuver the handpiece to avoid irradiating through any frost that remains from previous sites.

Overall, the DCD offers the greatest selectivity as far as confining cooling to the epidermis and upper dermis. Svaasand and Nelson suggest that the DCD may be the most capable tool for rapid and selective epidermal cooling. Air cooling, for example, will require about 20 seconds to cool the DE junction to the same temperature as a 40 ms spurt; moreover the cooling will extend to about 1600 μm below the surface with air versus 100 μm with DCD.

A cooling protection factor (CPF) can be defined as the ratio of the minimal fluence that causes epidermal injury without cooling and with cooling. It can be evaluated from the following equation:

$$\mathrm{CPF} = \frac{T_c - T_{ic}}{T_c - T_i}$$

In the above equation, T_{ic} and T_i are basal layer temperatures before laser irradiation with and without cooling, respectively. T_c is the critical temperature at which thermal injury occurs. In the authors' experience the CPF is 1.8 for DCD, 1.5 for the sapphire window, and 1.3 for cold air (e.g. when using the KTP or PDL in vascular lesions).

Applications of Cooling

It is helpful to examine real life applications and the use of cooling types described above.

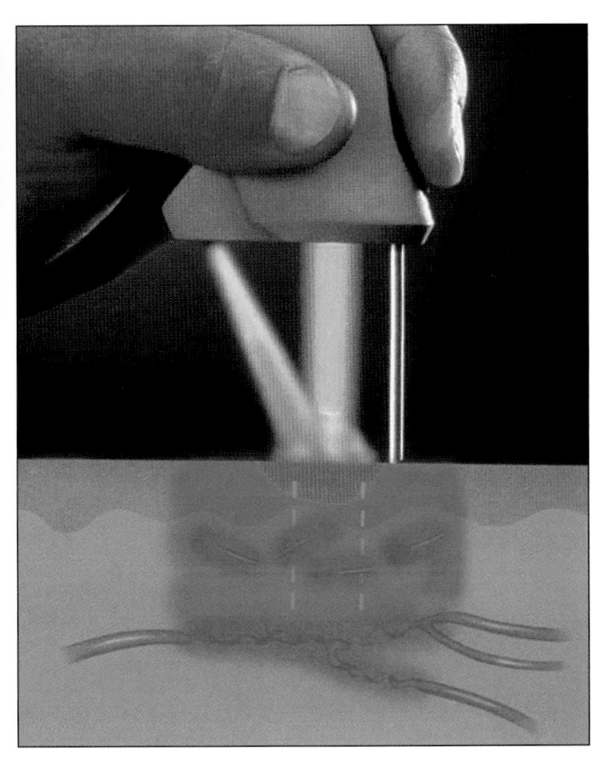

Fig. 9.4 Cryogen spray cooling used in treatment of leg veins with a Nd : YAG laser

Hair removal

Hair removal presents an excellent opportunity for surface cooling. Because the distance between the DE junction (epidermal melanin) and the bulb is great (2–5 mm), most cooling methods will be effective, particularly when the contrast between hair and skin color is great. Cold air and contact cooling are more likely to achieve some bulk cooling. DCD will provide excellent epidermal protection but little bulk cooling. One advantage of parallel contact cooling is that the handpiece can be pressed against the skin to reduce the surface–hair bulb distance. The maneuver increases the energy density at the bulb.

Vascular lesions

This is another application where cooling methods have proven to increase safety and efficacy, particularly in PWS and leg veins. Typically the vessel is 300–1300 μm beneath the skin. In mathematical models, the DCD will outperform the contact chiller which will in turn outperform cold air. However, as a practical matter, all of these methods have been found to achieve marked epidermal protection. Cold air was the least protective but also achieved the greatest analgesia. It has been suggested that cold air and contact cooling are prone to overcool the vessel and render it difficult to heat with laser. However, perfusion helps to maintain the blood vessel at body temperature. It should be noted that with all of the cooling devices, vessel clearing with a cooling device may require a slightly higher fluence than without cooling.

Epidermal pigmented lesions

With millisecond domain laser devices, contact with gel or sapphire achieves gentler heating of epidermal dyschromias. Cooling allows for preservation of the stratum corneum so that mild desquamation is delayed and associated with less inflammation. The DCD, which is the most efficient chiller, often chills 'too well' for epidermal pigmented lesions and typically needs to be turned off for their removal. However, some clinicians are achieving good results by using a bit of DCD with the alexandrite laser and increasing the fluence.

Nonablative remodeling with mid-infrared lasers

With MIR lasers, cooling and heating must be choreographed very tightly, since there is no intrinsic selectivity. It follows that the boundaries of the cooled volume will partly determine what 'slab' of skin is heated. For example, in wrinkle treatment, most solar elastosis resides from 100–600 μm below the surface. Presumably one wants to create a wound in this 'band' if the wrinkle is to be improved. With contact cooling with typical contact times (0.2–1.5 s), the upper dermis tends to be overcooled, and significant temperature elevation tends to be deeper than the zone of solar elastosis. In other words, when the volume to be heated is juxtaposed with the volume to be protected (the case with most MIR rejuvenation devices), confinement of spatial cooling is highly desirable.

Cooling and Pain

Surface cooling devices vary in their ability to reduce pain. On the one hand, cooling can act as a distracter, where cold mitigates pain by 'confusing' the cutaneous nerves. This phenomenon can be seen when using the 1064 nm laser with DCD and light skin. Both the laser and the cryospray cause discomfort, but the combination seems to make the procedure more tolerable. In this case, the epidermis is relatively spared due to the lack of melanin, and lack of bulk cooling argues against the DCD actually 'anesthetizing' the dermis. The DCD induced cold layer and heat generated by the laser are far apart in this scenario. On the other hand, pain generated by epidermal heating can certainly be mitigated by DCD. For example, the DCD reduces pain in vascular applications with PDL. Protecting the epidermis very efficiently, pain that would otherwise derive from the DE junction is diminished. Therefore, in treating deeper leg veins with a 1064 nm laser, the excellent spatial confinement of DCD cooling is a drawback, as there is a lack of bulk cooling. This should be contrasted with cold air cooling. Here cooling sometimes reduces postopertive edema and erythema but does not tend to alter the immediate surface tissue effects nor does it change clinical efficacy. It has been observed when treating leg veins with a 1064 nm laser that while the DCD, copper plate, and sapphire window achieve excellent epidermal protection, the cold air device affords the greatest pain alleviation. Most likely this is because the patient feels 'bathed' in cold. The low heat transfer coefficient demands long contact times for cold air, which subsequently enlarges the volume of tissue cooled.

In practice, the most commonly asked questions in the realm of laser cooling are:

1. Does one need to increase the laser fluence when applying surface cooling? For superficial vascular lesions and epidermal pigmented lesions, often the fluence must be increased. However, the increases are usually small. The basis for the increase is inadvertent cooling of the target. For deeper targets like hair, fluences normally do not need to be increased.
2. When one considers pre-, parallel, and post-cooling, which is most important? Because of the instantaneous nature of tissue heating, precooling is almost always required. Parallel cooling is most important for longer pulse durations. For pulse durations less than 10 ms, it is of minimal value. With regards to postcooling, once the epidermis is heated beyond some critical temperature (with whitening), much like 'unringing a bell', the skin cannot be 'rescued', no matter how heroically one applies ice packs. On the other hand, in some applications, immediate postcooling (also known as thermal quenching) can mitigate epidermal damage. Postcooling is most important when one heats a large volume of tissue just subjacent to the epidermis (i.e. using a MIR laser or a NIR laser at a high fluence) or treats a large blood vessel just beneath the epidermis (this vessel might take seconds to cool, and some heat diffusion will invariably proceed toward the epidermis). In addition, delayed postcooling measures such as icepacks may reduce inflammation mediated extension of laser induced injury.

Summary of the Pros and Cons of Six Cooling Strategies

Ice

Ice has the advantage of easy availability. It can, for example, be put in plastic and placed on the skin for minutes before treatment. Ice does provide for bulk cooling and therefore good analgesia if left on the surface long enough. This will aid in minimizing collateral damage. If simply placed on the skin for a few seconds prior to exposure, it provides some epidermal protection. A drawback is the lack of predictability in cooling. For example, if one leaves it in contact with the skin for 1 minute versus 10 seconds, the change in protection will be significant. Also, the provider will tend to interrupt treatment and rechill at irregular intervals, such that the cooling will not be uniform from place to place.

Cool gel alone

A problem with cool gel is that it becomes warm rather quickly. To cool the skin, it must be replaced with fresh cold gel every few seconds. Cool gel does provide for epidermal sinking, that is, the gel, so long as it is cooler than the skin temperature, will extract heat away better than air, a good insulator. Also, it allows for optical damping, allowing the escape of some laser energy that would otherwise accumulate at the surface.

Cold air

Cold air (Fig. 9.5) has few drawbacks—the main one being the long contact time required for adequate epidermal protection. However, it does

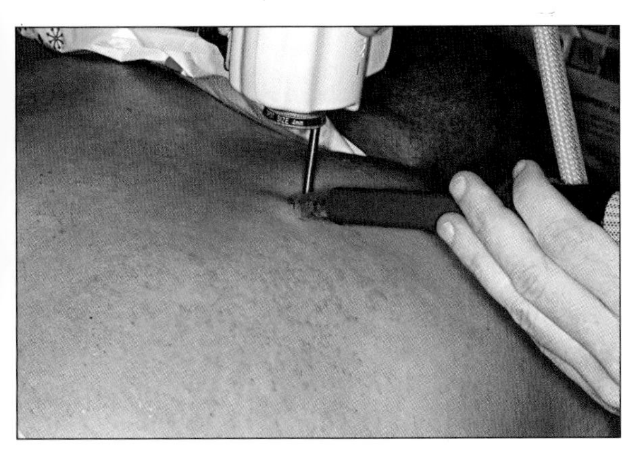

Fig. 9.5 Cold air used with 810 nm diode laser in laser hair reduction on the back

not interfere with the beam, does not involve a consumable, and other than working near the nose or ear, is well tolerated by the patient. There is almost no risk of cryoinjury. If one is using the device for comfort only, the patient can hold the tip and direct it in the treated area. If one is using it for epidermal protection, then the provider should hold the nozzle close to the skin to maximize the convective flow.

Contact with sapphire

This form of cooling is effective and allows for visualization of the target, and minimal beam interference (5–10% unless there is considerable condensation on the lens). Some intense pulsed light sources (IPLs) use active cooling with a quartz or sapphire crystal. Although not allowing for direct visualization of the target, the other attributes of contact cooling are preserved.

DCD

The advantage of DCD is rapid and reproducible cooling. Dai et al have shown that the PDL fluence ex vivo could safely be increased by up to 5 J/cm^2 with DCD. This finding is consistent with clinical experience, where one may find fluences as high as 9 J/cm^2 on a dark Hispanic patient with a setting of 40 ms spray and 30 ms delay. Without the DCD, settings might be limited to 5–6 J/cm^2. The disadvantages are the need to purchase a consumable (the spray), the potential for cryoinjury under certain conditions, and the potential for beam interference under certain conditions.

CoolRoller

The previously described CoolRoller acts as an easy-to-use ice cube. Its excellent thermal conductivity allows for rapid skin chilling. However, the number of times it is rolled across the skin determines the temperature reduction. Also one must pay attention to the temperature of the roller. After about 20 minutes, its cooling capacity decreases as it warms.

Complications of Cooling

Although cooling has revolutionized skin laser surgery, the reliance on it is a mixed blessing. In particular in cases where epidermal protection is critical (i.e. treating a dark skinned patient with a PWS), a lack of cooling when one expects it can be perilous. It is advisable to look, listen, and feel when using cooling technologies. All devices, no matter how well manufactured, can fail. Likewise, attention to detail is a prerequisite for the operator. Below are listed some potential problems associated with cooling:

- **DCD.** There have been instances when the cryogen spray canister may be empty but continued to 'fire'. The lack of the characteristic 'hiss' might be noted just prior to the laser pulse. Newer DCD models have more refined modules that are unlikely to allow an empty canister to fire.
- **Sapphire window.** One must check that the chiller is 'on' and the reservoir is full. If not, the handpiece will become increasingly warm and epidermal damage can occur (Fig. 9.6).
- **Passive cooling.** In the case of passively cooled IPLs, the handpiece must dissipate heat from reflected light that re-enters the closed loop system. With repeated pulses the handpiece temperature can increase up to 2°C per pulse. If the treatment is not interrupted often enough to rechill the handpiece tip, intense erythema may be noted. This might be followed by vesiculation and mild long term hypopigmentation.
- **Cold air device.** If the nozzle is directed toward the skin but there is no flowing air at the site, the tube might have become crimped.
- **Cold roller.** If the patient complains of increasing pain as the treatment proceeds, one should check the temperature of the roller. After about 20 minutes its protective and analgesic properties diminish as it warms to room temperature.

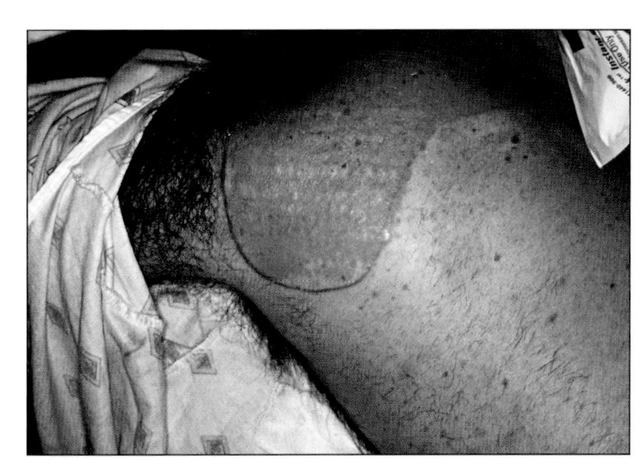

Fig. 9.6 Blister noted shortly after Nd : YAG treatment. The chiller was not turned on

- **Copper plate.** One must maintain the path of the handpiece along its longitudinal axis (Fig. 9.3); also, over a convex surface care must be taken to make contact between the plate and the skin.

Methods to Optimize Cooling

Before any pulse, one should, depending on the method of cooling utilized, either feel the handpiece tip to ensure a sapphire window is cool, or purge the DCD to ensure there is cryogen in the canister. With any other cooling devices, check the equipment and make sure any cooling apparatus, particularly if it is an external one, is properly attached to the laser and turned on.

Conditions change during laser surgery. In particular when treating large vascular lesions or areas prone to flushing, there is a tendency for the skin surface temperature to approach body temperature. This obliges the cooling device to extract more heat than at the beginning of treatment. For example, it might be noticed that when treating poikiloderma of the neck, the fluences utilized at baseline result in the reduction of telangiectasia. However, the same parameters may, after several minutes, result in mild whitening, suggestive of epidermal injury. Reducing the laser settings could be considered in this situation.

Manufacturers strive to ensure that their chosen cooling apparatus will always work. Some indicator that the chilling mechanism is not working is useful on the apparatus. There might also be warning indicators or temperature monitors on the handpiece tip. These indicators disable the laser if the cooling is malfunctioning.

Tanned skin, by definition, is injured skin. With the exception of the Nd : YAG or MIR lasers, even when good cooling is utilized, treatments may not be safe. A constitutively dark patient's skin is much more 'stable' and predictable to treat. If one must treat a tanned patient, one should hold the contact cooler on for longer, increase the DCD spray, or increase the cold air speed.

Test spots may be helpful, but only if utilized on skin with equivalent pigmentation to the area being treated. If intense redness or early graying is observed after 15 minutes, the fluence should be lowered or the cooling should be increased.

With the exception of the Nd : YAG laser, most epidermal cooling devices, even DCD, will not offer enough protection for very dark type VI skin.

Passive cooling devices must be used carefully, when the goal is not only pain relief but also epidermal protection.

A longer pulse duration is sometimes desirable due to the epidermal protection that it provides (a longer pulse permits cooling of the thin epidermis as the pulse slowly heats deeper structures). However, this can be a double edged sword—a longer pulse duration also leads to conductive losses from the target structures such as hair or blood vessels and hence to reduced peak temperatures of these structures upon laser heating. Thus, longer pulse durations may lead to a reduction in efficacy of treatment of hair or blood vessels, especially of smaller hair follicles or blood vessels.

Understanding the principles of cutaneous cooling will enable the physician to use modern 'chillers' more creatively and consistently. Almost all aspects of cutaneous laser surgery depend on the proper use of cold and hot effects. By choreographing hot and cold expertly, results will be optimized.

Further Reading

Aguilar G, Majaron B, Karapetian E, Lavernia EJ, Nelson JS 2003 Experimental study of cryogen spray properties for application in dermatologic laser surgery. IEEE Transactions on Biomedical Engineering 50:863–869

Aguilar G, Wang GX, Nelson JS 2003 Dynamic behavior of cryogen spray cooling: effects of spurt duration and spray distance. Lasers in Surgery and Medicine 32:152–159

Aguilar G, Wang GX, Nelson JS 2003 Effect of spurt duration on the heat transfer dynamics during cryogen spray cooling. Physics in Medicine and Biology 48:2169–2181

Altshuler GB, Zenzie HH, Erofeev AV, et al 1999 Contact cooling of the skin. Physics in Medicine and Biology 44:1003–1023

Buscher BA, McMeekin TO, Goodwin D 2000 Treatment of leg telangiectasia by using a long pulse dye laser at 595 nm with and without dynamic cooling device. Lasers in Surgery and Medicine 27:171–175

Chang CJ, Nelson JS 1999 Cryogen spray cooling and higher fluence pulsed dye laser treatment improve port wine stain clearance while minimizing epidermal damage. Dermatologic Surgery 25:767–772

Chang CW, Reinisch L, Biesman BS 2003 Analysis of epidermal protection using cold air versus chilled sapphire window with water or gel during 810 nm diode laser application. Lasers in Surgery and Medicine 32:129–136

Chess C 2000 Regarding the use of contact cooling devices during laser treatment of spider leg veins. Dermatologic Surgery 26:92–93 [comment]

Dai T, Pikkula BM, Tunnell JW, Chang DW, Anvari B 2003 Thermal response of human skin epidermis to 595 nm laser irradiation at high incident dosages and long pulse durations in conjunction with cryogen spray cooling: an ex vivo study. Lasers in Surgery and Medicine 33:16–24

Edris A, Choi B, Aguilar G, Nelson JS 2003 Measurements of laser light attenuation following cryogen spray cooling spurt termination. Lasers in Surgery and Medicine 32:143–147

Greve B, Hammes S, Raulin C 2001 The effect of cold air cooling on 585 nm pulsed dye laser treatment of port-wine stains. Dermatologic Surgery 27:633–636

Kao B, Kelly KM, Aguilar G, et al 2004 Evaluation of cryogen spray cooling exposure on in vitro model human skin. Lasers in Surgery and Medicine 34:146–154

Kauvar AN, Frew KE, Friedman PM, Geronemus RG 2002 Cooling gel improves pulsed KTP laser treatment of facial telangiectasia. Lasers in Surgery and Medicine 30:149–153

Kelly KM, Svaasand LO, Nelson JS 2003 Optimization of laser treatment safety in conjunction with cryogen spray cooling. Archives of Dermatology 139:1372–1373

Kelly KM, Svaasand LO, Nelson JS 2004 Further investigation of pigmentary changes after alexandrite laser hair removal in conjunction with cryogen spray cooling. Dermatologic Surgery 30(4 Pt 1):581–582

Majaron B, Svaasand LO, Aguilar G, Nelson JS 2002 Intermittent cryogen spray cooling for optimal heat extraction during dermatologic laser treatment. Physics in Medicine and Biology 47:3275–3288

Meyers G 1971 Analytical methods in conduction heat transfer. McGraw-Hill, New York

Nelson JS, Majaron B, Kelly KM 2000 Active skin cooling in conjunction with laser dermatologic surgery. Seminars in Cutaneous Medicine and Surgery 19:253–266

Pfefer TJ, Smithies DJ, Milner TE, et al 2000 Bioheat transfer analysis of cryogen spray cooling during laser treatment of port wine stains. Lasers in Surgery and Medicine 26:145–157

Raulin C, Greve B, Hammes S 2000 Cold air in laser therapy: first experiences with a new cooling system. Lasers in Surgery and Medicine 27:404–410

Ross EV, Sajben FP, Hsia J, Barnette D, Miller CH, McKinlay JR 2000 Nonablative skin remodeling: selective dermal heating with a mid-infrared laser and contact cooling combination. Lasers in Surgery and Medicine 26:186–195

Svaasand LO, Nelson JS 2004 On the physics of laser induced selective photothermolysis of hair follicles: influence of wavelength, pulse duration, and epidermal cooling. Journal of Biomedical Optics 9:353–361

Svaasand LO, Randeberg LL, Aguilar G, et al 2003 Cooling efficiency of cryogen spray during laser therapy of skin. Lasers in Surgery and Medicine 32:137–142

Zenzie HH, Altshuler GB, Smirnov MZ, Anderson RR 2000 Evaluation of cooling methods for laser dermatology. Lasers in Surgery and Medicine 26:130–144

10 Anesthesia

Suzanne Kilmer

Introduction

Contrary to popular lay opinion, most laser procedures are associated with some discomfort. Although a few are virtually pain-free, most are associated with sensations that range from mild warmth, to the 'the snap of a rubber band' or 'bacon grease spatter', to severe burning pain. In many cases, topical anesthetic preparations alleviate most of the discomfort. For more invasive treatments, the pain can be quite intense, necessitating use of anesthetics, analgesics and/or anxiolytics.

The use of topical anesthetics, local infiltration, regional blocks, and systemic analgesics will be discussed. Conscious sedation and general anesthesia require specific state-determined certifications for both the building that it is performed in as well as for the nurse anesthetist or physician providing the anesthesia. Training for conscious sedation and/or general anesthesia is beyond the scope of this chapter and will not be covered further here. Finally, concomitant cooling methods help protect the epidermis from unwanted thermal injury as well as diminish pain and will be described in detail later in this chapter.

Topical Anesthetics

There are now several agents utilized for topical anesthesia. Viscous lidocaine has long been used for mucosal surfaces and, once applied, acts within a few minutes. In contrast, when topical agents are applied to an intact epidermis, the stratum corneum, the main barrier slows, if not blocks, penetration. The vehicle is important and various delivery systems to traverse the epidermis have been used. In addition, the thickness of the stratum corneum varies in different anatomic locations, or a break in this barrier can occur with trauma, disease states, or can be chemically or mechanically induced with various peeling agents or microdermabrasion. Once through the epidermis, the topical anesthetics target the free dermal nerve endings and interfere with sodium channels to block nerve impulse conduction. Occlusion with plastic wrap enhances penetration and delivery to the dermis. Therefore, the time to adequate anesthesia and its duration depends upon the agent in use, state of the epidermis, and whether occlusion is used.

EMLA (AstraZeneca, USA), a 5% eutectic mixture of lidocaine (2.5%) and prilocaine (2.5%) in an oil and water emulsion, has been available in the USA for over a decade. EMLA provides excellent anesthesia, especially when longer application times and occlusion are employed, and is more efficacious than 2% lidocaine gel on mucosal surfaces. Multiple studies have demonstrated its significant efficacy for a variety of cutaneous procedures, including laser treatments. It has been shown to provide adequate anesthesia for pulsed-dye laser treatment of port wine stains (PWSs) without affecting the laser treatment's efficacy. Location and presence of a stratum corneum affect time to onset. Mucosal surfaces are often sufficiently anesthetized within 5–10 min, whereas the typical application required for intact skin is 30–60 min. Of interest, sufficient anesthesia to perform a punch biopsy to a depth of 6 mm can be achieved (EMLA was applied for 2.5 h under occlusion), supporting its use for procedures such as ablative laser resurfacing. Application with occlusion also hydrates the skin, which may explain the lower incidence of side effects when used for carbon dioxide laser resurfacing.

EMLA is associated with relatively few side effects but these may include erythema and/or blanching, pruritus, burning, purpura, allergy, methemoglobinemia and chemical eye injury. EMLA is initially vasoconstrictive (peaking at about 1.5 h) but after 2–3 h vasodilation is noted. Interestingly, EMLA did not affect the efficacy of pulsed-dye laser treatment of PWSs, likely due to defective vessel innervation.

Although comprised of anesthetics in the amide group, rare contact hypersensitivity to the prilocaine component has been proven by patch testing. The most concerning potential adverse effect from EMLA is methemoglobinemia, also a known side effect of prilocaine. It is more likely in neonates, especially premature infants, due to immaturity of the methemoglobinemia reductase pathway, but can also be seen in those with glucose-6-phosphate deficiency or with patients on medications that compromise these pathways. Limiting the amount of EMLA applied and the surface area covered, decreases this risk. It is recommended to limit the application to 2 g and cover an area of less than 100 cm^2 in those infants who weigh less than 10 kg and limit it to 10 g in those weighing from 10–20 kg.

Finally, caution must be used when EMLA is applied near the eye as the sodium hydroxide used in it to enhance penetration can lead to corneal abrasion or ulceration if not rinsed out quickly and thoroughly, should it inadvertently get into the eye. However, in over 3000 laser resurfacing cases where it was used in the periorbital region, the current author has had only a rare complaint of burning in the eye and, with a quick normal saline rinse, burning was relieved and no further sequaelae occurred.

LMX (Ferndale Laboratories Inc, Michigan, USA), one of the earliest topical anesthetics, is compounded as 4% or 5% lidocaine in a liposomal delivery system. This vehicle both facilitates penetration, thereby enhancing delivery, as well as lengthens its duration of action. The 5% cream is more effective and has a faster onset, and although marketed for anorectal pain, it can be used anywhere on the skin; it is best to forewarn the patient about this labeling information so as to not lead to inadvertent confusion as to how to apply it. It is not vasoactive and is faster acting than EMLA, but equal in anesthetic ability. After 30–60 min of application, anesthesia is adequate for most of the mild to moderately painful laser treatments.

Topicaine, betacaine-LA, and tetracaine are other frequently used topical anesthetics but are not as easily obtained or understood. Topicaine is a rapidly acting microemulsion of 4% lidocaine that has been available for over 5 years now. Betacaine-LA contains lidocaine, prilocaine, and a vasoconstrictor in a proprietary gel formulation that has a rapid onset (within 30 min) and significant anesthesia. Tetracaine, also with a rapid onset of 30 min, has been used in 4% cream and gel formulations but must be obtained from a manufacturer or compounded by a pharmacist. Although similar in efficacy to EMLA, when each was used as directed (30- vs. 60-minute application times), it was greater in anesthetic ability when applied for equal durations of 40, 60, or 120 min in one study but less efficacious than EMLA or ELA-max in another study, suggesting the formulation is important. EMLA was noted to cause blanching whereas tetracaine was associated with erythema of the skin.

S-Caine (Zars Inc, Salt Lake, UT, USA) is a 1:1 mixture of lidocaine and tetracaine. It is delivered either via a patch or as a cream that is applied to the skin, allowed to dry and then peeled off 15–60 min later. Although not yet FDA approved, several clinical studies have demonstrated excellent anesthetic efficacy. Longer application times are better for leg veins, likely due to their greater depth and that these lesions are typically more painful to treat. S-Caine may lead to vasodilation, which could be beneficial for treating vascular lesions.

Local Injections and Facial Nerve Blocks

Local infiltration of an anesthetic can be used for laser treatments associated with more pain and/or as an adjunct to nerve blocks. Unfortunately the anesthetic itself burns, but this discomfort can be minimized by slowly injecting pre-warmed, buffered lidocaine (1:10 ratio of 8.4% sodium bicarbonate to 1–2% lidocaine) through a 30 gauge needle. Of note, buffered lidocaine reduces the average anesthesia time from 50 min to 30 min and the unused portion must be refrigerated. In a sensitive patient, a topical anesthetic or ice can be used on the skin as well as vibration or pinching of the area to minimize pain perception. Use of 2% lidocaine without epinephrine avoids the 'adrenaline rush and heart pounding' that many patients find disconcerting, but the duration of anesthesia will be shorter.

As shown in Figure 10.1, many of the facial nerves can be easily accessed either percutaneously or, in some cases, intraorally. If the intraoral route is used then application of viscous lidocaine or other topical anesthetic can further reduce injection discomfort, although the actual puncture is rarely that uncomfortable.

The supraorbital, infraorbital, and mental nerves are vertically aligned along the midpupillary line. The supratrochlear and infratrochlear nerves are located 1.5 cm medial to the supraorbital nerve. These latter

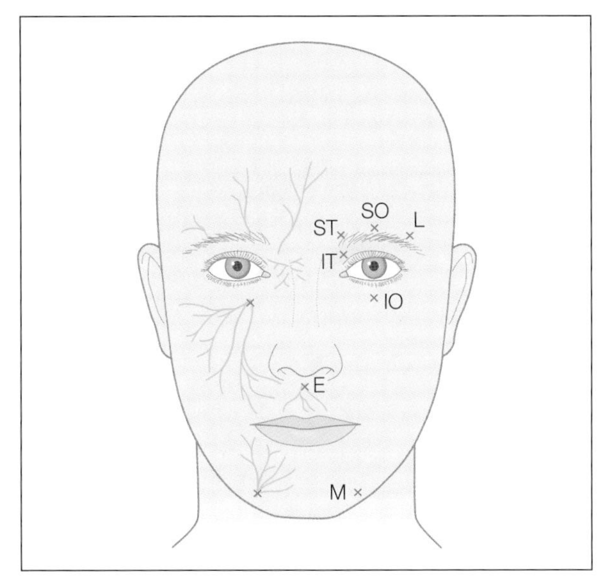

Fig. 10.1 Drawing of face with marked sites for nerve blocks. ST = supratrochlear nerve, SO = supraorbital nerve, L = lacrimal nerve, IT = infratrochlear nerve, IO = infraorbital nerve, E = ethmoid nerve, M = mental nerve

three nerves can be blocked with a single injection using a 30 gauge 1 in needle. The procedure is to enter just lateral to the supraorbital notch and advance medially 2 cm to just medial to the medial canthus, then inject 2 cc while withdrawing the needle.

For the infraorbital nerve, injection can be made from an intraoral position, going through the sulcus at the apex of the canine tooth and aiming for the infraorbital foramen (palpable on the infraorbital rim) (Fig. 10.2A). Injecting 2 cc in a fan-like distribution provides the best results. For the percutaneous route, injection should be made about 1 cm below the infraorbital rim in the midpupillary line. To block the mental nerve intraorally, the needle should be inserted 5 mm at the apex of the bicuspid and 2 cc injected (Fig. 10.2B). Percutaneously, injection should be in the midpupillary line halfway between the oral commissure and the mandibular margin. In addition, for full-face procedures, it may be helpful to block the lacrimal and ethmoid nerves, and locally infiltrate the corners of the mouth.

Systemic Medications

Systemic medications are frequently used in combination with the other modalities. Oral and/or intramuscular medications can help 'take the edge off' laser treatments. They may be used alone, but more frequently are used in conjunction with

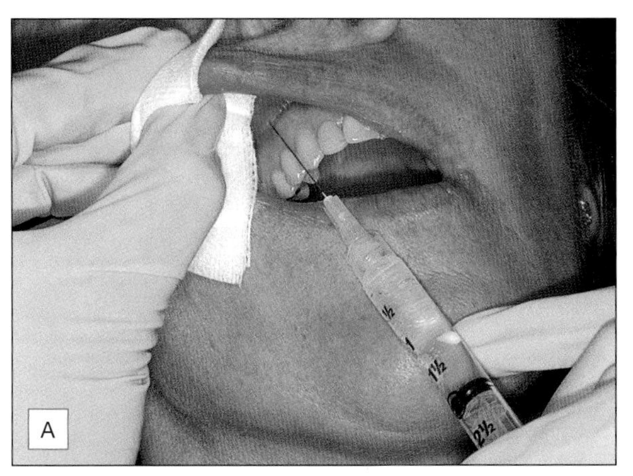

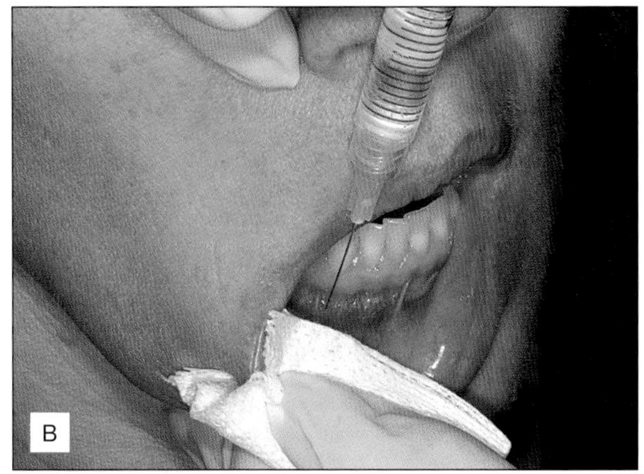

Fig. 10.2 Intraoral approach to infraorbital nerve (**A**) and mental nerve (**B**) blocks

topical, local, or regional anesthesia. Codeine and its derivatives are the most frequently used medications. In addition, anxiolytics are helpful in that they decrease the patient's perception of pain by decreasing anxiety level, thereby increasing their pain tolerance. Lorazepam is shorter acting but does not provide as good an amnestic effect as diazapam.

Finally, nonsteroidal anti-inflammatory drugs (NSAIDs) can be utilized for most laser procedures as bleeding is not typically a concern, although the purpura threshold may be decreased when using lasers to target vascular lesions. The most commonly used NSAIDs are ibuprofen and naproxen. In addition, ketolorac is an excellent alternative for more painful procedures and is typically given in doses of 60 mg i.m., but can be given orally as well. For patients over 60 years of age, the dose must be dropped to 30 mg i.m. This, as well as other NSAIDs, should be avoided in patients with a history of asthma, aspirin allergy, gastrointestinal (GI) bleeding, or ulcer.

Procedure: Anesthesia of Choice

The choice of anesthesia will depend on the laser procedure to be performed. The main considerations will be how fast the onset of the anesthetic needs to be, potential vasoactivity of the anesthetic, and depth of anesthesia required to perform the procedure.

Tattoos, hair removal, and pigmented lesions

For laser treatment of tattoos, hair, and pigmented lesions, the most practical choice will be LMX 4–5%. This can be prescribed ahead of time, allowing the patient to apply it prior to the appointment. If it is a first-time appointment and treatment is going to be performed, it may be more practical to use one of the faster onset topical anesthetics. These anesthetics are typically more difficult to obtain, hence the use of LMX or EMLA for subsequent treatments. Vasoactivity of the anesthetic agent is not an issue for treatment of these conditions.

Nonablative rejuvenation

Nonablative rejuvenation will have similar considerations to the earlier mentioned category, however if there is a vascular component present, consider the vasoactivity of the agent. Vasoconstrictive agents will diminish the target chromophore, hemoglobin, therefore it is best to utilize either a vasoinactive or vasodilating agent. Consideration for speed of onset is similar to that mentioned earlier in that for new patients who may decide to do the treatment on that first day, the faster acting agents will be better, whereas for subsequent appointments LMX can be used. There are many nonablative treatments that do not require the use of an anesthetic. On the first visit, a test spot can be delivered to assess the patient's discomfort level prior to application of anesthetic. They may be able to tolerate the treatment without the potentially confounding variables introduced by placement of the anesthetic, such as vasoactive changes and rare allergy.

Vascular lesions

For vascular lesions LMX would be the current topical anesthetic of choice because of its lack of vasoactivity. Again, S-Caine has the potential added advantage of some vasodilation. In a FDA clinical trial at the current author's facility, S-Caine was used in infants with PWSs or hemangiomas and compared to LMX. This study demonstrated excellent efficacy with no vasoconstriction and vasodilation at the treatment site was even noted in some patients.

Ablative laser resurfacing

There are a variety of anesthesia options for laser resurfacing. Although in many cases conscious sedation and even general anesthesia is used, ablative resurfacing can be performed quite successfully with topical anesthesia in conjunction with oral and/or i.m. medication. In addition, nerve blocks can be utilized to anesthetize the central portion of the face, the area most likely to receive additional passes for greater efficacy. Although there are several topical anesthetics available for use, the current author has found that EMLA provides the greatest anesthesia. As noted earlier, successful anesthesia to a depth of 6 mm was obtained when EMLA was applied with occlusion for 2.5 h. For the past 9 years this author has successfully performed ablative laser resurfacing utilizing EMLA in conjunction with systemic medications (not to the level of conscious sedation) with occasional nerve blocks. See Box 10.1 for her technique of applying EMLA for resurfacing (Fig. 10.3). In addition to the greater depth of anesthesia, the concomitant hydration seems to have a protective effect on the skin. The amount of superficial coagulative necrosis is thinner, whereas the depth of thermal injury appears to be the same when EMLA is used, although it leaves a greater number of normal collagen bundles amidst the thermally denatured collagen. This likely explains the high efficacy and patient satisfaction noted, in addition to the lower incidence of side effects such as hypo- and hyperpigmention, and scarring. In addition, patients

EMLA topical anesthesia protocol

- Wash the area with hot soapy water for 5–10 min.
- Apply a thick layer of EMLA to the treatment area and cover with plastic wrap.
- 45 min prior to the procedure, Valium (usually 10 mg) and pain medication (usually 2 Vicodin, Darvocet, Maxidone or Percocet) is given. The second tube of EMLA is added right over the same area (as the skin has usually absorbed most of it), and the plastic wrap is reapplied.
- The area is treated in sections and each section is wiped off immediately prior to being treated. All passes are done before moving on to the next section.

Box 10.1 EMLA topical anesthesia protocol

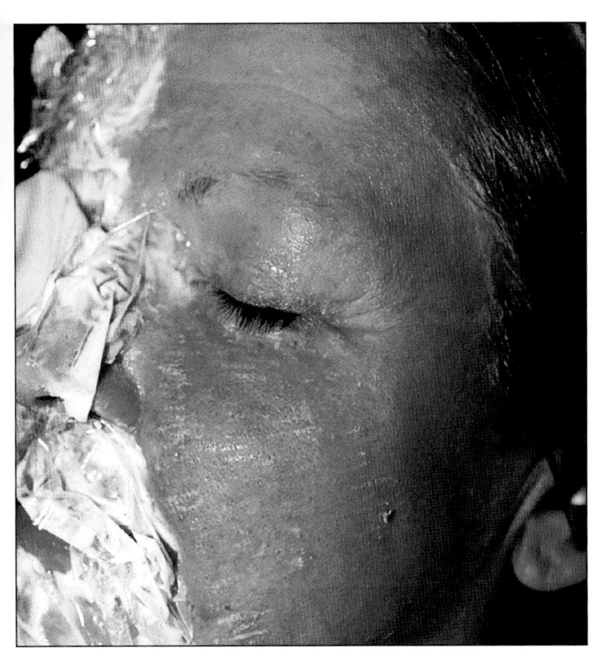

Fig. 10.3 EMLA applied

have minimal postoperative pain. The decreased superficial thermal damage is also associated with faster re-epithialization (6–7 d) and less prolonged erythema, which greatly decreases the downtime.

Summary

The optimum anesthetic choice will depend on the laser procedure to be performed, type of lesion being treated, patient's pain threshold, and physician's familiarity with the various anesthetic modalities described. Many options are available and can often be used in conjunction to maximize the patient's comfort.

Further Reading

Alster TS, Lupton JR 2002 Evaluation of a novel topical anesthetic agent for cutaneous laser resurfacing: a randomized comparison study. Dermatologic Surgery 28:1004–1006

Ashinoff R, Geronemus RG 1990 Effect of the topical anesthetic EMLA on the efficacy of pulsed dye laser treatment of port-wine stains. Journal of Dermatological Surgery and Oncology 16:1008–1011

Bryan HA, Alster TS 2002 The S-Caine peel: a novel topical anesthetic for cutaneous laser surgery. Dermatologic Surgery 28:999–1003

Chen JZ, Alexiades-Armenakas MR, Bernstein LJ, Jacobson LG, Friedman PM, Geronemus RG 2003 Two randomized, double-blind, placebo-controlled studies evaluating the S-Caine Peel for induction of local anesthesia before long-pulsed Nd:YAG laser therapy for leg veins. Dermatologic Surgery 29:1012–1018

Doshi SN, Friedman PM, Marquez DK, Goldberg LH 2003 Thirty-minute application of the S-Caine peel prior to nonablative laser treatment. Dermatologic Surgery 29:1008–1011

Eaglstein NF 1999 Chemical injury to the eye from EMLA cream during erbium laser resurfacing. Dermatologic Surgery 25:590–591

Friedman PM, Fogelman JP, Nouri K, Levine VJ, Ashinoff R 1999 Comparative study of the efficacy of four topical anesthetics. Dermatologic Surgery 25:950–954

Friedman PM, Mafong EA, Friedman ES, Geronemus RG 2001 Topical anesthetics update: EMLA and beyond. Dermatologic Surgery 27:1019–1026

Kilmer SL, Chotzen V, Zelickson BD, et al 2003 Full-face laser resurfacing using a supplemented topical anesthesia protocol. Archives of Dermatology 139:1279–1283

Ramos-Zabala A, Perez-Mencia MT, Fernandez-Garcia R, Cascales-Nunez MR 2004 Anesthesia technique for outpatient facial laser resurfacing. Lasers in Surgery and Medicine 34:269–272

Taddio A, Gurguis MG, Koren G 2002 Lidocaine-prilocaine cream versus tetracaine gel for procedural pain in children. Annals of Pharmacotherapy 36:687–692 [Review]

Subject Index

Notes
Index entries in **bold** refer to information in tables or boxes: index entries in *italics* refer to figures.

A

ablative laser resurfacing *see* laser ablation
absorption, photons, 4, *4*
acitretin, **109**
acne, 89–101
  equipment, 90–91
  expected benefits, 90
  patient selection, 89
  Propionibacterium acnes, 89, 93, 94
  remission, 90, 98
  sebaceous follicle
    anatomy, 89, *91–92*
    damage, 94
  side effects, 90–91
  therapy, 91, 93–100
    anatomical approaches, 91, 93, *94*
    costs, 90
    electromagnetic wave therapy, 91, 93–100
    intense pulsed light, 90, 96–97, *97,* 98
    isotretinoin, 100
    targets, *91–92,* 93
    ultraviolet light, 93, 94, 95
acroinfunfibulum, sebaceous follicle, 89
actinic chelitis, 75
  clinical features, 75
  diagnosis, **75**
  progression to SCC (risk), 75
  therapy, **77,** 80–81
  vermilectomy, 81
actinic keratoses (AK), 75, *76*
  anesthesia, 86
  complications, 87–88
  cosmetic concerns, 82
  costs, 77, 82
  diagnosis, 75, **75**
  patient interviews, 84
  patient selection, 76–78, 86
  squamous cell carcinoma progression, 75
  therapy
    ablation, *see* laser ablation, actinic keratoses
    advanced techniques, 88
    cryosurgery, 80, **83**
    light and laser, 80
    methyl 5-ALA, 80
    options, 77, **77**
    photodynamic therapy, *see* photodynamic therapy, actinic keratoses
    strategy, 82, **83**
  see also nonmelanoma skin cancer
air cooling *see* cold air cooling
alefacept, **109**
alexandrite laser, 3
  facial telangiectasias, 22–24
  hair reduction, 8
  hemangiomas, 15, **15**
  leg veins/venules, 7
  long pulsed, *see* long pulsed alexandrite laser
  vascular lesions, 7, 13
aluminium rollers, 129, *129*
  complications, 133
amateur tatoos *see* tattoo removal
ambulatory phlebectomy, leg veins/venules, 29
aminolevulinic acid (ALA)
  acne, 90, 93, 94
  application, 79
aminolevulinic acid photodynamic therapy (ALA-PDT)
  acne, 96, 97–98
  actinic keratoses, 79, 80, 84, *85*
  adverse effects, 79
  basal cell carcinoma, 81–82
  nonmelanoma skin cancer, 79, 84, *85*
  psoriasis, 107, 113, 119–120
  squamous cell carcinoma, 82
  see also photodynamic therapy
anesthesia, 137–141
  children, 25, 138
  hair removal, 140
  laser ablation, 86, 140–141
  local injections, 138–139
  neonates, 138
  nerve blocks, 138–139, *139*
  nonablative rejuvenation, 140
  nonmelanoma skin cancer, 86
  pigmented lesion removal, 61–62, 140
  psoriasis therapy, 110, 120, **121,** 122
  scar therapy, 72
  systemic medication, 139
  tattoo removal, 61–62, 140
  topical, 25, 137–138
  varicose veins, 38
  vascular lesions, 140
angiogenesis, scar formation, 67
angiography, arteriovenous vascular malformations, 25
anthralin, **108**
antibiotics, prophylactic
  actinic keratoses, laser ablation, 86
  laser ablation, nonmelanoma skin cancer, 86
  nonmelanoma skin cancer, 86

antivirals, prophylactic
  actinic keratoses laser ablation, 86
  laser ablation, nonmelanoma skin cancer, 86
  nonmelanoma skin cancer, 86
anxiolytic drugs, 139
areola tattoo removal, 65
argon lasers
  hemangiomas, 15
  history, 1
  vascular lesions, 12
argon pumped tunable dye laser, 12
arterial vascular malformation, 17
arteriovenous vascular malformation (AVMs), 17, 24–25
arthritis, psoriatic, 103
atoms, 1

B

basal cell carcinoma (BCC), 76, *76*
  diagnosis, **75,** 76
  laser therapy, 81–82
  light therapy, 81–82
  morpheaform, 81
  nodular, 81, 82
  pigmented, 81
  subtypes, 76, 81, 82
  superficial, 81
  therapy, **77,** 82, **83–84**
  see also nonmelanoma skin cancer
Beer's law, 4
benzoyl peroxide, 100
betacaine-LA, 138
blackheads, 89
blistering
  cooling complication, 133, *134*
  psoriasis therapies, 122, 123, 124, 125
blue and violet light, acne, 93, 95
blue light, acne, 90
BLU-U light
  acne, 90, 98
  actinic keratoses, 79, *79,* 85, *85, 86*
  nonmelanoma skin cancer, 85, *85, 86*
  photodynamic therapy, 79, *79,* 84, 85, *85, 86*
Bowen's disease, 82, 86
broad band ultraviolet B (BB-UVB), psoriasis, 103, **110**
bruits, 24
bulk cooling, 38

C

café au lait macules (CALMs), 41, 61
  complications, *49,* 61
  darker-skin types, 61
  expected benefits, 46
  ruby laser, 8
  study results, **51**
  therapy technique, 61
calcipotriene, **108**
capillary cavernous hemangiomas, 14
capillary (strawberry) hemangiomas, 14
capillary vascular malformation *see* port wine stains
carbon dioxide (CO_2) laser, 2, 3
  ablative resurfacing, 8–9
  actinic chelitis, 80–81
  actinic keratoses, 78, 80, 86
  basal cell carcinoma, 81
  history, 1
  lymphatic malformations, 25
  nevoid basal cell carcinoma syndrome, 75
  nonmelanoma skin cancer, 78, 86
  psoriasis therapy, 103, 110–111, 118, 120–122
    anesthesia, 110, 120, **121**
    complications, 111, **111,** 121–122
    cost, **111**
    equipment, **119**
    expected outcome, **110**
    mechanism of action, *106,* **107**
    postoperative care, 121, **121**
    pretherapy, 120, **121**
    reimbursement, **111**
    remission, 110
    side effects, 121–122
    technique, 120–121
  scar therapy, 68, 69
  squamous cell carcinoma, 82
  tattoo granulomas, 55, *57,* 65
  tattoo removal, 66
cavernous hemangiomas, 14
cherry angioma, 12, 24, 26
children, anesthesia, 25, 138
chromophores
  absorber, 6
  absorption, 4, *5*
  endogenous, 4
  exogenous, 4
  vascular lesion removal, 11, 12
coagulation necrosis, nonspecific, 12
codeine, 139
coherence of light, 2
cold air cooling, 6, 129
  complications, 133
  hair removal, 131
  leg veins/venules, 38, 132
  pros/cons, 132–133
  vascular lesions, 131
cold gels, 129, 131, 132
collagen
  absorption, 4
  light scattering properties, 4
  remodelling, 8–9
  wound healing, 67
collagen vascular disease, 21
collimation of light, 2, *2*
complement factors, wound healing, 67
compound nevi, 63, *63*
compression sclerotherapy, 29
congenital nevi, 63, *64*
contact cooling, 6, 128–129
  hair removal, 131
  nonablative remodeling, 131
  vascular lesions, 131
continuous pulse lasers, 3
continuous wave laser, vascular lesions, 12
cooling, 6–7, 127–135
  active, 128
  applications, 130–131

cooling (*cont'd*)
complications, 133–134
contact, *see* contact cooling
contraindications, 128
cutaneous nerve confusion, 131–132
epidermal damage, 6, 133, *134*
laser fluence, 132
methods, 128–130, 134
objectives, 128
pain, 131–132
passive, 128, 133
test spots, 134
timing, 128
see also specific types
cooling protection factor (CPF), 130
CoolRoller, 128, 129, *129*
pros/cons, 133
copper bromide laser, 12
copper plate cooling, 129, *130,* 134
copper vapor laser, 12
corneal abrasion, EMLA, 138
corticosteroids
psoriasis, **108**
scar therapy, 69–70, 73
cosmetic tattoos, 41
pigment darkening, *64,* 65
removal, 65
crusting
cherry angioma, 26
scar therapy complication, 73
venous lakes, 26
cryogen spray cooling, 6–7, 38, 129–130
frost formation, 129
see also dynamic cooling device
cryosurgery/cryotherapy
actinic keratoses, 80, **83**
basal cell carcinoma, 81
hemangiomas, 15
nonmelanoma skin cancer, 77, **77,** 82, **83**
scar tissue, 71
squamous cell carcinoma, 82
cyclosporin, **109**
cystic hygromas, 25

D

DCD *see* dynamic cooling device
decorative tattoo removal, 41
Demodex, 97
diazapam, 139
diclofenac (topical), **83**
diffuse neonatal hemangiomatosis, 14
diode lasers, 3
acne, 98
facial telangiectasias, 22–24, 24
hair reduction, 8
leg veins/venules, 35, **35**
varicose veins, 39
Doppler ultrasound, leg veins/venules, 30, *31*
duplex ultrasound, *32*
leg veins/venules, 31, *32*
varicose veins, 38, 39
dynamic cooling device (DCD), 129–130, *131*
complications, 133
cutaneous nerve confusion, 132
pigmented lesions, 131
pros/cons, 133
selectivity, 130
vascular lesions, 131

E

efalizumab, **109**
electrocautery
contraindication, 77–78, 82
facial telangiectasias, 21
electrodessication and curettage, 82, **83**
electromagnetic wave (EM) therapy, acne, 91, 93–100
photochemical tissue interactions, 94–96
photosensitizer assisted, 94, 97–99
EMLA, 137–138
application protocol, **140,** 141
patch testing, 138
side effects, 137–138
emollients, **108**
endogenous chromophores, 4
endovenous ablation, leg veins/venules, 31
energy fluence, 6, 12
epidermal damage
ablative laser resurfacing, 8
cooling, 6
pulsed dye laser, 26, 64, 127
vascular lesions therapy, 26
erbium:YAG (Er:YAG) laser, 3, 9, 103, 107
actinic keratoses, 78, 80, 86, 87, *87*
lymphatic malformations, 25
nonmelanoma skin cancer, 78, 86, 87, *87*
psoriasis therapy, 110–111, 118
anesthesia, 120, **121**
complications, 111, **111,** 121–122
costs, **111**
endpoints, 110, *112*
equipment, 118, **119**
expected outcome, **110**
mechanism of action, *106,* **107**
postoperative care, 121, **121**
pretherapy, 120, **121**
reimbursement, **110**
side effects, 121–122
technique, 120–121
erythema
acne therapy side effect, 90
port wine stain, 19
psoriasis, 125
vascular lesions, 25
erythroplasia of Queyrat (SCC in situ of the penis), 82
etanercept, **109**
ethmoid nerve block, 139
excimer laser, psoriasis therapy, 107, *107,* 113–114, *115,* 120, 123–125
anesthesia, **121**
combination therapy, 124
complications, **111,** 124, 125
cost, **111**
equipment, **120**
expected outcome, **110**

excimer laser, psoriasis therapy (*cont'd*)
inverse psoriasis, *117*
mechanism of action, *106,* **107**
minimal erythema dose testing, 123, *123,* **123**
postoperative care, **121,** 125
pretherapy, **121,** 123–125
reimbursement, **111**
scalp psoriasis, *117*
side effects, 125
technique, *124,* 124–125
see also high intensity ultraviolet B, psoriasis therapy
excisional surgery *see* surgery, excisional
exogenous chromophores, 4
eyebrow tattoo removal, 65
eye protection
laser ablation, 86
photodynamic therapy, 84
pigmented lesion removal, 62
scar therapy, 72
tattoo removal, 62

F

facial telangiectasias, 12, 21–24
collagen vascular disease, 21
postoperative care, **21**
rosacea association, 21
spider, 21, 22
therapy, 15, 21–24
fiberoptic cables, 3
fibroblasts, scarring, 67
Fitzpatrick skin types
cooling, 134
leg vein therapy, 36
pigmented lesion removal, 46, 58
port wine stains, 18
scar therapy, 68–69, 72
types IV-VI, 69, 72
tattoo removal, 45, *46,* 58, 65
blue/black ink, 59, 60
vascular lesions, 12
flash lamp pulsed dye laser
hemangiomas, 15–16
port wine stain, 18
vascular lesions, 7
wavelength, 6
see also intense pulsed light (IPL)
5-fluorouracil (5-FU)
actinic keratoses, 80, **83**
nonmelanoma skin cancer, **83**
scar therapy, 69–70, 73
squamous cell carcinoma, 82
foam sclerotherapy, varicose veins, 38, *38*
freckles, ruby laser, 8
full face photorejuvenation, 61

G

glaucoma, port wine stains, 18
granulomas
pyogenic, 12, 17
tattoo, 55, *57,* 65
greater saphenous vein (GSV), 29, *30,* 39
green light, acne, 93

H

hair removal/reduction, 8
anesthesia, 140
cooling, 131
light assisted, 6
thermal relaxation time, 6
heavy metal vapor lasers, 12
hemangiomas, 14–17
associated conditions, 14
classification, 14
clinical features, 14
complications, 14–15, 17
diagnosis, **13,** 14
involuting, 14
prevalence, 14
proliferating, 14
therapy, **15,** 15–17
steroids, 15
surgery, 15
ulcerated, 14–15
hemoglobin, absorption, 4
herpes simplex virus
pigmented lesion removal, 58
tattoo removal, 58
high intensity ultraviolet B, psoriasis therapy, 107, *108,* 113–114, *116,* 120
combination therapy, 124
comparison with other therapies, **118**
complications, **111,** 124, 125
costs, **111**
equipment, **120**
expected outcome, **110**
inflammatory T lymphocyte apoptosis, 113, *114*
mechanism of action, *106,* **107**
minimal erythema dose testing, 123, *123,* **123**
postoperative care, 125
pretherapy, 123–124
reimbursement, **111**
technique, *124,* 124–125
high peak power lasers, 3
hydrogel dressing, psoriasis therapies, 119, 122
hydroxyurea, **109**
hyperpigmentation
pigmented lesion removal, 63
post-inflammatory, pigmented lesion removal, 46, *49*
hyperpigmentation, post-therapy
acne therapy, 90
actinic keratoses, 88
café au lait macules, 61
nonmelanoma skin cancer, 79, 88
pigmented lesion removal, 63
psoriasis, 122, 123
psoriasis therapy, 125
scar therapy, 72, 73
tattoo removal, 43, 58, 60, *61,* 63
hypertrophic scars, 67–68, *68*
hypopigmentation, pigmented lesion removal, 63
hypopigmentation, post-therapy
actinic keratoses, 77, 82, 88
nonmelanoma skin cancer, 77, 79, 88
pigmented lesion removal, 63
pulsed dye lasers, 26

hypopigmentation, post-therapy (*cont'd*)
tattoo removal, 43, 60, 63
vascular lesions, 26

I

ibuprofen, 139
ice, 129, 132
imiquimod (topical)
actinic keratoses, **83**
nonmelanoma skin cancer, **83**
indocyanine green (ICG) dye, acne, 98–99
inflammation, wound healing, 67
inflammatory T-lymphocyte reduction
high intensity UVB, 113, *114*
pulse dye laser, 111, *113*
infliximab, **109**
infrainfundibulum, sebaceous follicle, 89
infraorbital nerve block, 139, *139*
infratrochlear nerve block, 138–139
infundibulum, sebaceous follicle, 89
acne therapy target, 93
mid-infrared lasers, 99, *100*
intense pulsed light (IPL)
acne, 90, 96–97, *97,* 98
actinic keratoses, 84
epidermal damage, 127
facial telangiectasias, 21, **23,** 24
hemangiomas, **15,** 16–17
lasers, 12–13
leg veins/venules, 36–37
lentigines, **50,** 61
light filters, 36
nonmelanoma skin cancer, 84
photorejuvenation, 96
Poikiloderma of Civatte, 24
port wine stain, 19
vascular lesions, 12–13
venous malformations, 20–21
interferon alpha, hemangiomas, 15
interleukins, wound healing, 72
inverse psoriasis, 114, 115, *117*
involuting hemangiomas, 14
isotretinoin, 100

K

Kasabach–Merritt syndrome, 14
keloids, 68, *68*
angiogenesis, 67
development, 67
excision, 70–71
fibroblasts, 67
location, 68
pulsed dye laser, 70–71, *71*
therapy history, 71
see also scar therapy
keratolytics, **108**
ketolorac, 139
Koebner phenomenon, 107
KTP lasers *see* potassium titanyl phosphate laser

L

lacrimal nerve block, 139
laser ablation, 8–9
actinic keratoses, 80, **83,** 86–88
anesthesia, 86
complications, 87–88
equipment, 86
eye protection, 86
full face, 86
postoperative care, 87
residual tumor, 87, *87*
side effects, 87–88
troubleshooting, 87
tumor-free dermis, 87, *87*
anesthesia, 86, 140–141
basal cell carcinoma, 81
collagen remodelling, 8–9
light–tissue interaction, 8–9
nerve blocks, 140
nonmelanoma skin cancer, **84,** 86–88
complications, 87–88
equipment, 86
full face resurfacing, 86
patients, 86
residual tumor, 87, *87*
side effects, 87–88
troubleshooting, 87
tumor-free dermis, 87, *87*
psoriasis, 103, 107
skin healing, 8–9
see also carbon dioxide (CO_2) laser; erbium:YAG (Er:YAG) laser
laser mediums, *2,* 2–3
lasers
delivery systems, 3
fiberoptic cables, 3
high peak power, 3
history, 1
light, 1–2
atom excitation, *1*
coherence, 2
collimation, 2, *2*
monochromacity, 2
simulated emission of radiation, *1,* 1–2
spontaneous emission of radiation, 1, *1*
mediums, *2,* 2–3
optical (resonator) cavity, 3
pulse characteristics, 3, *3,* 3–4
pulsed, 3
quality-switched (Q-switched), 3–4
superpulsing, 3
resinator cavity, 3
see also specific types
lateral subdermic venous system (LSVS), 29, *31*
leg veins/venules, 29–40
anatomy, 29, *30*
cooling, 33, 37–38, 132
diagnostic tools, **30,** 30–31
expected benefits, 29
matting, 31, *32*
patient evaluation, 29

leg veins/venules (*cont'd*)
  prevalence, 29
  sclerotherapy, 7, 31
    vs. lasers, 37
  side effects, 29
  therapy, 31, 33–37
    advanced techniques, 37–39
    laser selection, 29, 33–37
      see also pulsed dye laser (PDL)
    parameter selection, 33, **33**
    target selection, 31, *32*
  thermal relaxation time, 6
  varicose, *see* varicose veins
lentigines, 41, 46, 61
  clearance/improvement rates, **50**
  full face photorejuvenation, 61
  new lesion development post-therapy, 46
  Peutz–Jeghers syndrome, 46–47, *51*
  therapy, *47, 48,* **50,** 61
lesser saphenous vein (LSV), 29, *30*
Levulan Kerastick^{TM}, 79, *79,* 84, *85*
lidocaine, 137, 138
light avoidance, photodynamic therapy, 85, 86
light filters
  flashlamps, 6
  intense pulsed light, 36
light–tissue interaction, 5–9
  ablative resurfacing, 8–9
  clinical relevance, 7–9
  energy fluence, 6
  hair removal, 8
  laser wavelengths, *5,* 5–6
  nonablative resurfacing, 9
  photodynamic reactions, 5
  photostimulation, 5
  photothermolytic/photomechanical reactions, 5–6
  pigmented lesions, 7–8
  thermal damage time, 6
  thermal relaxation time, 5, 6
  vascular lesions, 7
lip tattoo removal, 65
LMX, 138, 140
long pulsed alexandrite laser
  facial telangiectasias, 22–24
  leg veins/venules, 34–35, **35**
lorazepam, 139
lymphangioma circumscriptum, 25
lymphatic malformations, 17, 25

M

magnetic resonance imaging, venous malformations, 20
malignant melanoma, 75, *75*
medical tattoo removal, 55
melanin
  absorption, 4, *5,* 6
  wavelength, 6
melanoma, 75, *75*
mental nerve block, 139, *139*
metastasis, squamous cell carcinoma, 76
methemoglobin, 36
methemoglobinemia, 138
methotrexate, **109**
mid-infrared (MIR) lasers
  acne, 93, *99,* 99–100, *100*
  cooling, 127, 131
minimal erythema dose (MED) testing
  excimer laser, 123, *123,* **123**
  high intensity UVB, 123, *123,* **123**
Mohs micrographic surgery
  nonmelanoma skin cancer, 82, **83**
  squamous cell carcinoma, 76
monochromacity of light, 2
mycophenolate motefil, **109**

N

nail, psoriatic changes, 103, *105*
naproxen, 139
narrow band ultraviolet B, psoriasis, 103, *106,* 107, **110**
Nd:YAG laser
  blue reticular veins, 24
  facial telangiectasias, 21–22, **22**
  frequency doubled, 13
  hair reduction, 8
  hemangiomas, 15, **15,** 16
  history, 1
  leg veins/venules, 7, **35,** 35–36, *36*
  port wine stain, 19
  Q-switched, *see* Q-switched (quality switched) laser(s), Nd:YAG
  scar therapy, 68, 69
  tattoo removal, 60–61, 65
  varicose veins, 39
  vascular lesions, 7, 13, 25, 26
  venous malformations, 20
near-infrared (NIR) lasers
  acne, 93
  cooling, 127
neodymium:yttrium-aluminium-garnet laser *see* Nd:YAG laser
neonates, anesthesia, 138
nerve blocks, 138–139, *139,* 140
nevi of Ito, 41, 46, **51–52,** 61
nevi of Ota, 7, 41, 46, **51–52,** 61
nevoid basal cell carcinoma syndrome, 81
nevus flammeus *see* port wine stains
nevus simplex (salmon patch, stork bite), 17, 24
nodular basal cell carcinoma, 81, 82
nodular port wine stain, 19
nonablative resurfacing, 9
  anesthesia, 140
  cooling, 9, 131
  light–tissue interaction, 9
  see also individual techniques
nonmelanoma skin cancer, 75–88
  anesthesia, 86
  comorbid conditions, 78
  costs, 77, 82
  electrocautery contraindication, 77–78
  major determinants, 82
  patient interviews, 84
  patient selection, 76–78
  therapy
    cosmetic concerns, 82
    cryotherapy, 77, **77,** 82, **83**
    electrodessication and curettage, 82, **83**

nonmelanoma skin cancer (*cont'd*)
excisional surgery, **83**
expected benefits, 78–82
laser ablation, *see* laser ablation
lasers used, **77, 78**
Mohs surgery, 82, **83**
options, 77, **77**
strategy, 82–84, **83**–84
surgery, 75
tips, 88
see also specific therapies
see also basal cell carcinoma (BCC); squamous cell carcinoma (SCC)
nonsteroidal anti-inflammatory drugs (NSAIDs), 139

O

Osler–Weber–Rendu syndrome, 17
oxyhemoglobin, 11, 12
absorption, 11, *11*

P

parallel cooling, 38, 128, 132
perforate invagination (PIN) stripping, 38
Peutz–Jeghers syndrome, 46–47, *51*
PHACES syndrome, 14
photochemical tissue interactions
acne, 93, 94–96
with photothermal interactions, 93, 96–98
photodynamic reactions, 5
photodynamic therapy (PDT), 5
acne, 96
actinic keratoses, 78–80, *79,* **83,** 84–86
complications, 86
efficacy, **78**
equipment, 84
light application, 85
patients, 84
postoperative care, 85
pretherapy, 84, 85
side effects, 86
troubleshooting, 85–86
waiting period, 85
aminolevulinic acid, *see* aminolevulinic acid photodynamic therapy (ALA-PDT)
basal cell carcinoma, 81–82
laser mediated, 80
light sources, **79**
nonmelanoma skin cancer, 75, 77, **77, 78,** 78–80, *79,* **84,** 84–86
adverse effects, 79
complications, 86
efficacy, **78**
equipment, 84
patients, 84
post therapy care, 85
protoporphyrin IX, 78
side effects, 86
troubleshooting, 85–86
photoprotective clothing, 85, 86
port wine stain, 19
psoriasis therapy, 107, 111–113, 119–120, 122–123
anesthesia, **121,** 122
complications, **111,** 122–123
cost, **111**
equipment, **120**
expected outcome, **110**
light sources, **120**
mechanism of action, **107**
porphyrin, 111, 113
postoperative care, **121,** 122
pretherapy, **121,** 122
protoporphyrin IX, 113
reimbursement, **111**
side effects, 122–123
technique, 122
photographs, pretherapy
scar therapy, 72
tattoo removal, 63
photomechanical reactions, 5–6
photoplethysmography, leg veins/venules, 30
photoprotective clothing, photodynamic therapy, 85, 86
photorejuvenation, full face, 61
photoselectivity, leg vein therapy, 37
photosensitizer, 5
photostimulation, 5
phototherapy, psoriasis, 103, *106,* **110**
photothermal tissue interactions
acne, 94, 99–100
with photochemical interactions, 93, 96–98
photothermolytic reactions, 5–6
phototoxicity
acne therapy side effect, 90–91
nonmelanoma skin cancer, 86
psoriasis therapy, 122, 124
pigmented lesion removal, 7–8, 41
anesthesia, 61–62, 140
café au lait macules, *see* café au lait macules (CALMs)
cold gels, 131
compound nevi, 63, *63*
congenital nevi, 63, *64*
cooling, 131
costs, 47
expected benefits, 46–47
eye protection, 62
Fitzpatrick skin types, 58
follow-up, 62
herpes simplex virus, 58
incomplete removal, 63
laser handpiece positioning, 62
lentigines, *see* lentigines
patient history, **60**
patient selection, 45–46
pigmentation alteration, 63
postoperative care, 62
Q-switched lasers, 41
side effects/complications, 63–65
tanned skin, 58
test spots, 58, *59, 60*
therapy, 58, 60–62
thermal injury/scarring, 64–65
thermal relaxation time, 41
troubleshooting, 63
Pityrosporum acnes, 5

plaque type psoriasis, 103, *104,* 115
  therapy limitations, 108–110
plethysmography, leg veins/venules, 30, *31*
Poikiloderma of Civatte, 21, 24
porphyrins, 111, 113
  absorption spectrum, *95*
  acne, 94
port wine stains (PWS), 7, 12, 17–19
  anesthesia, 137
  diagnosis, **13**
  glaucoma risk, 18
  hypertrophic, 19
  limb hypertrophy, 18
  nodular, 19
  prevalence, 17
  skin types, 18
  therapy, 18–20
  thermal relaxation time, 12
postcooling, 38, 128, 132
post-inflammatory hyperpigmentation, 46, *49*
potassium titanyl phosphate (KTP) laser
  acne, 90, 97
  acne vulgaris, 97
  cooling, 33
  epidermal damage, 127
  facial telangiectasias, 21, *23*
  hemangiomas, 15, **15,** 16
  leg veins/venules, 33, **33**
  purpura, 7
  rosacea, 97
  vascular lesions, 7, 13, 25
  venous malformations, 20
precooling, 38, 128, 129, 132
  vascular lesions, 12
professional tattoos, 41
proliferation, wound healing, 67
prophylactic antibiotics *see* antibiotics, prophylactic
prophylactic antivirals *see* antivirals, prophylactic
Propionibacterium acnes, 89
  acne therapy target, 93
  photoinactivation, 94
protoporphyrin IX (PpIX)
  acne, 93, 96, 97
  nonmelanoma skin cancer, 78
  psoriasis, 113
pruritus, scar therapy, 72
psoralens and ultraviolet A (PUVA), 103, **110**
psoriasis, 103–125
  action spectrum, 103
  biological agents, **109**
  biopsy, **104,** *105*
  complications, **111**
  diagnosis, 103, **104**
  differential diagnosis, **104**
  equipment, 118–125
  expected benefits, 110, **110,** 115
  intralesional agents, **108**
  inverse, 114, 115, *117*
  Koebner phenomenon, 107
  laser therapy, 103, *106,* 107, **107,** 115
    costs, **111**
    pulsed dye laser, *see* pulsed dye laser (PDL)
  light sources, 103, *106,* 107, **107**
  nail changes, 103, *105*
  patient evaluation, 114, **118**
  patient selection, 107–110, 115, 118, **118**
  phototherapy, 103, *106,* **110**
  preprocedure planning, 120
  reverse Koebner phenomenon, 103, 106, 110
  scalp, 114, *117*
  systemic agents, **109**
  therapy techniques, 114–125, *119,* 120, **121**
    comparison, **118**
  topical agents, **108**
psoriasis area and severity index (PASI), *123*
psoriatic arthritis, 103
pulsed dye laser (PDL), 3
  acne, 90, 96, 98
  actinic keratoses, 80
  cooling, 127, 132
  epidermal damage, 26, 64, 127
  facial telangiectasias, 12, 21, *22*
  hemangiomas, 12, 15, **15,** 16, *16*
  keloids, 70–71, *71*
  leg veins/venules, 7, 33–34, *34,* **34**
    pulse duration, 33, 34, **34**
  limitations, 13
  penetration depth, 13
  port wine stains, 7, 12, **18,** 18–19, *19, 20,* 33
  psoriasis, 107, 111, 118–119
    anesthesia, **121,** 122
    clearance, 111, *113*
    complications, **111**
    cost, **111**
    equipment, **119**
    expected outcome, **110**
    inflammatory T-lymphocyte reduction, 111, *113*
    mechanism of action, *106,* **107**
    postoperative care, **121,** 122
    pretherapy, **121,** 122
    reimbursement, **111**
    side effects, 122
    technique, 122
  scar therapy, 68, 69–71, 72
  telangiectases, 34
  thermal injury/scarring, 64
  vascular lesions, 7, 12, 25–26
  venous malformations therapy, 20
purpura
  hemangiomas, 17
  port wine stain, 20
  scar therapy, 69, 73
  vascular lesions, 25
PUVA (psoralens and ultraviolet A), 103, **110**
pyogenic granuloma, 12, 17

Q

Q-switched (quality switched) laser(s), 3–4
  cooling, 128
  pigmented lesion removal, 41
  short pulse, 3
  tattoo removal, 41, 45
Q-switched (quality switched) laser(s), alexandrite
  nevi of Ito, 61

Q-switched (quality switched) laser(s), alexandrite (*cont'd*)
nevi of Ota, 61
tattoo removal, 59, 65
Q-switched (quality switched) laser(s), Nd:YAG
café au lait macules, *49,* 61
frequency-doubled, 61
lentigines, *47, 48,* 61
nevi of Ito, 61
nevi of Ota, 7, 8
pigmented lesion removal, 7–8, *59, 60*
tattoo removal, 7–8
amateur tattoo, *42, 43, 46*
dark blue/black ink, 59, 60
pigment darkening, 64
professional tattoo, *53, 54*
red ink, 60
test spots, *59, 60*
traumatic tattoo, *56, 57*
Q-switched (quality switched) laser(s), ruby
compound nevi, *63*
congenital nevi, *64*
nevi of Ito, 61
nevi of Ota, *49,* 61
Peutz–Jeghers syndrome, *51*
post-inflammatory hyperpigmentation, *49*
tattoo removal
amateur tattoo, *42*
cosmetic tattoo, *64*
green ink therapy, 60
lighter skin, dark blue/black ink, 59
multicolored, 65
professional tattoo, *42, 44, 45*
quality-switched lasers *see* Q-switched (quality switched) laser(s)

R

radiation
spontaneous emission, 1, *1*
stimulated emission, *1,* 1–2
radiofrequency therapy
acne, 100
acne vulgaris, 100
varicose veins, 38–39, *39*
Rayleigh scatter, 4
red light, acne, 93
reflection, 4, *4*
remodelling, wound healing, 67
resurfacing *see* laser ablation; nonablative resurfacing
reticular veins, *32*
blue, 24
facial, 24
therapy, 31, 36
retinoids
pigmented lesion removal, 58
psoriasis, **108**
tattoo removal, 58
reverse Koebner phenomenon, 103, 107, 110
rhytide correction, 61
'road rash', 55
rosacea
facial telangiectasias, 21
intense pulsed light, 96
potassium titanyl phosphate laser, 97
ruby laser
acne, 99
café au lait macules, 8
freckles, 8
hair reduction, 8
history, 1
lentigines, 61
Q-switched, *see* Q-switched (quality switched) laser(s), ruby

S

saphenous vein reflux, 38
sapphire window cooling, *128,* 129
complications, 133
leg vein therapy, 38
pigmented lesions, 131
pros/cons, 133
S-Caine, 138, 140
scalp psoriasis, 114, *117*
scars/scarring
actinic keratoses, 77, 88
angiogenesis, 67
formation, 67
hypertrophic, 67–68, *68*
incidence, 67
keloids, *see* keloids
nonmelanoma skin cancer, 77, 88
pigmented lesion removal, 64–65
psoriasis, 122
tattoo removal, 63, 64–65
therapy, *see* scar therapy
vascular lesions, 26
scar therapy, 67–73
anesthesia, 72
complications, 73
drug therapy, 69–70, 73
equipment, 72
expected benefits, 69
eye protection, 72
Fitzpatrick skin type
determination, 72
IV-VI, 69, 72
laser handpiece positioning, 72
patient history, 71
patient interviews, 71–72
patient selection, 68–69
postoperative care, 72
side effects, 69, 72–73
skin tone, 68–69
strategy, 69–73, *70*
techniques, 72–73
test spots, 69
young scars, 69, *70*
scattering, light, 4
sclerotherapy
contraindications, 37
facial telangiectasias, 21
hemangiomas, 15
leg veins/venules, 7, 29, 31
varicose veins, 38, *38*

sclerotherapy (*cont'd*)
venous malformations, 20
vs. lasers therapy, 37
sebaceous follicle, 89, *91–92*
sebaceous gland
absorption curve, 93, *94*
acne therapy target, 93
damage in acne therapy, 94
indocyanine green dye, 98
selective photothermolysis, 5, 11
extended theory, 6, 8
vascular lesions, 11
skin cooling *see* cooling
skin crusting *see* crusting
skin types *see* Fitzpatrick skin types
spider nevi (spider telangiectasias), 21, 22
spider telangiectasias (spider nevi), 21, 22
spontaneous emission of radiation, 1, *1*
squamous cell carcinoma (SCC), 75, 76, *76*
cryotherapy, 82
diagnosis, **75**
erythroplasia of Queyrat, 82
5-fluorouracil, 82
in situ (Bowen's disease), 82, 86
laser therapy, 82
metastasis, 76
Mohs micrographic surgery, 76
surgical excision, 76
therapy options, **77**
see also nonmelanoma skin cancer
steroid therapy, hemangiomas, 15
stimulated emission of radiation, *1,* 1–2
strawberry (capillary) hemangiomas, 14
stripping, varicose veins, 38
Sturge–Weber syndrome, 17
sun avoidance, photodynamic therapy, 85, 86
sunblock, photodynamic therapy, 85
superpulsing lasers, 3
supraorbital nerve block, 138–139
supratrochlear nerve block, 138–139
surface cooling *see* cooling
surgery, excisional
hemangiomas, 15
keloids, 70–71
nonmelanoma skin cancer, **83**
squamous cell carcinoma, 76

T

tanned skin
cooling, 134
pigmented lesion removal, 58
tattoo removal, 45
tanning, psoriasis therapy side effect, 125
tar, **108**
tattoo removal, 7–8, 8, 41, 58, *58,* 59–61
alternative approaches, 65
amateur tattoos, 41, *42, 43, 46*
anesthesia, 61–62, 140
before/after photographs, *42, 44, 45, 53, 54*
blue/black ink removal, 8, 59, 60
carbon dioxide laser, 66
clearance/improvement rates, **54–55**
complications, 63–65
cosmetic tattoos, 41, *64,* 65
costs, 55
exogenous chromophores, 4
expected benefits, 47, 52, 55
eye protection, 62
Fitzpatrick skin types, 58
IV-VI, 45, 60, 65
follow-up therapy, 62
granulomas, 55, *57,* 65
green ink removal, 8, 60–61
herpes simplex virus, 58
incomplete, 41, *44, 45,* 63
ink colour variation, 52, *53,* 58
laser handpiece positioning, 62
light–tissue interaction, 7–8
medical tattoos, 55
multicolored tattoos, 65
patient history, **60**
patient selection, 41–43, *46*
postoperative care, 62
Q-switched lasers, *see* Q-switched (quality switched) laser(s)
red ink removal, 8, 60
side effects, 63–65
study results, **54–55**
tattoo pigment darkening, 64, *64*
test spots, 58, *59, 60,* 65
thermal injury/scarring, 64–65
thermal relaxation time, 6, 41
traumatic tattoo, *see* traumatic tattoo removal
troubleshooting, 62–63
telangiectasias
facial, *see* facial telangiectasias
matting, 31, *32*
therapy, 34, 35, 36
tetracaine, 138
tetrafluoroethane, 129
thermal damage time (TDT), 6, 8
thermal injury
pigmented lesion removal, 64–65
tattoo removal, 64–65
thermal quenching, 132
thermal relaxation time (TRT), 5, 6
hair follicle, 6
light assisted hair removal, 6
pigmented lesion removal, 41
port wine stain, determination, 11–12
tattoo removal, 41
thermokinetic selectivity, 6
thermokinetic selectivity, 6
6-thioguanine, **109**
tissue cooling *see* cooling
tissue interaction with light *see* light–tissue interaction
tissue–light interaction *see* light–tissue interaction
tissue optics, *4,* 4–5
absorption, 4, *4*
reflection, 4, *4*
scattering, 4
transmission, *4,* 5
titanium:sapphire laser
pigmented lesion removal, 41
tattoo removal, 41

T lymphoctes *see* inflammatory T-lymphocyte reduction
topicaine, 138
topical anesthesia, 25, 137–138
transmission, light, *4,* 5
traumatic tattoo removal, 55, *56, 57*
  Q-switched Nd:YAG laser, *56, 57*
  road rash, 55
  tattoo granulomas, 55, *57,* 65
triamcinolone (TAC), scar therapy, 73

U

ulcerated hemangiomas, 14–15
UltraPulse laser, 3
ultraviolet A (UVA)
  acne, 93, 94, 95
  with psoralens, 103, **110**
ultraviolet B (UVB)
  acne, 94
  broad band, 103, **110**
  high intensity, *see* high intensity ultraviolet B
  narrow band, 103, *106,* 107, **110**
ultraviolet (UV) light
  acne, 93, 94, 95
  psoriasis, 103, *106*

V

Vancouver Scar Scale, 72
varicose veins
  anesthesia, 38
  duplex ultrasound guidance, 38, 39
  endovenous ablation, 38–39
  laser and radiofrequency therapy, 38–39
  ligation, 38
  perforate invagination stripping, 38
  sclerotherapy, 38, *38*
  stripping, 38
  target selection, 31
vascular lesions, 7, 11–27
  anesthesia, 25, 140
  complications, 12, 26
  cooling, 12, 25, 131
  facial telangiectasias, *see* facial telangiectasias
  Fitzpatrick skin types, 12
  fluence, 12
  hemangiomas, *see* hemangiomas
  malformations, *see* vascular malformations
  nonspecific coagulation necrosis, 12
  oxyhemoglobin, 11, *11,* 12
  port wine stain, *see* port wine stains
  pyogenic granuloma, 12, 17
  side effects, 26
  therapy recommendations, 11, 25–26
vascular malformations, 17–18
  arterial, 17
  arteriovenous, 17, 24–25
  associated syndromes, 17
  capillary, *see* port wine stains
  categorization, 17
  definition, 14
  diagnosis, **13**
  lymphatic, 17, 25
  venous, 17, 20–21
veins, legs *see* leg veins/venules
venous lakes, 24, 26
venous malformations, 17, 20–21
vermilectomy, actinic chelitis, 81
veulectasia, legs *see* leg veins/venules
violet-blue light, acne, 93, 94

W

water, light absorption, 4
wavelengths, light, *5,* 5–6
  scattering, 4
Wood's light, acne, 90
wound healing, 67

Y

yellow light, acne, 93

Z

Zimmer, 129

ELSEVIER DVD-ROM LICENSE AGREEMENT

PLEASE READ THE FOLLOWING AGREEMENT CAREFULLY BEFORE USING THIS DVD-ROM PRODUCT. THIS DVD-ROM PRODUCT IS LICENSED UNDER THE TERMS CONTAINED IN THIS DVD-ROM LICENSE AGREEMENT ("Agreement"). BY USING THIS DVD-ROM PRODUCT, YOU, AN INDIVIDUAL OR ENTITY INCLUDING EMPLOYEES, AGENTS AND REPRESENTATIVES ("You" or "Your"), ACKNOWLEDGE THAT YOU HAVE READ THIS AGREEMENT, THAT YOU UNDERSTAND IT, AND THAT YOU AGREE TO BE BOUND BY THE TERMS AND CONDITIONS OF THIS AGREEMENT. ELSEVIER INC. ("Elsevier") EXPRESSLY DOES NOT AGREE TO LICENSE THIS DVD-ROM PRODUCT TO YOU UNLESS YOU ASSENT TO THIS AGREEMENT. IF YOU DO NOT AGREE WITH ANY OF THE FOLLOWING TERMS, YOU MAY, WITHIN THIRTY (30) DAYS AFTER YOUR RECEIPT OF THIS DVD-ROM PRODUCT RETURN THE UNUSED, PIN NUMBER PROTECTED, DVD-ROM PRODUCT, AND ALL ACCOMPANYING DOCUMENTATION TO ELSEVIER FOR A FULL REFUND.

DEFINITIONS As used in this Agreement, these terms shall have the following meanings:

"Proprietary Material" means the valuable and proprietary information content of this DVD-ROM Product including all indexes and graphic materials and software used to access, index, search and retrieve the information content from this DVD-ROM Product developed or licensed by Elsevier and/or its affiliates, suppliers and licensors.

"DVD-ROM Product" means the copy of the Proprietary Material and any other material delivered on DVD-ROM and any other human-readable or machine-readable materials enclosed with this Agreement, including without limitation documentation relating to the same.

OWNERSHIP This DVD-ROM Product has been supplied by and is proprietary to Elsevier and/or its affiliates, suppliers and licensors. The copyright in the DVD-ROM Product belongs to Elsevier and/or its affiliates, suppliers and licensors and is protected by the national and state copyright, trademark, trade secret and other intellectual property laws of the United States and international treaty provisions, including without limitation the Universal Copyright Convention and the Berne Copyright Convention. You have no ownership rights in this DVD-ROM Product. Except as expressly set forth herein, no part of this DVD-ROM Product, including without limitation the Proprietary Material, may be modified, copied or distributed in hardcopy or machine-readable form without prior written consent from Elsevier. All rights not expressly granted to You herein are expressly reserved. Any other use of this DVD-ROM Product by any person or entity is strictly prohibited and a violation of this Agreement.

SCOPE OF RIGHTS LICENSED (PERMITTED USES) Elsevier is granting to You a limited, non-exclusive, non-transferable license to use this DVD-ROM Product in accordance with the terms of this Agreement. You may use or provide access to this DVD-ROM Product on a single computer or terminal physically located at Your premises and in a secure network or move this DVD-ROM Product to and use it on another single computer or terminal at the same location for personal use only, but under no circumstances may You use or provide access to any part or parts of this DVD-ROM Product on more than one computer or terminal simultaneously.

You shall not (a) copy, download, or otherwise reproduce the DVD-ROM Product in any medium, including, without limitation, online transmissions, local area networks, wide area networks, intranets, extranets and the Internet, or in any way, in whole or in part, except for printing out or downloading nonsubstantial portions of the text and images in the DVD-ROM Product for Your own personal use; (b) alter, modify, or adapt the DVD-ROM Product, including but not limited to decompiling, disassembling, reverse engineering, or creating derivative works, without the prior written approval of Elsevier; (c) sell, license or otherwise distribute to third parties the DVD-ROM Product or any part or parts thereof; or (d) alter, remove, obscure or obstruct the display of any copyright, trademark or other proprietary notice on or in the DVD-ROM Product or on any printout or download of portions of the Proprietary Materials.

RESTRICTIONS ON TRANSFER This License is personal to You, and neither Your rights hereunder nor the tangible embodiments of this DVD-ROM Product, including without limitation the Proprietary Material, may be sold, assigned, transferred or sublicensed to any other person, including without limitation by operation of law, without the prior written consent of Elsevier. Any purported sale, assignment, transfer or sublicense without the prior written consent of Elsevier will be void and will automatically terminate the License granted hereunder.

TERM This Agreement will remain in effect until terminated pursuant to the terms of this Agreement. You may terminate this Agreement at any time by removing from Your system and destroying the DVD-ROM Product. Unauthorized copying of the DVD-ROM Product, including without limitation, the Proprietary Material and documentation, or otherwise failing to comply with the terms and conditions of this Agreement shall result in automatic termination of this license and will make available to Elsevier legal remedies. Upon termination of this Agreement, the license granted herein will terminate and You must immediately destroy the DVD-ROM Product and accompanying documentation. All provisions relating to proprietary rights shall survive termination of this Agreement.

LIMITED WARRANTY AND LIMITATION OF LIABILITY NEITHER ELSEVIER NOR ITS LICENSORS REPRESENT OR WARRANT THAT THE DVD-ROM PRODUCT WILL MEET YOUR REQUIREMENTS OR THAT ITS OPERATION WILL BE UNINTERRUPTED OR ERROR-FREE. WE EXCLUDE AND EXPRESSLY DISCLAIM ALL EXPRESS AND IMPLIED WARRANTIES NOT STATED HEREIN, INCLUDING THE IMPLIED WARRANTIES OF MERCHANTABILITY AND FITNESS FOR A PARTICULAR PURPOSE. IN ADDITION, NEITHER ELSEVIER NOR ITS LICENSORS MAKE ANY REPRESENTATIONS OR WARRANTIES, EITHER EXPRESS OR IMPLIED, REGARDING THE PERFORMANCE OF YOUR NETWORK OR COMPUTER SYSTEM WHEN USED IN CONJUNCTION WITH THE DVD-ROM PRODUCT. WE SHALL NOT BE LIABLE FOR ANY DAMAGE OR LOSS OF ANY KIND ARISING OUT OF OR RESULTING FROM YOUR POSSESSION OR USE OF THE SOFTWARE PRODUCT CAUSED BY ERRORS OR OMISSIONS, DATA LOSS OR CORRUPTION, ERRORS OR OMISSIONS IN THE PROPRIETARY MATERIAL, REGARDLESS OF WHETHER SUCH LIABILITY IS BASED IN TORT, CONTRACT OR OTHERWISE AND INCLUDING, BUT NOT LIMITED TO, ACTUAL, SPECIAL, INDIRECT, INCIDENTAL OR CONSEQUENTIAL DAMAGES. IF THE FOREGOING LIMITATION IS HELD TO BE UNENFORCEABLE, OUR MAXIMUM LIABILITY TO YOU SHALL NOT EXCEED THE AMOUNT OF THE LICENSE FEE PAID BY YOU FOR THE SOFTWARE PRODUCT. THE REMEDIES AVAILABLE TO YOU AGAINST US AND THE LICENSORS OF MATERIALS INCLUDED IN THE SOFTWARE PRODUCT ARE EXCLUSIVE.

If this DVD-ROM Product is defective, Elsevier will replace it at no charge if the defective DVD-ROM Product is returned to Elsevier within sixty (60) days (or the greatest period allowable by applicable law) from the date of shipment.

Elsevier warrants that the software embodied in this DVD-ROM Product will perform in substantial compliance with the documentation supplied in this DVD-ROM Product. If You report a significant defect in performance in writing to Elsevier, and Elsevier is not able to correct same within sixty (60) days after its receipt of Your notification, You may return this DVD-ROM Product, including all copies and documentation, to Elsevier and Elsevier will refund Your money.

YOU UNDERSTAND THAT, EXCEPT FOR THE 60-DAY LIMITED WARRANTY RECITED ABOVE, ELSEVIER, ITS AFFILIATES, LICENSORS, SUPPLIERS AND AGENTS, MAKE NO WARRANTIES, EXPRESSED OR IMPLIED, WITH RESPECT TO THE DVD-ROM PRODUCT, INCLUDING, WITHOUT LIMITATION THE PROPRIETARY MATERIAL, AND SPECIFICALLY DISCLAIM ANY WARRANTY OF MERCHANTABILITY OR FITNESS FOR A PARTICULAR PURPOSE.

If the information provided on this DVD-ROM Product contains medical or health sciences information, it is intended for professional use within the medical field. Information about medical treatment or drug dosages is intended strictly for professional use, and because of rapid advances in the medical sciences, independent verification of diagnosis and drug dosages should be made.

IN NO EVENT WILL ELSEVIER, ITS AFFILIATES, LICENSORS, SUPPLIERS OR AGENTS, BE LIABLE TO YOU FOR ANY DAMAGES, INCLUDING, WITHOUT LIMITATION, ANY LOST PROFITS, LOST SAVINGS OR OTHER INCIDENTAL OR CONSEQUENTIAL DAMAGES, ARISING OUT OF YOUR USE OR INABILITY TO USE THE DVD-ROM PRODUCT REGARDLESS OF WHETHER SUCH DAMAGES ARE FORESEEABLE OR WHETHER SUCH DAMAGES ARE DEEMED TO RESULT FROM THE FAILURE OR INADEQUACY OF ANY EXCLUSIVE OR OTHER REMEDY.

U.S. GOVERNMENT RESTRICTED RIGHTS The DVD-ROM Product and documentation are provided with restricted rights. Use, duplication or disclosure by the U.S. Government is subject to restrictions as set forth in subparagraphs (a) through (d) of the Commercial Computer Restricted Rights clause at FAR 52.22719 or in subparagraph (c)(1)(ii) of the Rights in Technical Data and Computer Software clause at DFARS 252.2277013, or at 252.2117015, as applicable. Contractor/Manufacturer is Elsevier Inc., 360 Park Avenue South, New York, NY 10010 USA.

GOVERNING LAW This Agreement shall be governed by the laws of the State of New York, USA. In any dispute arising out of this Agreement, You and Elsevier each consent to the exclusive personal jurisdiction and venue in the state and federal courts within New York County, New York, USA.